INTRODUCTORY
TEXTBOOK OF
PSYCHIATRY

FIFTH EDITION

INTRODUCTORY
TEXTBOOK OF
PSYCHIATRY

FIFTH EDITION

Donald W. Black, M.D.
Nancy C. Andreasen, M.D., Ph.D.

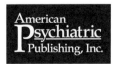

American Psychiatric Publishing, Inc.

Washington, DC
London, England

Note: The authors have worked to ensure that all information in this book is accurate at the time of publication and consistent with general psychiatric and medical standards, and that information concerning drug dosages, schedules, and routes of administration is accurate at the time of publication and consistent with standards set by the U.S. Food and Drug Administration and the general medical community. As medical research and practice continue to advance, however, therapeutic standards may change. Moreover, specific situations may require a specific therapeutic response not included in this book. For these reasons and because human and mechanical errors sometimes occur, we recommend that readers follow the advice of physicians directly involved in their care or the care of a member of their family.

Manufactured in the United States of America on acid-free paper
14   13   12   11   10   5   4   3   2   1
Fifth Edition

Typeset in Adobe's Palatino and Kabel

American Psychiatric Publishing, Inc.
1000 Wilson Boulevard
Arlington, VA 22209-3901
www.appi.org

Bulk discounts of 20% are available on purchases of 25–99 copies of this or any other APPI title; please contact APPI Customer Service at appi@psych.org or 800-368-5777. To purchase 100 or more copies of the same title, please e-mail us at bulksales@psych.org for a price quote.

Library of Congress Cataloging-in-Publication Data
Black, Donald W., 1956–
   Introductory textbook of psychiatry / Donald W. Black, Nancy C. Andreasen.—5th ed.
       p. ; cm.
   Andreasen's name appears first on the 4th ed.
   Includes bibliographical references and index.
   ISBN 978-1-58562-382-2 (alk. paper) — ISBN 978-1-58562-400-3 (pbk. : alk. paper) 1. Psychiatry. I. Andreasen, Nancy C. II. Title.
   [DNLM: 1. Mental Disorders. 2. Psychiatry. WM 100 B6275i 2011]
   RC454.A427 2011
   616.89—dc22

                                                        2010000533

British Library Cataloguing in Publication Data
A CIP record is available from the British Library.

CONTENTS

PART I
BACKGROUND

P A R T I I
PSYCHIATRIC DISORDERS

P A R T   I I I
Special Topics

Disclosures of Competing Interests

The authors of this book have indicated a financial interest in or other affiliation with a commercial supporter, a manufacturer of a commercial product, a provider of a commercial service, a nongovernmental organization, and/or a government agency, as listed below:

Nancy C. Andreasen, M.D., Ph.D. *Advisory Board Member and Research Support:* Johnson & Johnson

Donald W. Black, M.D. *Research Support:* AstraZeneca, Forest Laboratories; *Stocks:* Johnson & Johnson

Preface

STUDENTS SOMETIMES BEGIN working in psychiatry with a set of preconceptions about what it is—preconceptions shaped by the fact that information about psychiatry is omnipresent in popular culture. Taxi drivers, CEOs, teachers, and ministers often feel qualified to offer information and advice about how to handle "psychiatric problems" even though they may be unaware of distinctions as fundamental as the difference between psychiatry and psychology. These two disciplines are blurred together in the popular mind, and the term *psychiatry* evokes a potpourri of associations—Freud's couch, Jack Nicholson receiving electroconvulsive therapy in *One Flew Over the Cuckoo's Nest*, Dr. Phil discussing sexual adjustment on television. These images and associations tend to cloak psychiatry with an aura of vagueness, imprecision, muddle-headedness, and mindless coercion. It is unfortunate that such preconceptions are so pervasive, but fortunate that most of them are in error, as students who use this book in conjunction with studying psychiatry in a clinical setting will soon discover.

What is psychiatry? It is the branch of medicine that focuses on the diagnosis and treatment of mental illnesses. Some of these illnesses are very serious, such as schizophrenia, Alzheimer's disease, and the various mood disorders. Others may be less serious, but still very significant, such as anxiety disorders and personality disorders. Psychiatry differs from psychology by virtue of its medical orientation. Its primary focus is illness or abnormality, as opposed to normal psychological functioning; the latter is the primary focus of psychology. Of course, abnormal psychology is a small branch within psychology, just as understanding normality is necessary for the psychiatrist to recognize and treat abnormal functioning. The primary purposes of psychiatry as a discipline within medicine are to define and recognize illnesses, to identify methods for treating them, and ultimately to develop methods for discovering their causes and implementing preventive measures.

There are several reasons why psychiatry may be the most exciting discipline within medicine. First, psychiatrists are specialists who work with the most interesting organ within the body, the brain. The brain is intrinsically fascinating because it controls nearly all aspects of functioning within the rest of the body as well as the way people interact with and relate to one another. Psychiatry has rapidly advanced in recent years through the burgeoning of neuroscience, which has provided psychiatrists with the tools by which they can understand brain anatomy, chemistry, and physiology, thereby gradually developing a scientific base that will permit them to understand human emotion and behavior and to develop methods for treating abnormalities in these domains.

Yet as psychiatry evolves into a relatively high-powered science, it remains a very clinical and human branch within medicine. It can be an especially rewarding field for students who have chosen medicine because they wish to have contact with patients. The clinician working in psychiatry must spend time with his or her patients and learn about them as human beings as well as individuals who have illnesses or problems. Learning a person's life story is fun and interesting; as one colleague once said, "It amazed me when I realized that I would get paid for asking people things that everybody always wants to know about anyway!"

Finally, psychiatry has enormous breadth. As a scientific discipline, it ranges from the highly detailed facts of molecular biology to the abstract concepts of the mind. As a clinical discipline, it ranges from the absorbingly complex disturbances that characterize illnesses such as schizophrenia to the understandable fearfulness shown by young children when they must separate from their parents and attend school or be left with a babysitter. It can be very scientific and technical, as in the frontier-expanding research currently occurring in molecular genetics or neuroimaging; but it can also be very human and personal, as when a clinician listens to a patient's story and experiences the pleasure of being able to offer help by providing needed insights or even simple encouragement and support.

This book is intended as a tool to help you learn from your patients and from your teachers. We have tried to keep it simple, clear, and factual. References are provided for students who want to explore in more depth the topics covered in the various chapters. We have written this book primarily for medical students and residents in their first several years of training, although we anticipate that it may also be useful to individuals seeking psychiatric training from the perspectives of other disciplines such as nursing or social work. We hope that, using this book as a tool, students of all ages and types will learn to enjoy working with psychiatric patients and with the art and science of contemporary psychiatry as much as we do.

We are grateful to the many readers who, over the years, have written to us with their useful suggestions. Medical students, psychiatry residents, and other trainees who have used the book have given us critical feedback that has helped shape this book. We thank our many colleagues who have provided help and guidance: Jennifer McWilliams, Linda Madson, Jon E. Grant, Jodi Tate, Jess Fiedorowicz, Robert Philibert, Laurie McCormick, Jerry Lewis, Anthony Miller, Wayne Bowers, Mark Granner, Vicki Kijewski, Susan Schultz, Del Miller, Tracy Gunter, Russell Noyes, and Scott Temple.

We also thank Robert E. Hales, Editor-in-Chief of American Psychiatric Publishing, and his dedicated staff who shared our vision for the book and brought it to fruition.

Introduction

You are not here merely to make a living.... You are here to enrich the world, and you impoverish yourself if you forget the errand.

Woodrow Wilson

MANY OF YOU reading this book will be getting your first introduction to psychiatry. You may not realize that, along with surgery, it is one of the oldest medical specialties. It emerged as a special branch of medicine in the eighteenth century, when a few general physicians decided to devote themselves exclusively to the care of the mentally ill. They were influenced by the humanistic and humane principles of the Enlightenment, which they shared with the American Founding Fathers who wrote the Declaration of Independence and the U.S. Constitution and with other great statesmen such as Woodrow Wilson.

Philippe Pinel, a leader of the French Revolution, is usually considered to be the founding father of modern psychiatry. In 1793, he was named director of the Bicêtre, the hospital in Paris for insane men. Soon afterward he instituted a grand, symbolic change by removing the chains that bound the patients to the walls at the Bicêtre and created a new type of treatment that he referred to as "moral treatment." (This meant treating patients in ways that were morally and ethically sensitive.) He was later made director of the corresponding hospital for women, the Salpêtrière. In addition to treating the mentally ill with kindness and decency, Pinel also tried to approach the study of mental illness scientifically. He described his efforts in his *Treatise on Insanity* (1806):

> I, therefore, resolved to adopt that method of investigation which has invariably succeeded in all the departments of natural history, viz. To notice successively every fact, without any other object than that of

collecting materials for future use; and to endeavor, as far as possible, to divest myself of the influence, both of my own prepossessions and the authority of others. (p. 2)

Thus a new specialty within medicine was created, consisting of those doctors who chose to specialize in the care of the mentally ill. They became known as "psychiatrists," which means literally "physicians who heal the mind."

What does that mean? What does a psychiatrist actually do? Why do people choose to study psychiatry, and why do some choose to make this their specialty? People study psychiatry and become psychiatrists because they are interested in what makes human beings tick. Some of us have chosen to become psychiatrists because we want to understand the human mind and spirit as well as the human brain. We chose to join a very clinical specialty because we are interested in people, and we like to work with them as individuals. We like to think about people within the context of the social matrix in which they live, to skillfully elicit a "life narrative" that summarizes their past and current experiences, and to use that information to better understand how their symptoms arise and can be treated. Each person we encounter is a new adventure, a new voyage of discovery, and a new life story. Patterns tend to generalize across individuals, yet each patient is unique. This is what makes psychiatry challenging, intellectually rich, complex, and even enjoyable—despite the fact that we often care for people who suffer intensely and for whom we wish we could offer even more help. We are privileged to explore the most private and personal aspects of people's lives and to help them achieve healthier lives.

Many people study psychiatry and become psychiatrists because they are fascinated by the human brain—the most complex and interesting organ in the human body. All of our emotions, thoughts, beliefs, and behaviors arise from the workings of that furrowed and folded chunk of tissue that is so carefully protected inside our skulls. Modern neuroscience has begun to unlock the secrets of the human brain using a variety of tools that reach from the molecular to the systems level. What we contain within our memory stores forms the essence of our human individuality. We have already learned a great deal about how memories are stored and retained at the molecular and cellular level. We are also unlocking the mysteries of brain development and aging and the complex ways that human thoughts are created. Understanding these processes, as well as many others, offers the opportunity for understanding the mechanisms of mental illness, for finding better treatments, and perhaps even for preventing them. These are exciting times to be studying the human brain!

Lastly, people study psychiatry and become psychiatrists because mental illnesses are among the most clinically important diseases from which human beings suffer. In 1996 two investigators at Harvard University, working in collaboration with the World Health Organization, published a pivotal book titled *The Global Burden of Disease*. This book captured the attention of leaders in the medical community because it provided the first objective summary of the costs of various types of illness to society throughout the world. One head-turning fact is the cost exacted by mental illnesses. For example, a mental illness—unipolar major depression—is the costliest illness in the world. Furthermore, four mental illnesses are among the top 10 diseases affecting people between ages 15 and 44 years: depression, alcohol misuse, bipolar disorder, and schizophrenia. Because self-inflicted injuries are also a consequence of mental illness, 5 of the 10 leading causes of disability in the world are attributable to psychiatric disorders. The message is clear: doctors can no longer afford to ignore mental illnesses. Every physician must learn to identify and diagnose mental illnesses and either provide treatment or referral to a specialist. Some must pursue a deeper understanding by becoming psychiatrists.

The study of *psychiatry*, the branch of medicine devoted to the study of mental illnesses, is therefore a discipline dedicated to the investigation of abnormalities in brain function manifested in diseases that afflict individuals in interesting and important ways. The clinical appearance of these abnormalities may be obvious and severe, as in the case of psychosis, or subtle and mild, as in the case of personality disorders. Ultimately the drive of modern psychiatry is to develop a comprehensive understanding of normal brain function at levels that range from mind to molecule and to determine how aberrations in these normal functions (produced either endogenously through genetic coding or exogenously through environmental influences) lead to the development of symptoms of mental illnesses.

PART I

BACKGROUND

ogy. By and large, a full understanding of etiology is limited to the infectious diseases, in which the etiology is exposure to some infectious agent to a degree sufficient that the body's immune mechanisms are overwhelmed. (Even in this instance, our knowledge of immune mechanisms is incomplete.)

For most diseases, however, our understanding is at the level of pathophysiology rather than etiology. Diseases are defined in terms of the mechanisms that produce particular symptoms, such as infarction in the myocardium, inflammation in the joints, or abnormal regulation of insulin production.

In the areas of pathophysiology and etiology, psychiatry has more uncharted territory than the rest of medicine. Most of the disorders or diseases diagnosed in psychiatry are *syndromes:* collections of symptoms that tend to occur together and that appear to have a characteristic course and outcome. Much of the current investigative research in psychiatry is directed toward the goal of identifying the pathophysiology and etiology of major mental illnesses, but this goal has been achieved for only a few disorders (Alzheimer's disease, vascular dementia, Huntington's disease, and substance-induced syndromes such as amphetamine-related psychosis or the Wernicke-Korsakoff syndrome).

■ Why Diagnose Patients?

Diagnoses in psychiatry serve a variety of important purposes and are not just a "label." Making a careful diagnosis is as fundamental in psychiatry as it is in the remainder of medicine.

Diagnosis introduces order and structure to our thinking and reduces the complexity of clinical phenomena. Psychiatry is a diverse field, and symptoms of mental illness encompass a broad range of emotional, cognitive, and behavioral abnormalities. The use of diagnoses introduces order and structure to this complexity. Disorders are divided into broad classes based on common features (e.g., psychosis, substance abuse, dementia, anxiety). Within each of the major classes, specific syndromes are then further delineated (e.g., dividing substance-related disorders in terms of the type of substance involved, dividing the dementias into Alzheimer's disease and vascular dementia). The existence of broad groupings, subdivided into specific disorders, creates a structure within the apparent chaos of clinical phenomena and makes mental illnesses easier to learn about and understand. Although diagnoses are not necessarily defined in terms of etiology or pathophysiology, they are typically defined in terms of syndromal features.

Diagnoses facilitate communication among clinicians. When psychiatrists give a patient's symptoms a specific diagnosis, such as bipolar disorder, they are making a specific statement about the clinical picture with which that particular patient presents. A diagnosis concisely summarizes information for all other clinicians who subsequently examine the patient's records or to whom the patient is referred. A diagnosis of bipolar disorder, for example, indicates that

- The patient has had at least one episode of mania.
- During that episode of mania, the patient experienced a characteristic group of symptoms such as elated mood, increased energy, racing thoughts, rapid speech, grandiosity, and poor judgment.
- The patient probably has had episodes of depression as well, characterized by sadness, insomnia, decreased appetite, feelings of worthlessness, and other typical depressive symptoms.

The use of diagnostic categories gives clinicians a kind of "shorthand" through which they can summarize large quantities of information relatively easily.

Diagnoses help to predict outcome. Many psychiatric diagnoses are associated with a characteristic course and outcome. For example, bipolar disorder is usually episodic, with periods of relatively severe abnormalities in mood interspersed with periods of near normality or complete normality. Thus, patients with bipolar disorder have a relatively good outcome. Some other types of disorders, such as schizophrenia or personality disorders, typically have a more chronic course. Diagnoses are a useful way of summarizing the clinician's expectations about the patient's future course of illness.

Diagnoses are often used to choose an appropriate treatment. As psychiatry has advanced clinically and scientifically, relatively specific treatments for particular disorders or groups of symptoms have been developed. For example, antipsychotic drugs are typically used to treat psychoses. Thus they are used for disorders such as schizophrenia, in which psychosis is typically prominent, as well as for forms of mood disorder in which psychotic symptoms occur. A diagnosis of mania suggests the use of mood stabilizers such as lithium carbonate or valproate. Some relatively targeted medications are now available, such as the selective serotonin reuptake inhibitors for obsessive-compulsive disorder.

Diagnoses are used to assist in the search for pathophysiology and etiology. Clinical researchers use diagnoses to reduce heterogeneity in their samples and to separate groups of patients who may share a common mechanism or cause that produces their symptoms. Patients who share a relatively specific set of symptoms, such as severe schizophrenia characterized by negative symptoms, are often hypothesized to have a disorder that is mechanistically or etiologically distinct. Knowledge about specific groupings of clinical symptoms can be related to knowledge about brain specialization and function in order to formulate hypotheses about the neurochemical or anatomical substrates of a particular disorder. Ideally, the use of diagnoses defined on the basis of the clinical picture will lead ultimately to diagnoses that serve the fundamental purpose of identifying causes.

■ Other Purposes of Diagnosis

Beyond these clinical uses, diagnostic systems also have other purposes. Although physicians prefer to conceptualize their relationships with patients in terms of care and treatment, diagnoses are used by other health care providers, attorneys, epidemiologists, and insurance companies. Each time a clinician makes a diagnosis and records it, he or she must do so with an awareness of the other, nonclinical uses to which it may be put.

Diagnoses are used to monitor treatment and to make decisions about reimbursement. As health care has become increasingly managed, diagnoses are often used to determine the length of a hospital stay or the choice of a treatment course for a specific condition. Physicians or their assistants sometimes must spend hours speaking on the telephone with insurers to request additional days, or in writing letters to insurers appealing their decisions for denial of care if the patient's course of treatment appears to exceed the preset guidelines. Depending on the insurer, some diagnoses may not be covered at all—for example, alcoholism and other drug use disorders. The range of diagnoses covered by insurers continues to change rapidly and may accelerate with the new health reform measures passed by the U.S. Congress in 2010.

Diagnoses are used by attorneys in malpractice suits and in other litigation. Although psychiatrists are the least frequently sued among medical specialists, lawsuits are a concern for all physicians in our litigious society. Some diagnoses, such as major depression, carry with them a clear set of risks, such as suicide. Clinicians must be aware of those risks and clearly document that they have provided appropriate care. As the *Diagnostic and Statistical Manual of Mental Disorders* (DSM) has made the diagnostic system of psychiatry more open and available, both lawyers and patients have learned much more about psychiatric classification. A physician called into court must expect to defend a recorded diagnosis with appropriate documentation that the various criteria have been assessed and are met.

Diagnoses are used by health care epidemiologists to determine the incidence and prevalence of various diseases throughout the world. Diagnoses recorded in hospital or clinic charts are translated into a standard system established by the World Health Organization (WHO), the International Classification of Diseases (ICD). This system is used to track regional differences in disease patterns as well as changes over time.

Diagnoses are used to make decisions about insurance coverage. A carelessly made diagnosis, be it of hypertension or major depression, may make it difficult for a patient to obtain life insurance or future health care insurance. Diagnoses also are sometimes used to make decisions about employment, admission to college, and other important opportunities. Because mental illnesses may be subject to discrimination and misunderstanding, these diagnoses involve a particular risk. The clinician obviously must walk a fine line—perhaps impossibly fine.

■ The History Behind DSM

The process of diagnosis in psychiatry is partially simplified by the fact that the national professional organization to which most psychiatrists in the United States belong, the American Psychiatric Association, has formulated a manual that summarizes all of the diagnoses used in psychiatry, specifies the symptoms that must be present to make a given diagnosis, and organizes these diagnoses together into a classification system. This manual is titled the *Diagnostic and Statistical Manual of Mental Disorders* (DSM).

The impetus to organize a DSM began during World War II. For the first time, psychiatrists from all over the United States were brought together in clinical settings that required them to communicate clearly with one another. It became apparent that diagnostic practices varied widely throughout the United States, no doubt reflecting a diversity of training. Shortly thereafter, the American Psychiatric Association convened a task force to develop a diagnostic manual for use in all of American psychiatry. The product was DSM-I, which was published in 1952. Over the years, the DSM has undergone three major revisions (DSM-II, DSM-III, and DSM-IV). Currently, diagnoses in psychiatry are based on DSM-IV, which was published in 1994, and its text revision, DSM-IV-TR, which was published in 2000. A fifth edition, DSM-5, is now being developed and is expected to be published in 2013.

Compared with DSM-III and DSM-IV, DSM-I and DSM-II were relatively simple. For example, the definition of manic-depressive illness in DSM-II was as follows:

> **Manic-Depressive Illnesses (Manic-Depressive Psychoses)**
> These disorders are marked by severe mood swings and a tendency to remission and recurrence. Patients may be given this diagnosis in the absence of a previous history of affective psychosis if there is no obvious precipitating event. This disorder is divided into three major subtypes: manic type, depressed type, and circular type. (p. 8)

These early handbooks were relatively small. DSM-I contained 132 pages, and DSM-II contained 119 pages. DSM-III, which came out in 1980, was the first effort by a medical specialty to provide a comprehensive and detailed diagnostic manual in which all disorders were defined by specific criteria. DSM-III was a hefty tome—494 pages.

DSM-III represented a major change, which was subsequently carried forward in the next revisions, DSM-IV and DSM-IV-TR. Because of their vagueness and imprecision, the definitions in DSM-I and DSM-II did not adequately fulfill many of the purposes for making a diagnosis. In particular, the descriptions were not specific enough to facilitate communication among clinicians and to delineate one disorder from another. Research investigations made it clear that different clinicians using DSM-I or DSM-II guidelines would give different diagnoses to the same patient. The authors of DSM-III agreed to formulate specific diagnostic criteria that would be as objective as possible to define each of the disorders; would make their decisions about defining criteria and overall organizational structure on the basis of existing research data whenever possible; and would not resort to anecdotal approaches or simple clinical opinion if at all possible.

For the first time, the methods by which a psychiatric diagnosis could be made were relatively clear. Most of the time, the criteria require that a specified subset from a listed group of symptoms be present in order to make a diagnosis.

Psychiatry is the only specialty in medicine that has so consistently and comprehensively formalized the diagnostic processes for the disorders within its domain. This precision and structure are particularly important in psychiatry because it lacks specific laboratory diagnostic tests and confirmed etiologies for most disorders. Consequently, a DSM diagnosis relies largely on the patient's presenting symptoms and history. Without the structure provided by diagnostic criteria, the diagnostic process could become imprecise and unclear.

The DSM system, as represented by all versions since DSM-III, has been an effective treatment for some of the previous lack of clarity of psychiatric diagnosis. But this treatment has not been without some untoward side effects as well.

■ Advantages and Disadvantages of the DSM System

Advantages

The advantages of the DSM system can be summarized as follows:

The DSM system has substantially improved the reliability of diagnosis. *Reliability,* a biometric concept, refers to the ability of two observers to agree on what they see. It is measured by a variety of statistical methods, such as percent agreement, correlation coefficients, and the kappa statistic, which corrects for chance agreement. The reliability of DSM-III was assessed in field trials and found to be relatively good. Even more extensive field trials and reliability studies were done for DSM-IV. These have been extensively summarized in the DSM sourcebooks. The kappa statistics for most diagnoses are approximately 0.8 or greater, which is considered very good.

The DSM system has clarified the diagnostic process and facilitated history taking. Because DSM-IV-TR specifies exactly which symptoms must be present to make a diagnosis, as well as the characteristic course of disorders whenever this is appropriate, it is highly objective. During the 1970s, many psychiatrists received predominantly psychodynamic training that de-emphasized a medical approach to diagnosis. This approach stressed the importance of recognizing underlying psychological processes rather than objective signs and symptoms. Although clinically useful, this approach was more subjective, was difficult to teach to beginners, and re-

cian with an indication of the patient's overall prognosis, because high-functioning individuals typically have a better outcome.)

■ How to Become Familiar With the DSM System

The DSM system is obviously large and complex. Beginning students and residents should not attempt to master everything at once. Rather, they should focus on the major and common conditions that are frequently seen either in psychiatric practice or in primary care settings. They should become very familiar with the diagnostic criteria for a few common conditions, such as schizophrenia, major depression, dementia, anxiety disorders, and personality disorders. A few sets of symptom criteria (e.g., major depression) should be committed to memory, simply because they are used so often in so many different clinical settings. The system is too vast to commit all of it to memory, however, so the clinician should not feel concerned about the need to refer back to the criteria when evaluating patients' symptoms and making diagnoses.

■ Self-Assessment Questions

1. What is the overall purpose of diagnosis and classification in medicine? Describe the extent to which it has been achieved in psychiatry.

2. Describe some of the specific purposes of psychiatric diagnosis.

3. Describe some of the changes introduced by DSM-III and carried forth to the present.

4. Define the concepts of reliability and validity. How is reliability measured?

5. Describe the advantages of the DSM approach. What are some of its disadvantages?

6. What is meant by the term *multiaxial*? List the five axes that are included in DSM-IV-TR.

CHAPTER 2

Interviewing and Assessment

Festina lente.
(Make haste slowly.)

A Latin proverb

THE FIRST ENCOUNTER with a patient begins with taking a clinical history, just as in other specialties. The novice may feel some anxiety about approaching and interviewing people with mental illnesses, but largely because they have been portrayed in the media in such disturbing ways. Think of Randall Patrick McMurphy in *One Flew Over the Cuckoo's Nest,* or John Nash in *A Beautiful Mind.* Furthermore, psychiatric history-taking requires the interviewer to ask uncomfortable questions such as "Do you hear voices when no one is around?" or to ask about areas of life that are especially private and intimate, such as sexual preferences and practices. However, it is a bit like learning to ski or swim. Once you head down the mountain (or get in the water), you will find history-taking to be surprisingly easy, interesting, and even fun. Demands placed on the interviewer will vary, of course, depending on the type of illness the patient has and its severity. Patients with milder syndromes, such as anxiety disorders or personality disorders, are usually more capable of describing their symptoms and history clearly and articulately. The severely ill depressed, manic, or psychotic patient presents a real challenge, and clinicians may have to depend on informants, such as family members or friends, in addition to the patient.

■ The Psychiatric Interview

An initial psychiatric evaluation serves several purposes. One is to formulate an impression as to the patient's diagnosis or differential diagnosis and to begin to generate a treatment plan. The second purpose is to produce a document for the patient's record that contains information organized in a standard, readable, and easily interpretable way. The initial interview is often therapeutic as well, in that it permits the clinician to establish a relationship with the patient and to reassure him or her that help will be provided.

The outline of that written record is summarized in Table 2–1. As the table indicates, a standard psychiatric evaluation is very similar to the evaluations used in the rest of medicine, with some minor modifications. The content of the present illness and past history is focused primarily on psychiatric symptoms, and the family history includes more information about psychiatric illnesses in family members. Family history and social history also include more social and personal information than is recorded in the standard medical history. An important part of the interview—the mental status examination—is typically included only in psychiatric and neurological evaluations.

Identification of Patient and Informants

Identify the patient by stating his or her age, race, gender, marital status, and occupational status. Indicate whether the patient was the sole informant or whether additional history was obtained from family members or previous psychiatric records. Indicate whether the patient was self-referred, was brought in at the request of family members, or was referred by a physician; if either of the latter two, specify which family members or physician. In addition, indicate how reliable the informant appears to be.

Chief Complaint

Begin by stating the patient's chief complaint in his or her own words, using quotation marks (e.g., "I'm thinking of killing myself" or "I get

TABLE 2–1. Outline of the psychiatric evaluation

Identification of patient and informants

Chief complaint

History of present illness

Past psychiatric history

Family history

Social history

General medical history

Mental status examination

General physical examination

Neurological examination

Diagnostic impression

Treatment and management plan

angry and want to hurt people"). An additional sentence or two of amplifying information also may be provided, particularly if the patient's
chief complaint is relatively vague.

History of Present Illness

Provide a concise history of the illness or problem that brought the patient in for treatment. Begin by describing the onset of the symptoms. If
this is the patient's first episode, first psychiatric evaluation, or first hospital admission, that should be stated early in the history of the present
illness. Indicate how long ago the first symptoms began, the nature of
their onset (e.g., acute, insidious), and whether the onset was precipitated by any particular life events or problems. If the latter, these events
or problems should be described in some detail. Likewise, medical conditions that may have served as precipitants should be described. If drug
or alcohol abuse was a potential precipitant, that also should be noted.

The evolution of the patient's various symptoms should be described. A systematic summary of all symptoms present, in a form useful for making a differential diagnosis of the present illness, should be
provided. This listing of symptoms should reflect the criteria included
in DSM-IV-TR and should specify both which symptoms are present
and which symptoms are absent. The description of symptoms should

not be limited to those included in the DSM-IV-TR diagnostic criteria, however, because these typically do not provide a full description of the range of symptoms that patients have (i.e., they are minimal, not comprehensively descriptive). The description of the present illness also should indicate the degree of incapacity that the patient is experiencing as a consequence of the symptoms, as well as the influence of the symptoms on personal and family life. Any treatments the patient has received for the present illness should be noted, including dosages, duration of treatment, and effectiveness of the specific medications, because these will often dictate the next step.

Past Psychiatric History

The past psychiatric history provides a summary of past illnesses, problems, and their treatment. In patients with complex histories and chronic psychiatric illnesses, this portion of the history will be quite extensive. It should begin by noting the age at which the patient was first seen for psychiatric evaluation and the number of past hospitalizations or episodes. Thereafter, past episodes should be described in chronological order, with some information about duration of episodes, types of symptoms present, severity of symptoms, treatments received, and response to treatment. If a characteristic pattern is present (e.g., episodes of mania are always followed by episodes of depression, or past depressive episodes have consistently responded to a particular medication), this should be noted because it provides useful prognostic treatment information. If the patient's memory for past symptoms is relatively poor, or the bulk of the past history is obtained from old records rather than from the patient himself or herself, this also should be recorded. Confirmation by family members of types and patterns of symptoms and number of episodes also should be noted.

Family History

The age and occupation of both parents and all siblings should be noted, as should the age and education or occupation of all children (if applicable). If any of these first-degree relatives (parents, siblings, children) has a history of any mental illness, the specific illness should be mentioned, along with information about treatment, hospitalization, and long-term course and outcome. It may be necessary to describe specific disorders because many patients will not recognize alcoholism or criminality, for example, as relevant problems: "Do any blood relatives have a history of alcoholism, criminality, drug abuse, severe depression, suicide attempts, or suicide? Have any ever been psychiatrically hospitalized or institutionalized? Do you know why? Have any ever taken 'nerve pills' or seen psychiatrists, psychologists, or counselors?" The interviewer should obtain as much information as possible about mental illness in the extended family as well. Any relevant information about the family's social, cultural, or educational background also may be included in this section of the interview. It is often helpful to draw pedigrees in complicated cases.

Social History

The social history provides a concise narrative description of the patient's life history. It includes information about where the patient was born, where he or she grew up, and the nature of his or her early life adjustment. Any problems during childhood, such as temper tantrums, school phobia, or delinquency, should be noted. The patient's relationships with his or her parents and siblings should be described. Psychosexual development, such as age at first sexual experience, also should be described. Information about familial religious or cultural attitudes that is relevant to the patient's condition should be noted. Educational history should be summarized, including information about how many years of school the patient completed, quality of school performance, and nature of academic interests. Some description should be provided of the patient's interest and participation in extracurricular activities and interpersonal relationships during adolescence and early adulthood. Work history and military history also should be summarized. Certain areas may need more emphasis and detail, depending on the chief complaint and diagnostic formulation.

This section also contains a summary of the patient's current social situation, including marital status, occupation, and income. With patients who are unemployed or disabled, it may be helpful to ask, "What was your usual (or past) occupation?" The location of the patient's residence should be described, as well as the specific family members who live with the patient. This section of the history should provide information about the various social supports currently available to the patient. Habits (e.g., smoking, use of alcohol) should be recorded as well.

General Medical History

The patient's current and past state of health should be summarized. Any existing illness for which the patient is currently receiving treatment should be noted, as well as the types of treatments, medications, and their dosages. Include vitamins, supplements, herbals, or other nontraditional treatments (e.g., acupuncture, chiropractic, dietary supplements). Allergies, past surgeries, traumatic injuries, or other serious medical illnesses should be summarized. Head injuries, headaches, seizures, and other problems involving the central nervous system are particularly relevant.

Mental Status Examination

The mental status examination is the psychiatric equivalent of the physical examination in medicine. It includes a comprehensive evaluation of the patient's appearance, thinking and speech patterns, memory, and judgment.

The components of the mental status examination are summarized in Table 2–2. Some domains are determined simply by observing the patient (e.g., appearance, affect). Other portions are determined by asking the patient relatively specific questions (e.g., mood, abnormalities in perception). Still others are assessed by asking the patient a specified set of questions (e.g., memory, general information). The interviewer should develop his or her own repertoire of techniques to assess functions such as memory, general information, and calculation. He or she should consistently use this same repertoire for all patients so that he or she develops a good sense of the range of normal and abnormal responses in individuals of various ages, educational levels, and diagnoses.

Appearance and Attitude

Describe the patient's general appearance, including grooming, hygiene, and facial expression. Note whether the patient looks his or her stated age, younger, or older. Note type and appropriateness of dress. Describe whether the patient's attitude is cooperative, guarded, angry, or suspicious.

Motor Activity

Note the patient's level of motor activity. Does he or she sit quietly, or is he or she physically agitated? Note any abnormal movements, tics, or mannerisms. If relevant, evaluate for and note any indications of catatonia, such as waxy flexibility (described later in the chapter under "Catatonic Motor Behavior"). Determine whether any indications of ab-

TABLE 2–2.   Outline of the mental status examination

Appearance and attitude	General information
Motor activity	Calculations
Thought and speech	Capacity to read and write
Mood and affect	Visuospatial ability
Perception	Attention
Orientation	Abstraction
Memory	Judgment and insight

normal movements are present, such as the oral-buccal movements seen in persons with tardive dyskinesia.

Thought and Speech

Psychiatrists often speak about "thought disorder" or "formal thought disorder." This concept refers to the patient's pattern of speech, from which abnormal patterns of thought are inferred. It is, of course, not possible to evaluate thought directly. Note the rate of the patient's speech—whether it is normal, slowed, or pressured. Note whether the patient's speech indicates a pattern of thought that is logical and goal directed or whether any of a variety of abnormalities in form of thought is present (e.g., derailment, incoherence, poverty of content of speech). Summarize the content of the thought, noting in particular any delusional thinking that is present. Delusions, when present, should be described in detail. (If already noted in the history of the present illness, this can be indicated with a simple statement such as "Delusions were present as described above.")

Mood and Affect

The term *mood* refers to an emotional attitude that is relatively sustained; it is typically determined through the patient's own self-report, although some inferences can be made from the patient's facial expression. Note whether the patient's mood is neutral, euphoric, depressed, anxious, or irritable.

Affect is inferred from emotional responses that are usually triggered by some stimulus. Affect refers to the way that a patient conveys his or her emotional state, as perceived by others. The examiner watches the response of the patient's face to a joke or a smile, determines whether the patient shows appropriate or inappropriate emotional reactions, and notes the degree of reactivity of emotion. Affect is typically described as full, flat, blunted, or inappropriate. *Flat* or *blunted affect* is inferred when the patient shows very little emotional response and seems emotionally dulled, whereas *inappropriate affect* refers to emotional responses that are not appropriate to the content of the discussion, such as silly laughter for no apparent reason.

Perception

Note any abnormalities in perception. The most common perceptual abnormalities are hallucinations: abnormal sensory perceptions in the absence of an actual stimulus. Hallucinations may be auditory, visual, tactile, or olfactory. Sometimes hypnagogic or hypnopompic hallucinations occur when the patient is falling asleep or waking from sleep; these are not considered true hallucinations. An *illusion* is a misinterpretation of an actual stimulus—for example, seeing a shadow and believing it is a man.

Orientation

Describe the patient's level of orientation. Normally, this includes orientation to time, place, and person. Orientation is assessed by asking the patient to describe the day, date, year, time, place where he or she is currently residing, his or her name and identity, and why he or she is in the hospital (or clinic).

Memory

Memory is divided into very short term, short term, and long term. All three types should be described. Very-short-term memory involves the immediate registration of information, which is usually assessed by having the patient repeat back immediately a series of digits or three pieces of information (e.g., the color green, the name Mr. Williams, and the address 1915 High Street). The examiner determines whether the patient can recall these items immediately after he or she is told them. If the patient has difficulty, he or she should be given the items repeatedly until he or she is able to register them. If he or she is unable to register them after three or four trials, this should be noted. The patient should then be warned that he or she will be asked to recall these items in 3–5 minutes. His or her ability to remember them after that time interval is an indication of his or her short-term memory. Long-term memory is assessed by asking the patient to recall events that occurred in the past several days, as well as events that occurred in the more remote past, such as months or years ago.

General Information

General information is assessed by asking the patient a specific set of questions covering topics such as the names of the last five presidents, current events, or information about history or geography (e.g., "Can you tell me what happened on September 11, 2001?"; "Who is our president?"). The patient's fund of general information should be noted in relation to his or her level of educational achievement. This is particularly important in assessing the possibility of dementia.

Calculations

The standard test of calculations is serial 7s. This test involves having the patient subtract 7 from 100, then 7 from that product, and so on for at least five subtractions. Some chronic patients become relatively well trained in this exercise, so it is a good idea to have other tools in one's repertoire. One that is quite useful involves asking the patient to make calculations necessary in daily living (e.g., "If I went to the store and bought six oranges, priced at three for a dollar, and gave the clerk a $10 bill, how much change would I get back?"). Calculations can be modified for the patient's educational level. Poorly educated patients may need to calculate serial 3s. Likewise, real-life calculations can be simplified or made more complex.

Capacity to Read and Write

The patient should be given a simple text and asked to read it aloud. He or she also should be asked to write down a specific sentence, either of the examiner's choice or of his or her own choice. The patient's ability to read and write should be assessed relative to his or her level of education.

Visuospatial Ability

The patient should be asked to copy a figure. This figure can be quite simple, such as a square inside a circle. An alternative task is to ask the patient to draw a clock face and set the hands at some specified time, such as 10 minutes past 11 o'clock.

Attention

Attention is assessed in part by several of the tasks just described, such as calculations or clock setting. Additional tests of attention can be used, such as asking the patient to spell a word backward (e.g., "world"). The patient also can be asked to name five things that start with a specific letter, such as *d*. The latter is a good test of cognitive and verbal fluency.

Abstraction

The patient's capacity to think abstractly can be assessed in a variety of ways. One favorite method is asking the patient to interpret proverbs, such as "A rolling stone gathers no moss" or "Don't cry over spilt milk." Alternatively, the patient can be asked to identify commonalities between two items (e.g., "How are an apple and an orange alike?"; "How are a fly and a tree alike?").

Judgment and Insight

Assess overall judgment and insight by noting how realistically the patient has appraised his or her illness and various life problems. Insight can be ascertained relatively directly—for example, by asking "Do you believe you are mentally ill?" or "Do you believe that you need treatment?" Judgment may not be as easily assessed, but the patient's recent choices and decisions will help in its determination. Sometimes simple questions may be helpful. The following are frequently used: "If you found a stamped, addressed envelope, what would you do?" and "If you were in a movie theater and smelled smoke, what would you do?"

General Physical Examination

The general physical examination should follow the standard format used in the rest of medicine, covering organ systems of the body from head to foot. Examinations of patients of the opposite sex (e.g., male physician examining a female patient) should always be chaperoned.

Neurological Examination

A standard neurological examination should be performed. A detailed neurological evaluation is particularly important in psychiatric patients to rule out focal signs that might help to explain the patient's symptoms.

Diagnostic Impression

The clinician should note his or her diagnostic impression based on all five DSM-IV-TR axes whenever possible. When appropriate, more than one diagnosis should be made. When the diagnosis is uncertain, the qualifier *provisional* should be added. Not infrequently, it is difficult to make a definitive diagnosis at the time of the index evaluation. When this situation occurs, differential diagnostic possibilities should be listed.

Treatment and Management Plan

The treatment and management section will vary, depending on the level of diagnostic certainty. If the diagnosis is quite uncertain, the first step in treatment and management will involve additional assessments to determine the diagnosis with more certainty. Thus the treatment and management plan may include a list of laboratory tests appropriate to assist in the differential diagnosis listed above. Alternatively, when the diagnosis is straightforward, a specific treatment plan can be outlined, including a proposed medication regimen, plans for vocational rehabilitation, a program for social skills training, occupational therapy, marital counseling, or other ancillary treatments appropriate to the patient's specific problems.

■ Interviewing Techniques

Although the demands of the interview may vary depending on the patient and his or her illness, some techniques are common to most interviewing situations.

Establish rapport as early in the interview as possible. It is often best to begin by asking the patient about him- or herself (e.g., What kind of work do you do? What do you do for fun? How old are you?). Questions about these topics should not be asked in a manner that seems to "grill" the patient but rather in a way that indicates that the interviewer is genuinely interested in getting to know the patient. Interest can be indicated through follow-up questions. The overall tone of the opening of the interview should convey warmth and friendliness. Once rapport has been established, the interviewer should then inquire about what kind of problem the patient has been having, and what brought him or her to the clinic or hospital.

Determine the patient's chief complaint. Sometimes this complaint will be helpful and explicit (e.g., "I've been feeling very depressed," or "I've been having a pain in my head that other doctors can't explain").

At other times, the chief complaint may be relatively vague and require several follow-up questions (e.g., "I don't know why I'm here—my family brought me," or "I've been having trouble at work"). When the replies are not particularly explicit, the interviewer will need to follow up his or her initial questions with others that will help determine the nature of the patient's problem (e.g., "What kinds of things have been bothering your family?" "What kind of trouble at work?"). The initial portion of the interview, devoted to eliciting the chief complaint, should take as long as is necessary to determine the patient's primary problem. When the patient is a clear, logical informant, he or she should be allowed to tell his or her story as freely as possible without interruption. When he or she is a relatively poor informant, the interviewer will need to be active and directive.

Use the chief complaint to develop a provisional differential diagnosis. As in the rest of medicine, once the patient's primary problem has been determined, the interviewer begins to construct in his or her mind a range of explanations as to the specific diagnosis that might lead to that particular problem. For example, if the patient indicates that he or she has been hearing voices, the differential diagnosis includes a variety of disorders that produce this type of psychotic symptom, such as schizophrenia, schizophreniform disorder, psychotic mania, substance abuse involving hallucinogens, or alcoholic hallucinosis. It may be comforting to realize that the fundamental process of interviewing and diagnosing is the same in psychiatry as it is in internal medicine or neurology.

Rule the various diagnostic possibilities in or out by using more focused and detailed questions. The existence of DSM-IV-TR is particularly helpful in this regard. If the patient's chief complaint has suggested three or four different possible diagnoses, the interviewer can determine which is most relevant by referring to the diagnostic criteria for those disorders. Thus the interviewer elicits additional symptoms beyond those already enumerated when discussing the chief complaint. The interviewer inquires about the course and onset of the symptoms and about the presence of physical or psychological precipitants, such as drugs, alcohol, or personal losses.

Follow up vague or obscure replies with enough persistence to accurately determine the answer to the question. Some patients, particularly psychotic patients, have great difficulty answering questions clearly and concisely. They may say "yes" or "no" to every question asked. When a pattern of this sort is observed, the patient should be re-

background. Although delusions are sometimes defined as *fixed false beliefs*, in their mildest form delusions may persist for only weeks to months, and the patient may question his or her beliefs or doubt them. The patient's behavior may or may not be influenced by the specific delusions. The assessment of the severity of delusions and of the global severity of delusional thinking should take into account their persistence, their complexity, the extent to which the patient acts on them, the extent to which the patient doubts them, and the extent to which the beliefs deviate from those that nonpsychotic people might have. Beliefs held with less than a delusional intensity are often referred to as *overvalued ideas*.

Persecutory delusions.   People with persecutory delusions believe that they are being conspired against or persecuted in some way. Common manifestations include the belief that one is being followed, that one's mail is being opened, that one's room or office is bugged, that the telephone is tapped, or that one is being harassed by police, government officials, neighbors, or fellow workers. Persecutory delusions are sometimes relatively isolated or fragmented, but in some cases the person has a complex system of delusions involving both a wide range of forms of persecution and a belief that there is a well-planned conspiracy behind them: for example, that the patient's house is bugged and that he or she is being followed because the government wrongly considers him or her a secret agent of a foreign government. This delusion may be so complex that at least to the patient, it explains almost everything that happens to him or her.

- Have you had trouble getting along with people?
- Have you felt that people are against you?
- Has anyone been trying to harm you in any way?
- (Do you think people have been conspiring or plotting against you? Who?)

Delusions of jealousy.   The patient believes that his or her spouse or partner is having an affair with someone. Random bits of information are construed as "evidence." The person usually goes to great effort to prove the existence of the affair, searching for hair in the bedclothes, the odor of shaving lotion or smoke on clothing, or receipts or checks indicating that a gift has been bought for the lover. Elaborate plans are often made to trap the two together.

- Have you worried that your (husband, wife, boyfriend, girlfriend) might be unfaithful to you?
- (What evidence do you have?)

that to the patient. At the end of the initial interview, if you are uncertain about diagnosis or treatment, indicate that you have learned a great deal but that you need to think about the problem some more and perhaps gather more information before arriving at a recommendation.

■ Definitions of Common Signs and Symptoms and Methods for Eliciting Them

A vast panoply of signs and symptoms characterizes major mental illnesses. The following are some of the more common ones seen in psychiatric patients. Where appropriate, some suggested questions are provided that can be used to probe for these symptoms. Follow-up questions appear in parentheses.

Symptoms That Frequently Occur in Psychotic Disorders

The term *psychosis* has several different meanings, which may be especially confusing to beginning students. In the broadest sense, the term refers to the group of symptoms that characterize the most severe mental illnesses, such as schizophrenia or mania, and that involve an impairment in the ability to make judgments about the boundaries between what is real and unreal (sometimes called "impaired reality testing"). At a more operational level, *psychosis* refers to a specific group of symptoms that are common in these severe disorders. In the narrowest sense, psychosis is synonymous with having delusions and hallucinations. A somewhat broader operational definition also includes bizarre behavior, disorganized speech ("positive formal thought disorder"), and inappropriate affect. This group of symptoms is also known as *positive symptoms;* they may occur in any psychotic disorder, but are most common in schizophrenia. A second group of symptoms, referred to as *negative symptoms,* occur primarily in schizophrenia; they include alogia, affective blunting, avolition-apathy, anhedonia-asociality, and attentional impairment.

Delusions

Delusions represent an abnormality in content of thought. They are false beliefs that cannot be explained on the basis of the patient's cultural

Do not be afraid to ask about topics that you or the patient might find difficult or embarrassing. Beginning interviewers sometimes find it difficult to ask about topics such as sexual relationships, sexual experiences, or even use of alcohol or drugs. Yet all this information is part of a complete psychiatric interview and must be included. Nearly all patients expect doctors to ask these questions and are not offended. Likewise, beginning interviewers are sometimes embarrassed to ask about symptoms of psychosis, such as hearing voices. To the interviewer, these symptoms seem so "crazy" that the patient might be insulted by being asked about them. Again, however, information of this type is basic and cannot be avoided. If the patient seems "obviously" not psychotic, questions about psychotic symptoms still should be asked—and in an unapologetic manner. If the patient seems amused or annoyed, then the interviewer can explain that it is necessary to cover all kinds of questions to provide a comprehensive evaluation of each patient.

Do not forget to ask about suicidal thoughts. This is another topic that may seem to fall into the "embarrassing" category. Nevertheless, suicide is a common outcome of many psychiatric illnesses, and it is incumbent on the interviewer to ask about it. The subject can be broached quite tactfully by a question such as "Have you ever felt life isn't worth living?" The topic of suicide can then be broached, leading to questions such as "Have you ever thought about taking your life?" Further tips on interviewing the suicidal patient are provided in Chapter 15.

Give the patient a chance to ask questions at the end. From the patient's point of view, there is nothing more frustrating than being interviewed for an hour and then ushered out of the office or examining room with his or her own questions unanswered. The questions that patients ask often tell a great deal about what is on their mind. A patient might be prompted by asking, "Is there anything you feel is important that we haven't talked about?" Even if their questions are not helpful to the diagnostic process, they are significant to the patient and therefore intrinsically important.

Conclude the initial interview by conveying a sense of confidence and, if possible, of hope. Thank the patient for providing so much information. Compliment him or her, in whatever way it can be done sincerely, on having told his or her story well. Indicate that you now have a much better understanding of his or her problems, and conclude by stating that you will do what you can to help him or her. If you already have a relatively good idea that his or her problem is one that is amenable to treatment, explain

peatedly asked to describe his or her experiences as explicitly as possible. For example, if the patient says that he or she hears voices, he or she should be asked to describe them in more detail—whether they are male or female, what they say, and how often they occur. The greater the level of detail the patient is able to provide, the more confident the clinician can feel that the symptom is truly present. Because making a diagnosis of schizophrenia or another major psychiatric disorder has important prognostic implications, the clinician should not hastily accept an answer that suggests vaguely that the patient may have a particular symptom of a disorder.

Let the patient talk freely enough to observe how tightly his or her thoughts are connected. Most patients should be allowed to talk for at least 3 or 4 minutes without interruption in the course of any psychiatric interview. The very laconic patient, of course, will not be able to do this, but most can. The coherence of the pattern in which the patient's thoughts are presented may provide major clues to the type of problem that he or she is experiencing. For example, patients with mania, schizophrenia, or depression may have any one of a variety of types of "formal thought disorder" (see section "Definitions of Common Signs and Symptoms and Methods for Eliciting Them" later in this chapter). Coherence of thought also may be helpful in making a differential diagnosis between dementia and depression.

Use a mixture of open and closed questions. Interviewers can learn a great deal about patients by mixing up their types of questions, just as a good pitcher mixes up his or her pitches. Open-ended questions permit the patient to ramble and become disorganized, whereas closed questions determine whether the patient can come up with the specifics when pressed. These are important indicators as to whether the patient is conceptually disorganized or confused, whether he or she is being evasive, or whether he or she is answering randomly or falsely. The content of the questions should be mixed as well. For example, at some point in the interview, the interviewer will probably want to drop his or her objective style of interviewing and focus on some personal topic that is affect laden, such as sexual or interpersonal relationships (e.g., "Can you tell me about your relationship with your mother?" or "Tell me about your marriage"). These questions will give the interviewer important clues about the patient's capacity to show emotional responsiveness. Evaluating the patient's mood and affect is a fundamental aspect of the psychiatric evaluation, just as is evaluating the coherence of his or her thinking and communication.

that to the patient. At the end of the initial interview, if you are uncertain about diagnosis or treatment, indicate that you have learned a great deal but that you need to think about the problem some more and perhaps gather more information before arriving at a recommendation.

■ Definitions of Common Signs and Symptoms and Methods for Eliciting Them

A vast panoply of signs and symptoms characterizes major mental illnesses. The following are some of the more common ones seen in psychiatric patients. Where appropriate, some suggested questions are provided that can be used to probe for these symptoms. Follow-up questions appear in parentheses.

Symptoms That Frequently Occur in Psychotic Disorders

The term *psychosis* has several different meanings, which may be especially confusing to beginning students. In the broadest sense, the term refers to the group of symptoms that characterize the most severe mental illnesses, such as schizophrenia or mania, and that involve an impairment in the ability to make judgments about the boundaries between what is real and unreal (sometimes called "impaired reality testing"). At a more operational level, *psychosis* refers to a specific group of symptoms that are common in these severe disorders. In the narrowest sense, psychosis is synonymous with having delusions and hallucinations. A somewhat broader operational definition also includes bizarre behavior, disorganized speech ("positive formal thought disorder"), and inappropriate affect. This group of symptoms is also known as *positive symptoms*; they may occur in any psychotic disorder, but are most common in schizophrenia. A second group of symptoms, referred to as *negative symptoms*, occur primarily in schizophrenia; they include alogia, affective blunting, avolition-apathy, anhedonia-asociality, and attentional impairment.

Delusions

Delusions represent an abnormality in content of thought. They are false beliefs that cannot be explained on the basis of the patient's cultural background. Although delusions are sometimes defined as *fixed false beliefs*, in their mildest form delusions may persist for only weeks to months, and the patient may question his or her beliefs or doubt them. The patient's behavior may or may not be influenced by the specific delusions. The assessment of the severity of delusions and of the global severity of delusional thinking should take into account their persistence, their complexity, the extent to which the patient acts on them, the extent to which the patient doubts them, and the extent to which the beliefs deviate from those that nonpsychotic people might have. Beliefs held with less than a delusional intensity are often referred to as *overvalued ideas*.

Persecutory delusions.   People with persecutory delusions believe that they are being conspired against or persecuted in some way. Common manifestations include the belief that one is being followed, that one's mail is being opened, that one's room or office is bugged, that the telephone is tapped, or that one is being harassed by police, government officials, neighbors, or fellow workers. Persecutory delusions are sometimes relatively isolated or fragmented, but in some cases the person has a complex system of delusions involving both a wide range of forms of persecution and a belief that there is a well-planned conspiracy behind them: for example, that the patient's house is bugged and that he or she is being followed because the government wrongly considers him or her a secret agent of a foreign government. This delusion may be so complex that at least to the patient, it explains almost everything that happens to him or her.

- Have you had trouble getting along with people?
- Have you felt that people are against you?
- Has anyone been trying to harm you in any way?
- (Do you think people have been conspiring or plotting against you? Who?)

Delusions of jealousy.   The patient believes that his or her spouse or partner is having an affair with someone. Random bits of information are construed as "evidence." The person usually goes to great effort to prove the existence of the affair, searching for hair in the bedclothes, the odor of shaving lotion or smoke on clothing, or receipts or checks indicating that a gift has been bought for the lover. Elaborate plans are often made to trap the two together.

- Have you worried that your (husband, wife, boyfriend, girlfriend) might be unfaithful to you?
- (What evidence do you have?)

Delusions of sin or guilt.   The patient believes that he or she has committed some terrible sin or done something unforgivable. Sometimes the patient is excessively or inappropriately preoccupied with things he or she did as a child that were perceived to be wrong, such as masturbating. Sometimes the patient feels responsible for causing some disastrous event, such as a fire or an accident, with which he or she in fact has no connection. Sometimes these delusions have a religious flavor, involving the belief that the sin is unpardonable and that the patient will suffer eternal punishment from God. Sometimes the patient simply believes that he or she deserves punishment by society. The patient may spend a good deal of time confessing these sins to whoever will listen.

- Have you felt that you have done some terrible thing?
- Is there anything that is bothering your conscience?
- (What is it?)
- (Do you feel you deserve to be punished for it?)

Grandiose delusions.   The patient believes that he or she has special powers or abilities or is a famous person, such as a rock star, Napoleon, or Christ. The patient may believe he or she is writing some definitive book, composing a great piece of music, or developing some wonderful new invention. The patient is often suspicious that someone is trying to steal his or her ideas and may become quite irritated if his or her abilities are doubted.

- Do you have any special powers, talents, or abilities? Great wealth?
- Do you feel you are going to achieve great things?

Religious delusions.   The patient is preoccupied with false beliefs of a religious nature. Sometimes these exist within the context of a conventional religious system, such as beliefs about the Second Coming, the Antichrist, or possession by the Devil. At other times, they may involve an entirely new religious system or a pastiche of beliefs from a variety of religions, particularly Eastern religions, such as ideas about reincarnation or Nirvana. Religious delusions may be combined with grandiose delusions (if the patient considers him- or herself a religious leader), delusions of guilt, or delusions of being controlled. Religious delusions must be outside the range of beliefs considered normal for the patient's cultural and religious background.

- Are you a religious person?
- Have you had any unusual religious experiences?
- Have you become closer to God?

Somatic delusions. The patient believes that somehow his or her body is diseased, abnormal, or changed. For example, the patient may believe that his or her stomach or brain is rotting, that his or her hands have become enlarged, or that his or her facial features are ugly or mis-shapen (this belief is referred to as dysmorphophobia). Sometimes somatic delusions are accompanied by tactile or other hallucinations, and when this occurs, both should be considered to be present. (For example, a patient believes that he has ball bearings rolling about in his head, placed there by a dentist who filled his teeth, and can actually hear them clanking against one another.)

- Is there anything wrong with the way your body is working?
- Have you noticed any change in your appearance?

Ideas and delusions of reference. The patient believes that insignificant remarks, statements, or events have some special meaning for him or her. For example, the patient walks into a room, sees people laughing, and suspects that they were just talking about him or her. Sometimes items read in the newspaper, heard on the radio, or seen on television are considered special messages to the person. In the case of *ideas of reference,* the patient is suspicious but recognizes that his or her idea may be erroneous. When the patient actually believes that the statements or events refer to him or her, then this is considered a delusion of reference.

- Have you walked into a room and thought that people were talking about you or laughing at you?
- Have you seen things in magazines or on TV that seem to refer to you or contain a special message for you?
- Have you received special messages in any other ways?

Delusions of passivity (being controlled). The patient has a subjective experience that his or her feelings or actions are controlled by some outside force. The central requirement for this type of delusion is an actual strong subjective experience of being controlled. It does not include simple beliefs or ideas, such as that the patient is acting as an agent of God or that friends or parents are trying to coerce him or her into doing something. Rather, the patient must describe, for example, that his or her body has been occupied by some alien force that is making it move in peculiar ways, or that messages are being sent to his or her brain by radio waves and causing him or her to experience particular feelings that the person recognizes are not his or her own.

- Have you felt that you were being controlled by some outside person or force?
- (Do you feel like a puppet on a string?)

Delusions of mind reading.　The patient believes that people can read his or her mind or know his or her thoughts—that is, the patient subjectively experiences and recognizes that others know his or her thoughts, but he or she does not think that they can be heard out loud.

- Have you had the feeling that people could read your mind or know what you are thinking?

Thought broadcasting/Audible thoughts.　The patient believes that his or her thoughts are broadcast so that he or she or others can hear them. Sometimes the patient experiences his or her thoughts as a voice outside his or her head; this is an auditory hallucination as well as a delusion. Sometimes the patient feels that his or her thoughts are being broadcast, although he or she cannot hear them him- or herself. Sometimes he or she believes that his or her thoughts are picked up by a microphone and broadcast on the radio, the television, or through the Internet.

- Have you heard your own thoughts out loud, as if they were a voice outside your head?
- Have you felt that your thoughts were broadcast so that other people could hear them?

Thought insertion.　The patient believes that thoughts that are not his or her own have been inserted into his or her mind. For example, the patient may believe that a neighbor is practicing voodoo and planting alien sexual thoughts into his or her mind. This symptom should not be confused with experiencing unpleasant thoughts that the patient recognizes as his or her own, such as delusions of persecution or guilt.

- Have you felt that thoughts were being placed into your head by some outside person or force?

Thought withdrawal.　The patient believes that thoughts have been taken away from his or her mind. He or she is able to describe a subjective experience of beginning a thought and then suddenly having it removed by some alien force. This symptom does not include the mere subjective recognition of alogia.

- Have you felt that your thoughts were taken away by some outside person or force?

Hallucinations

Hallucinations represent an abnormality in perception. They are false perceptions occurring in the absence of an identifiable external stimulus. They may be experienced in any of the sensory modalities, including hearing, touch, taste, smell, and vision. True hallucinations should be distinguished from illusions (which involve a misperception of an external stimulus), hypnagogic and hypnopompic experiences (which occur when a patient is falling asleep and waking up, respectively), or normal thought processes that are exceptionally vivid. If the hallucinations have a religious quality, then they should be judged within the context of what is normal for the patient's social and cultural background.

Auditory hallucinations. The patient reports hearing voices, noises, or sounds. The most common auditory hallucinations involve hearing voices speaking to the patient or calling his or her name. The voices may be male or female, familiar or unfamiliar, and critical or complimentary. Typically, patients with schizophrenia experience the voices as unpleasant and negative. Less frequently patients report that the voices are comforting or provide companionship. Hallucinations involving sounds other than voices, such as noises or music, should be considered less characteristic and less severe.

- Have you heard voices or other sounds when no one was around or when you could not account for them?
- (What did they say?)

Voices commenting. These hallucinations involve hearing a voice that makes a running commentary on the patient's behavior or thought as it occurs (e.g., "Carl is brushing his teeth. Carl is about to eat breakfast").

- Have you heard voices commenting on what you are thinking or doing?
- (What do they say?)

Voices conversing. These hallucinations involve hearing two or more voices talking with each other, usually discussing something about the patient.

- Have you heard two or more voices talking with each other?
- (What do they say?)

Somatic or tactile hallucinations. Somatic or tactile hallucinations involve experiencing peculiar physical sensations in the body. They include burning, itching sensations, or tingling sensations or the perception that the body has changed in shape or size.

- Have you had burning sensations or other strange sensations in your body?
- (What were they?)

Olfactory hallucinations. The patient experiences unusual smells that are typically quite unpleasant. Sometimes the patient may believe that he or she smells bad. This belief should be considered a hallucination if the patient can actually smell the odor but should be considered a delusion if he or she believes that only others can smell the odor.

- Have you experienced any unusual smells or smells that others do not notice?
- (What were they?)

Visual hallucinations. The patient sees shapes or people that are not actually present. Sometimes these are shapes or colors, but most typically they are figures of people or humanlike objects. They also may be characters of a religious nature, such as the Devil or Christ. As always, visual hallucinations involving religious themes should be judged within the context of the patient's cultural background.

- Have you had visions or seen things that other people cannot?
- (What did you see?)

Bizarre or Disorganized Behavior

The patient's behavior is unusual, bizarre, or fantastic. The information for this symptom will sometimes come from the patient, sometimes come from other sources, and sometimes come from direct observation. Bizarre behavior due to the immediate effects of intoxication with alcohol or drugs should not be considered a symptom of psychosis. Social and cultural norms must be considered in making the determination of bizarre behavior, and detailed examples should be elicited and noted.

Clothing and appearance. The patient dresses in an unusual manner or does other strange things to alter his or her appearance. For example, the patient may shave off all his or her hair or paint body parts different colors. The patient's clothing may be quite unusual; for example, he or she may choose to wear some outfit that appears generally inappropriate and unacceptable, such as a baseball cap backward with rubber galoshes and long underwear covered by denim overalls. The patient may dress in a fantastic costume representing some historical personage or a person from outer space. He or she may wear clothing completely inappropriate to the climatic conditions, such as heavy wools in summer.

- Has anyone made comments about the way you dress?
- (What did they say?)

Social and sexual behavior.   The patient may do things that are considered inappropriate according to usual social norms. For example, he or she may masturbate in public, urinate or defecate in inappropriate receptacles, walk along the street muttering to him- or herself, or begin talking to people whom he or she has never before met about intimate personal matters (as when riding on a subway or standing in some public place). He or she may drop to his or her knees praying and shouting or suddenly assume a fetal position when in the midst of a crowd. He or she may make inappropriate sexual overtures or remarks to strangers.

- Have you done anything that others might think is unusual or that has called attention to yourself?
- Has anyone complained or commented about your behavior?
- (What were you doing at the time?)

Aggressive and agitated behavior.   The patient may behave in an aggressive, agitated manner, often quite unpredictably. He or she may start arguments inappropriately with friends or members of his or her family or accost strangers on the street and begin haranguing them angrily. He or she may write letters or send e-mails of a threatening or angry nature to government officials or others with whom he or she has some quarrel. Occasionally, patients may perform violent acts, such as injuring or tormenting animals or attempting to injure or kill human beings.

- Have you been unusually angry or irritable with anyone?
- (How did you express your anger?)
- Have you done anything to try to harm animals or people?

Ritualistic or stereotyped behavior.   The patient may develop a set of repetitive actions or rituals that he or she must perform over and over. Sometimes he or she will attribute some symbolic significance to these actions and believe that they are either influencing others or preventing himself or herself from being influenced. For example, he or she may

eat jelly beans every night for dessert, assuming that different consequences will occur depending on the color of the jelly beans. He or she
may have to eat foods in a particular order, wear particular clothes, or
get dressed in a certain order. He or she may have to write messages to
him- or herself or to others over and over, sometimes in an unusual or
occult language.

* Are there any things that you do over and over?
* Are there any things that you have to do in a certain way or in a par-
  ticular order?
* (Why do you do it?)
* (Does it have any special meaning or significance to you?)

Disorganized Speech (Positive Formal Thought Disorder)

Disorganized speech, which is also referred to as *positive formal thought disorder,* is fluent speech that tends to communicate poorly for a variety of
reasons. The patient tends to skip from topic to topic without warning;
is distracted by events in the nearby environment; joins words together
because they are semantically or phonologically alike, even though they
make no sense; or ignores the question asked and answers another. This
type of speech may be rapid, and it frequently seems quite disjointed.
Unlike alogia (negative formal thought disorder; see subsection "Alogia" later in this chapter), a wealth of detail is provided, and the flow of
speech tends to have an energetic rather than an apathetic quality to it.

To evaluate thought disorder, the patient should be permitted to talk
without interruption for as long as 5 minutes. The interviewer should
observe closely the extent to which the patient's sequencing of ideas is
well connected. Close attention should also be paid to how well the patient can reply to various types of questions, ranging from simple
("When were you born?") to more complicated ("Why did you come to
the hospital?"). If the ideas seem vague or incomprehensible, the interviewer should prompt the patient to clarify or elaborate.

Derailment (loose associations).   The patient has a pattern of spontaneous speech in which the ideas slip off the track onto another that is
clearly but obliquely related or onto one completely unrelated. Things
may be said in juxtaposition that lack a meaningful relationship, or the
patient may shift idiosyncratically from one frame of reference to another. At times, there may be a vague connection between the ideas, and
at other times, none will be apparent. This pattern of speech is often
characterized as sounding "disjointed." Perhaps the most common
manifestation of this disorder is a slow, steady slippage, with no single

derailment being particularly severe, so that the speaker gets farther and farther off the track with each derailment without showing any awareness that his or her reply no longer has any connection with the question that was asked. This abnormality is often characterized by lack of cohesion between clauses and sentences and by unclear pronoun references.

> **Interviewer:** Did you enjoy college?
> **Subject:** Um-hm. Oh hey well I, I oh, I really enjoyed some communities. I tried it, and the, and the next day when I'd be going out, you know, um, I took control, like, uh, I put, um, bleach on my hair in, in California. My roommate was from Chicago and she was going to the junior college. And we lived in the Y.W.C.A., so she wanted to put it, um, peroxide on my hair, and she did, and I got up and I looked at the mirror and tears came to my eyes. Now do you understand it—I was fully aware of what was going on but why couldn't I, I…why the tears? I can't understand that, can you?

Tangentiality. The patient replies to a question in an oblique, tangential, or even irrelevant manner. The reply may be related to the question in some distant way, or the reply may be unrelated and seem totally irrelevant.

> **Interviewer:** What city are you from?
> **Subject:** Well, that's a hard question to answer because my parents… I was born in Iowa, but I know that I'm white instead of black, so apparently I came from the North somewhere and I don't know where, you know, I really don't know whether I'm Irish or Scandinavian, or I don't, I don't believe I'm Polish, but I think I'm, I think I might be German or Welsh.

Incoherence (word salad, schizophasia). The patient has a pattern of speech that is essentially incomprehensible at times. Incoherence is often accompanied by derailment. It differs from derailment in that with incoherence the abnormality occurs at the level of the sentence or clause, which contains words or phrases that are joined incoherently. The abnormality in derailment involves unclear or confusing connections between larger units, such as sentences or clauses. This type of language disorder is relatively rare. When it occurs, it tends to be severe or extreme, and mild forms are quite uncommon. It may sound quite similar to Wernicke's aphasia or jargon aphasia, and in these cases the disorder should only be called incoherence definitively when history and laboratory data exclude the possibility of a past stroke and clinical testing for aphasia has negative results.

> **Interviewer:** What do you think about current political issues like the energy crisis?

Subject: They're destroying too many cattle and oil just to make soap. If we need soap when you can jump into a pool of water, and then when you go to buy your gasoline, my folks always thought they should, get pop but the best thing to get, is motor oil, and, money. May, may as, well go there and, trade in some, pop caps and, uh, tires, and tractors to grup, car garages, so they can pull cars away from wrecks, is what I believed in.

Illogicality. The patient has a pattern of speech in which conclusions are reached that do not follow logically. Illogicality may take the form of non sequiturs (meaning "it does not follow"), in which the patient makes a logical inference between two clauses that is unwarranted or illogical. It may take the form of faulty inductive inferences. It may also take the form of reaching conclusions based on faulty premises without any actual delusional thinking.

Subject: Parents are the people that raise you. Anything that raises you can be a parent. Parents can be anything—material, vegetable, or mineral—that has taught you something. Parents would be the world of things that are alive, that are there. Rocks—a person can look at a rock and learn something from it, so that would be a parent.

Circumstantiality. The patient has a pattern of speech that is very indirect and delayed in reaching its goal ideas. In the process of explaining something, the speaker brings in many tedious details and sometimes makes parenthetical remarks. Circumstantial replies or statements may last for many minutes if the speaker is not interrupted and urged to get to the point. Interviewers will often recognize circumstantiality on the basis of needing to interrupt the speaker to complete the process of history taking within an allotted time. When not called circumstantial, these people are often referred to as long-winded.

Although it may coexist with instances of poverty of content of speech or loss of goal, circumstantiality differs from poverty of content of speech in containing excessive amplifying or illustrative detail and from loss of goal in that the goal is eventually reached if the person is allowed to talk long enough. It differs from derailment in that the details presented are closely related to some particular goal or idea and that the particular goal or idea must, by definition, eventually be reached (unless the patient is interrupted by an impatient interviewer).

Pressure of speech. The patient has an increase in the amount of spontaneous speech as compared with what is considered ordinary or socially customary. The patient talks rapidly and is difficult to interrupt. Pressured speech is often seen in mania but can be found in other syndromes as well. Some sentences may be left uncompleted because of eagerness to get on to a new idea. Simple questions that could be answered in only a few words or sentences are answered at great length so that the answer takes minutes rather than seconds and indeed may not stop at all if the speaker is not interrupted. Even when interrupted, the speaker often continues to talk. Speech tends to be loud and emphatic. Sometimes speakers with severe pressure will talk without any social stimulation and talk even though no one is listening. When patients are receiving antipsychotics or mood stabilizers, their speech is often slowed down by medication, and then it can be judged only on the basis of amount, volume, and social appropriateness. If a quantitative measure is applied to the rate of speech, then a rate greater than 150 words per minute is usually considered rapid or pressured. This disorder may be accompanied by derailment, tangentiality, or incoherence, but it is distinct from them.

Distractible speech.   During the course of a discussion or an interview, the patient stops talking in the middle of a sentence or idea and changes the subject in response to a nearby stimulus, such as an object on a desk, the interviewer's clothing or appearance, and so forth.

> **Subject:** Then I left San Francisco and moved to…where did you get that tie? It looks like it's left over from the '50s. I like the warm weather in San Diego. Is that a conch shell on your desk? Have you ever gone scuba diving?

Clanging.   The patient has a pattern of speech in which sounds rather than meaningful relations appear to govern word choice, so that the intelligibility of the speech is impaired and redundant words are introduced in addition to rhyming relationships. This pattern of speech also may include punning associations, so that a word similar in sound brings in a new thought.

> **Subject:** I'm not trying to make a noise. I'm trying to make sense. If you can make sense out of nonsense, well, have fun. I'm trying to make sense out of sense. I'm not making sense [cents] anymore. I have to make dollars.

Catatonic Motor Behavior

Catatonic motor symptoms are not common and should only be considered present when they are obvious and have been directly observed by the clinician or some other professional.

Stupor.   The patient has a marked decrease in reactivity to the environment and reduction of spontaneous movements and activity. The patient may appear to be aware of the nature of his or her surroundings.

Rigidity. The patient shows signs of motor rigidity, such as resistance to passive movement.

Waxy flexibility (catalepsy). The patient maintains postures into which he or she is placed for at least 15 seconds.

Excitement. The patient has apparently purposeless and stereotyped excited motor activity not influenced by external stimuli.

Posturing and mannerisms. The patient voluntarily assumes an inappropriate or a bizarre posture. Manneristic gestures or tics also may be observed. These involve movements or gestures that appear artificial or contrived, are not appropriate to the situation, or are stereotyped and repetitive. (Patients with tardive dyskinesia may have manneristic gestures or tics, but these should not be considered manifestations of catatonia.)

Inappropriate Affect

The patient's affect expressed is inappropriate or incongruous, not simply flat or blunted. Most typically, this manifestation of affective disturbance takes the form of smiling or assuming a silly facial expression while talking about a serious or sad subject. For example, the patient may laugh inappropriately when talking about thoughts of harming another person. (Occasionally, patients may smile or laugh when talking about a serious subject that they find uncomfortable or embarrassing. Although their smiling may seem inappropriate, it is due to anxiety and therefore should not be rated as inappropriate affect.)

Alogia

Alogia is a general term coined to refer to the impoverished thinking and cognition that often occur in patients with schizophrenia (from the Greek *a*, "no"; *logos*, "mind, thought"). Patients with alogia have thinking processes that seem empty, turgid, or slow. Because thinking cannot be observed directly, it is inferred from the patient's speech. The two major manifestations of alogia are nonfluent empty speech (poverty of speech) and fluent empty speech (poverty of content of speech). Blocking and increased latency of response also may reflect alogia.

Poverty of speech. The patient has a restricted *amount* of spontaneous speech, so that replies to questions tend to be brief, concrete, and unelaborated. Unprompted additional information is rarely provided. Replies may be monosyllabic, and some questions may be left unanswered altogether. When confronted with this speech pattern, the inter-

viewer may find him- or herself frequently prompting the patient, to encourage elaboration of replies. To elicit this finding, the examiner must allow the patient adequate time to answer and to elaborate his or her answer.

> **Interviewer:** Can you tell me something about what brought you to the hospital?
> **Subject:** A car.
> **Interviewer:** I was wondering about what kinds of problems you've been having. Can you tell me something about them?
> **Subject:** I dunno.

Poverty of content of speech.   Although the patient's replies are long enough so that speech is adequate in amount, it conveys little information. Language tends to be vague, often overabstract or overconcrete, repetitive, and stereotyped. The interviewer may recognize this finding by observing that the patient has spoken at some length but has not given adequate information to answer the question. Alternatively, the patient may provide enough information but require many words to do so, so that a lengthy reply can be summarized in a sentence or two. This abnormality differs from circumstantiality in that the circumstantial patient tends to provide a wealth of detail.

> **Interviewer:** Why is it, do you think, that people believe in God?
> **Subject:** Well, first of all because He, uh, He are the person that is their personal savior. He walks with me and talks with me. And, uh, the understanding that I have, um, a lot of people, they don't readily, uh, know their own personal self. Because, uh, they ain't, they all, just don't know their personal self. They don't, know that He, uh—seemed like to me, a lot of 'em don't understand that He walks and talks with 'em.

Blocking.   The patient's train of speech is interrupted before a thought or an idea has been completed. After a period of silence, which may last from a few seconds to minutes, the person indicates that he or she cannot recall what he or she has been saying or meant to say. Blocking should be judged to be present only if a person voluntarily describes losing his or her thought or if, on questioning by the interviewer, the person indicates that that was his or her reason for pausing.

> **Subject:** So I didn't want to go back to school so I...(1-minute silence while the patient stares blankly)
> **Interviewer:** What about going back to school? What happened?
> **Subject:** I dunno. I forgot what I was going to say.

Increased latency of response. The patient takes a longer time to reply to questions than is usually considered normal. He or she may seem distant, and sometimes the examiner may wonder whether he or she has heard the question. Prompting usually indicates that the patient is aware of the question but has been having difficulty formulating his or her thoughts to make an appropriate reply.

> **Interviewer:** When were you last in the hospital?
> **Subject:** (30-second pause) A year ago.
> **Interviewer:** Which hospital was it?
> **Subject:** (30-second pause) This one.

Perseveration. The patient persistently repeats words, ideas, or phrases so that once a patient begins to use a particular word, he or she continually returns to it in the process of speaking. Perseveration differs from "stock words" in that the repeated words are used in ways inappropriate to their usual meaning. Some words or phrases are commonly used as pause-fillers, such as "you know" or "like," and these should not be considered perseverations.

> **Interviewer:** Tell me what you are like—what kind of person you are.
> **Subject:** I'm from Marshalltown, Iowa. That's 60 miles northwest, northeast of Des Moines, Iowa. And I'm married at the present time. I'm 36 years old; my wife is 35. She lives in Garwin, Iowa. That's 15 miles southeast of Marshalltown, Iowa. I'm getting a divorce at the present time. And I am at present in a mental institution in Iowa City, Iowa, which is 100 miles southeast of Marshalltown, Iowa.

Affective Flattening or Blunting

Affective flattening or blunting manifests itself as a characteristic impoverishment of emotional expression, reactivity, and feeling. Affective flattening can be evaluated by observation of the patient's behavior and responsiveness during a routine interview. The evaluation of affective expression may be influenced by the patient's use of prescription drugs, because the parkinsonian side effects of antipsychotics may lead to mask-like facies and diminished associated movements. Other aspects of affect, such as responsivity or appropriateness, will not be affected, however.

Unchanging facial expression. The patient's face does not change expression, or changes less than normally expected, as the emotional content of the discourse changes. His or her face appears wooden, me-

chanical, and frozen. Because antipsychotics may partially mimic this effect, the interviewer should be careful to note whether the patient is taking medication.

Decreased spontaneous movements.   The patient sits quietly throughout the interview and shows few or no spontaneous movements. He or she does not shift position, move his or her legs, or move his or her hands or does so less than normally expected.

Paucity of expressive gestures.   The patient does not use his or her body as an aid in expressing his or her ideas through means such as hand gestures, sitting forward in his or her chair when intent on a subject, or leaning back when relaxed. Paucity of expressive gestures may occur in addition to decreased spontaneous movements.

Poor eye contact.   The patient avoids looking at others or using his or her eyes as an aid in expression. He or she appears to be staring into space even when he or she is talking. The interviewer should consider the quality as well as the quantity of eye contact.

Affective nonresponsivity.   The patient fails to smile or laugh when prompted. This function may be tested by smiling or joking in a way that would usually elicit a smile from a psychiatrically normal individual.

Lack of vocal inflections.   While speaking, the patient fails to show normal vocal emphasis patterns. Speech has a monotonic quality, and important words are not emphasized through changes in pitch or volume. The patient also may fail to change volume with changes of content, so that he or she does not drop his or her voice when discussing private topics or raise it as he or she discusses things that are exciting or for which louder speech might be appropriate.

Avolition-Apathy

Avolition-apathy manifests itself as a characteristic lack of energy and drive. Patients become inert and are unable to mobilize themselves to initiate or persist in completing many different kinds of tasks. Unlike the diminished energy or interest of depression, the avolitional symptom complex in schizophrenia usually is not accompanied by saddened or depressed affect. The avolitional symptom complex often leads to severe social and economic impairment.

Grooming and hygiene.   The patient pays less attention to grooming and hygiene than is normal. Clothing may appear sloppy, outdated, or

soiled. He or she may bathe infrequently and not care for his or her hair, nails, or teeth—leading to manifestations such as greasy or uncombed hair, dirty hands, body odor, or unclean teeth and bad breath. Overall, the appearance is dilapidated and disheveled. In extreme cases, the patient may even have poor toilet habits.

Impersistence at work or school. The patient has difficulty in seeking or maintaining employment (or doing schoolwork) as appropriate for his or her age and gender. If a student, he or she does not do homework and may even fail to attend class. Grades will tend to reflect this. If a college student, he or she may have registered for courses but dropped several or all of them. If of working age, the patient may have found it difficult to work at a job because of an inability to persist in completing tasks and apparent irresponsibility. He or she may go to work irregularly, wander away early, fail to complete expected assignments, or complete them in a disorganized manner. He or she may simply sit around the house and not seek any employment or seek it only in an infrequent or desultory manner. If a homemaker or a retired person, the patient may fail to complete chores, such as shopping or cleaning, or complete them in a careless and half-hearted way. If in a hospital or an institution, he or she does not attend or persist in vocational or rehabilitative programs effectively.

- Have you been able to (work, go to school) during the past month?
- Have you been attending vocational rehabilitation or occupational therapy sessions (in the hospital)?
- What have you been able to do?
- (Do you have trouble finishing what you start?)
- (What kinds of problems have you had?)

Physical anergia. The patient tends to be physically inert; he or she may sit in a chair for hours at a time and not initiate any spontaneous activity. If encouraged to become involved in an activity, he or she may participate only briefly and then wander away or disengage him- or herself and return to sitting alone. He or she may spend large amounts of time in some relatively mindless and physically inactive task such as watching television or playing solitaire. Family members may report that the patient spends most of his or her time at home "doing nothing except sitting around." Either at home or in an inpatient setting, he or she may spend much of his or her time sitting unoccupied.

- How have you been spending your time?
- Do you have any trouble getting yourself going?

Anhedonia-Asociality

Anhedonia-asociality encompasses the patient's difficulties in experiencing interest or pleasure. It may express itself as a loss of interest in pleasurable activities, an inability to experience pleasure when participating in activities normally considered pleasurable, or a lack of involvement in social relationships of various kinds.

Recreational interests and activities.   The patient may have few or no interests, activities, or hobbies. Although this symptom may begin insidiously or slowly, there will usually be some obvious decline from an earlier level of interest and activity. Patients with relatively milder loss of interest will engage in some activities that are passive or nondemanding, such as watching television, or will show only occasional or sporadic interest. Patients with the most extreme loss will appear to have a complete and intractable inability to become involved in or enjoy activities. The evaluation in this area should take both the quality and the quantity of recreational interests into account.

- What do you do for enjoyment?
- (How often do you do those things?)
- Have you been attending recreational therapy?
- (What have you been doing?)
- (Do you enjoy it?)

Sexual interest and activity.   The patient may show a decrement in sexual interest and activity or enjoyment as compared to what would be judged healthy for the patient's age and marital status. Individuals who are married may manifest disinterest in sex or may engage in intercourse only at the partner's request. In extreme cases, the patient may not engage in sex at all. Single patients may go for long periods without sexual involvement and make no effort to satisfy this drive. Whether married or single, patients may report that they subjectively feel only minimal sex drive or that they take little enjoyment in sexual intercourse or in masturbatory activity even when they engage in it.

- What has your sex drive been like?
- Have you been able to enjoy sex lately?
- (What is your usual sexual outlet?)
- (When was the last time you engaged in sexual activity?)

Ability to feel intimacy and closeness.   The patient may be unable to form intimate and close relationships of a type appropriate for his or her

age, gender, and family status. In the case of a younger person, this area should be evaluated in terms of relationships with the opposite sex and with parents and siblings. In the case of an older person who is married, the relationship with the spouse and with children should be evaluated, whereas unmarried individuals should be judged in terms of opposite- or same-sex relationships or relationships with family members who live nearby. Patients may show few or no feelings of affection to available family members, or they may have arranged their lives so that they are completely isolated from any intimate relationships, live alone, and make no effort to initiate contacts with family or others.

- Do you feel close to your family (husband, wife, partner, children)?
- Is there anyone outside your family to whom you feel especially close?
- (How often do you see [them, him, her]?)

Relationships with friends and peers.   Patients also may be relatively restricted in their relationships with friends and peers of either gender. They may have few or no friends, make little or no effort to develop such relationships, and choose to spend all or most of their time alone.

- Do you have many friends?
- (Are you very close to them?)
- (How often do you see them?)
- (What do you do together?)
- Have you gotten to know any patients in the hospital?

Attention

Attention is often poor in patients with severe mental illnesses. The patient may have trouble focusing his or her attention or may be able to focus only sporadically and erratically. He or she may ignore attempts to converse with him or her, wander away while in the middle of an activity or a task, or appear to be inattentive when engaged in formal testing or interviewing. He or she may or may not be aware of the difficulty in focusing attention.

Social inattentiveness.   While involved in social situations or activities, the patient appears inattentive. He or she looks away during conversations, does not pick up the topic during a discussion, or appears uninvolved or disengaged. He or she may abruptly terminate a discussion or a task without any apparent reason. He or she may seem "spacey" or "out of it." He or she may seem to have poor concentration when playing games, reading, or watching television.

the death of a loved one. If the patient has not lost a loved one, ask him or her to compare the feelings with those after some significant personal loss appropriate to his or her age and experience.

- The feelings of (sadness) you are having now—are they the same as the feelings you would have had when someone close to you died, or are they different?
- (How are they similar or different?)

Nonreactivity of mood.   The patient does not feel much better, even temporarily, when something good happens.

- Do your feelings of depression go away or get better when you do something you enjoy, such as talking with friends, visiting your family, or playing with a pet (engaging in some other favorite activity)?

Diurnal variation.   The patient's mood shifts during the course of the day. Some patients feel terrible in the morning but feel steadily better as the day goes on and even near normal in the evening. Others feel good in the morning and worse as the day progresses.

- Is there any time of the day that is especially bad for you?
- (Do you feel worse in the morning? In the evening? Or is it about the same all the time?)

Anxiety Symptoms

Panic attacks.   The patient has discrete episodes of intense fear or discomfort in which a variety of symptoms occur, such as shortness of breath, dizziness, palpitations, or shaking.

- Have you ever experienced a sudden attack of panic or fear, in which you felt extremely uncomfortable?
- (How long did it last?)
- (Did you notice any other symptoms occurring at the same time?)
- (Did you feel as if you were going to die or go crazy?)

Agoraphobia.   The patient has a fear of going outside (literally "a fear of the marketplace"). In many patients, however, the fear is more generalized and involves being afraid of being in a place or situation from which escape might be difficult.

- Have you ever been afraid of going outside, so that you tended to just stay home all the time?

- Have you been afraid of getting caught or trapped somewhere so that you would be unable to escape?

Social phobia. The patient has a fear of being in some social situation in which he or she will be seen by others and may do something that he or she might find to be humiliating or embarrassing. Some common social phobias include fear of public speaking, fear of eating in front of others, and fear of using public bathrooms.

- Do you have any special fears, such as a fear of public speaking?
- Of eating in front of others?

Specific phobia. The patient is afraid of some specific circumscribed stimulus, such as animals (e.g., snakes, insects), seeing blood, being at high places, or being afraid to fly on airplanes.

- Are you afraid of snakes?
- The sight of blood?
- Air travel?
- Do you have any other specific fears?

Obsessions. The patient experiences persistent ideas, thoughts, or impulses that are unwanted and experienced as unpleasant. The patient tends to ruminate and worry about them. The patient may try to ignore or suppress them but typically finds this difficult. Some common obsessions include repetitive thoughts of performing some violent act or becoming contaminated by touching other people or inanimate objects, such as a doorknob.

- Are you ever bothered by persistent ideas that you can't get out of your head, such as being dirty or contaminated?
- (Can you give me some specific examples?)

Compulsions. The patient has to perform specific acts over and over in a way that he or she recognizes to be senseless or inappropriate. The compulsions are usually performed to ease some worry or obsession or to prevent some feared event from occurring. For example, a patient may have the worry that he or she has left the door unlocked and must return to check it repeatedly. Obsessions about contamination may lead to repetitive hand washing. Obsessions about thoughts of violence may lead to ritualistic behavior designed to prevent injury to the person about whom violence has been imagined.

- Are there any types of actions that you have to perform over and over, such as washing your hands or checking the stove?
- (Can you give me some examples?)

■ Self-Assessment Questions

1. Describe the way in which the patient's chief complaint can be used to take a history and to develop a differential diagnosis.

2. Describe several techniques that are important for concluding the initial interview with a patient.

3. Enumerate the components of a standard psychiatric history, giving each of the main headings of the overall outline.

4. Summarize the major components of the mental status examination.

5. Enumerate and describe at least four of the positive symptoms of psychosis. Give examples of some typical kinds of delusions and hallucinations.

6. Enumerate and describe at least four negative symptoms.

7. Enumerate and define some of the symptoms observed in depression.

8. Enumerate and define some of the symptoms observed in mania.

9. Enumerate and define some of the symptoms observed in anxiety disorders.

CHAPTER 3

The Neurobiology and Genetics of Mental Illness

Men ought to know that from the brain, and from the brain only, arise our pleasures, joys, laughter, and jests, as well as our sorrows, pains, griefs, and fears. Through it, in particular, we think, see, hear....

Hippocrates

STUDENTS OF PSYCHIATRY are privileged to study diseases that affect the most interesting and important organ in the body: the miraculous human brain. The human brain has created and invented the myriad achievements that surround us every day—skyscrapers, computers, complex economic markets, advances in medical science ranging from vaccines to antibiotics to magnetic resonance scanners, an understanding of quantum mechanics and chaos theory, and art, music, and literature. These achievements have been accomplished because the human brain is one of the most complex systems in the universe. Composed of more than 100 billion neurons (more nerve cells than the stars in the Milky Way), the brain expands its communicating and thinking power by multiplying connectivity through an average of 1,000–10,000 synapses per nerve cell. The synapses are "plastic" in that they remodel themselves continuously in response to changes in their environment and the inputs that they receive. The whole human brain system is composed of feedback loops and circuits composed of multiple neurons, further expanding the fine-tuning and thinking capacities. The abilities that we all have to think, feel emotions, and relate to other people in normal ways depend on the activity of this complex organ. The disturbances in thought, emotion, and behavior that we observe in the mentally ill also are ultimately due to aberrations in the brain. Understanding those brain aberrations—and correcting them—is our ultimate challenge.

Modern psychiatry stretches from mind to molecule and from clinical neuroscience to molecular biology as it attempts to understand how aberrations in thinking and behavior are rooted in underlying biological mechanisms. During the past several decades neuroscience has grown to become one of the largest domains of scientific research. This chapter provides a selective overview of a few topics from neurobiology that are relevant to understanding either the symptoms or treatment of mental illnesses.

■ Anatomical and Functional Brain Systems

The human brain may be divided into a variety of systems that mediate many different cognitive, emotional, and perceptual functions, such as the motor system, the visual system, the auditory system, and the somatosensory system. The systems that are of special interest to psychiatry are those that represent circuitry or functions that are particularly disturbed in mental illnesses. These systems represent some of the "last frontiers" in the study of the human brain. Three important anatomical systems are the prefrontal system, the limbic system, and the basal ganglia system. Important functional systems include the executive function, memory, language, attention, and reward systems.

Any method for dividing the brain into parts or systems is somewhat arbitrary because the three anatomical systems are all interconnected with one another and work interactively. The functional systems are also highly interdependent with one another and with the prefrontal, limbic, and basal ganglia systems as well. Furthermore, the division of the brain into "functional and anatomical systems" and "neurochemical systems" is also arbitrary. These oversimplifications are introduced purely for conceptual convenience, providing a strategy for reducing the overwhelming complexity of the central nervous system (CNS) to a level that permits discussion and analysis. Ultimately, however, a full understanding of the brain can only occur by an ongoing process of analysis (or breakdown and simplification) as well as synthesis (or rebuilding and unifying).

One must add a word of caution about our existing level of ignorance. We do not as yet have a complete map of the human brain, summarizing accurately its various neural circuits and chemical anatomy. This process is ongoing and becoming much more sophisticated, particularly with the aid of neuroimaging techniques such as structural and functional magnetic resonance imaging (sMRI and fMRI), diffusion tensor imaging (DTI), magnetic resonance spectroscopy (MRS), magnetoencephalography (MEG), and positron emission tomography (PET). These technologies permit in vivo study of the anatomy and physiology of the human brain in ways that were previously impossible. Prior to the availability of neuroimaging, our knowledge about circuitry and functional systems was based primarily on lesion and postmortem studies. Directly visualizing how the brain performs mental work with fMRI or PET imaging is clearly more accurate than trying to infer indirectly how it works by observing what it cannot do when parts are missing.

The Prefrontal System and Executive Functions

The prefrontal system, or prefrontal cortex, is one of the largest cortical subregions in the human brain. It constitutes 29% of the cortex in human beings, compared with 17% in chimpanzees, 7% in dogs, and 3.5% in cats. The relative development of the prefrontal cortex in various animal species is shown in Figure 3–1.

This huge association region in the brain integrates input from much of the neocortex, limbic regions, hypothalamic and brainstem regions, and (via the thalamus) most of the rest of the brain. Its high degree of development in human beings suggests that it may mediate a variety of specifically human functions often referred to as *executive functions,* such as high-order abstract thought, creative problem solving, and the temporal sequencing of behavior. Lesion and trauma studies, supplemented by experimental studies in nonhuman primates, have substantially added to this view of the functions of the prefrontal cortex. It is now clear that the prefrontal cortex mediates a large variety of functions, including attention and perception, moral judgment, temporal integration, and affect and emotion.

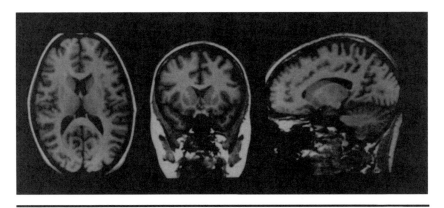

FIGURE 3–3.   The basal ganglia as seen with magnetic resonance imaging.
The triplanar resampling and visualization, achieved through locally developed software for image analysis (BRAINS, or Brain Research: Analysis of Images, Networks, and Systems), permits viewing of structures with a complex shape such as the caudate from three different angles, thus enhancing our capacity to understand brain anatomy three-dimensionally.
Source.   Copyright © 1993 Nancy C. Andreasen.

The Memory System

The memory system is a major functional brain system that may be impaired in some mentally ill patients. Deficits in learning and memory are the hallmark of the dementias. Although patients with psychotic disorders do not typically have severe memory deficits, some investigators have speculated that the neural mechanisms of delusions and hallucinations might be based on either abnormal excitability or abnormal connectivity in the neural circuitry used for the encoding, retrieval, and interpretation of memories. Within psychoanalytic theory, it has long been believed that the various "neuroses," such as anxiety disorders or hysteria (i.e., somatization disorder), might represent the painful stimulus of repressed memories that have not been psychologically integrated. The process of psychotherapy involves the process of learning, which is based in turn on memory; patients who successfully complete a course of psychotherapy have learned new ways of understanding their past experiences and relating to other people.

Memory is in fact a diverse set of functions that are mediated in different ways. Typically, memory is now thought of as a two-stage process. The first stage involves working memory; this is the form we use when we "learn" a telephone number long enough to dial it or a driver's license number long enough to write it down. This type of memory is accessible in short-term storage and is used as a mental scratchpad that we call on when we perform mental operations such as arithmetic calculations from numbers that have been quoted to us. Long-term memory, on the other hand, consists of information that we have learned and retained for periods of time greater than a few minutes. This type of memory is sometimes referred to as "consolidated" memory and is currently being employed by the students reading this textbook.

Normal human experience, as well as research in neuroscience, indicates that a variety of techniques can be used to facilitate learning, or consolidation of memory. These include such things as repetition, rehearsal, or mnemonic devices. This type of memory is mediated by a different set of mechanisms that lead to long-term storage of information. The work of Eric Kandel, using the gill withdrawal reflex in the snail *Aplysia* as a model, has shown that long-term memory depends on the synthesis of proteins in neurons that are synaptically connected during the time that short-term learning has been occurring; this process creates a molecular consolidation of memory that is more permanently stored. Kandel, a psychiatrist, received the Nobel Prize in Physiology or Medicine in 2000 for this work, which explains the extraordinary capacity of the human brain for neuroplastic remodeling throughout the lifespan.

The Language System

As far as we know, the capacity to communicate in a highly developed and complex language is limited to human beings. Although porpoises, dolphins, and a few other creatures are believed to communicate specific messages to one another, human beings alone appear to have a syntactically complex language that exists in both oral and written forms. The ability to record our history and to communicate scientifically and culturally has permitted us to repeatedly build complex civilizations and social systems, and to destroy them as well.

The capacity to communicate in oral and written language is facilitated by dedicated brain regions that probably occur only in human beings. These language systems are localized in the neocortex. A simplified schematic diagram of the human brain circuitry traditionally considered to mediate language functions appears in Figure 3–4. Lesion studies suggest that this system is located primarily in the left hemi-

Attention is mediated through multiple brain systems. Input to the brain is first provided by the reticular activating system, which arises in the brainstem. Midline circuitry passes this information through the thalamus, which plays a major role in "gating" or "filtering." Many other brain regions also play a major role in attention, including the cingulate gyrus, the hypothalamus, the hippocampus and amygdala, and the prefrontal, temporal, parietal, and occipital cortices. Neuroimaging studies using both fMRI and PET have demonstrated that the cingulate gyrus shows increases in activity during tasks that place heavy demands on the attentional system, such as those that involve competition and interference between stimuli. Attention is impaired in many mental illnesses, ranging from schizophrenia to attention-deficit/hyperactivity disorder (ADHD) to the mood disorders.

The Reward System

As behaviorists have noted for many years, human beings are strongly motivated by positive reinforcement. Put more simply, they are prone to seek pleasure and to avoid pain. Therefore, it is not surprising that the brain also possesses a reward system—a network that is used for the experience of pleasure. Its major components are the ventral tegmental area, the nucleus accumbens, the prefrontal cortex (particularly the anterior cingulate and ventral frontal cortex), the amygdala, and the hippocampus.

The reward system is relevant to many types of psychiatric disorders. It is often said that substance abuse develops when exposure to a drug such as cocaine "hijacks the brain reward system" by inducing an intense experience of pleasure that stimulates craving and repeated drug-seeking behavior. This system has been implicated in all types of dependence on both illegal (e.g., amphetamines, opiates) and legal (e.g., nicotine, alcohol) substances. It is also thought to provide the basis for other types of pleasure-seeking or addictive behaviors and their consequences, such as pathological gambling or compulsive overeating and obesity.

■ Neurochemical Systems

In addition to the functional and anatomical systems described earlier, the brain also consists of a grouping of neurochemical systems. These systems provide the "fuel" that permits the functional and anatomical systems to run (or run poorly, when an abnormality occurs). The neuro-

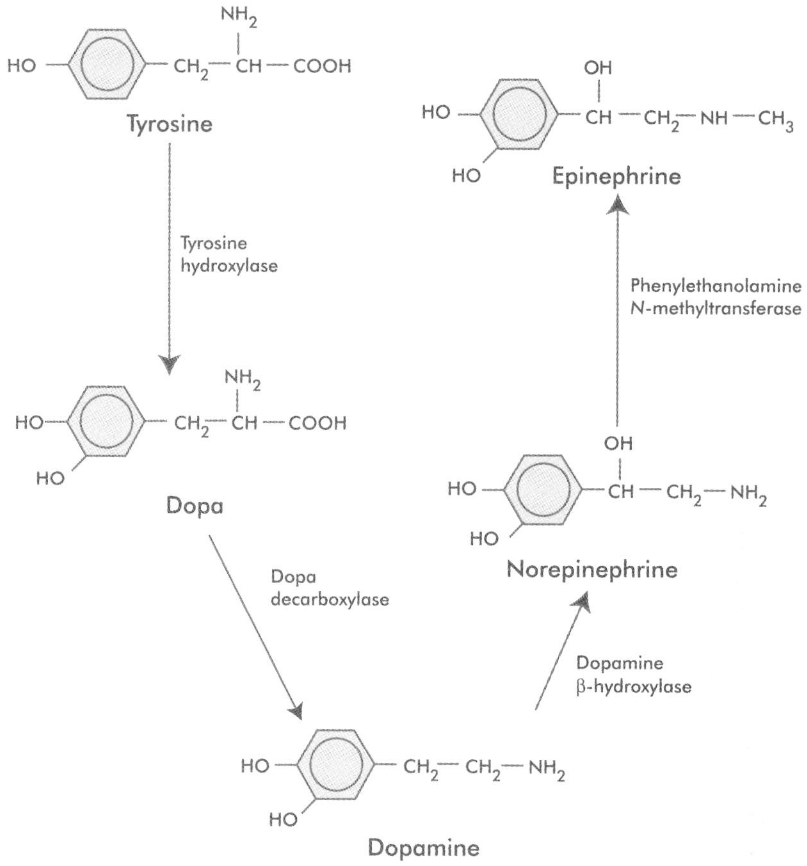

FIGURE 3–5. Synthetic pathway of dopamine.

chemical systems are interwoven and interdependent with the anatomical and functional systems. Any anatomic subsystem within the brain usually runs on multiple classes of neurotransmitters. Clearly, this complexity of anatomic and neurochemical organization permits much greater fine tuning of the entire system.

The Dopamine System

Dopamine, a catecholamine neurotransmitter, is the first product synthesized from tyrosine through the enzymatic activity of tyrosine hydroxylase. Its synthetic pathway, as well as the subsequent ones of norepinephrine and epinephrine, is shown in Figure 3–5.

There are three subsystems within the brain that use dopamine as their primary neurotransmitter. These all arise in the ventral tegmental area. One group, arising in the substantia nigra, projects to the caudate and putamen and is referred to as the nigrostriatal pathway. Its terminations appear to be rich in both D_1 and D_2 receptors. A second major tract, called the mesocortical or mesolimbic (or mesocorticolimbic), arises in the ventral tegmental area and projects to the prefrontal cortex and temporolimbic regions such as the amygdala and hippocampus. The concentration of D_2 receptors in these regions is minimal, whereas D_1 receptors predominate. The third component of the dopamine system originates in the arcuate nucleus of the hypothalamus and projects to the pituitary. The first two of these dopamine subsystems are summarized in Figure 3–6. As the figure indicates, the dopamine system is fairly specifically localized in the human brain. Because its projections include only a limited part of the cortex and focus primarily on brain regions important to cognition and emotion, it is considered to be one of the most important neurotransmitter systems for the understanding of these functions and potentially for the understanding of their disturbances in many types of mental illnesses.

For many years schizophrenia, the most important among the various psychotic disorders, was explained by the *dopamine hypothesis,* which proposed that the symptoms of this illness were due to a functional excess of dopamine. Because the efficacy of many of the antipsychotic drugs used to treat psychosis is highly correlated with their ability to block D_2 receptors, the dopamine hypothesis also suggested that the abnormality in this illness might specifically lie with D_2 receptors. There is a modest but much weaker correlation with their ability to block D_1 receptors. The dopamine hypothesis is currently being reappraised, however, in the light of several new lines of evidence that have emerged. First, the distribution of D_1 and D_2 receptors has been more specifically mapped, and there appears to be a rather sparse density of D_2 receptors in critical brain regions that mediate cognition and emotion, such as the prefrontal cortex, amygdala, and hippocampus. These regions are, however, high in D_1 and serotonin type 2 receptors (5-HT$_2$). These observations, coupled with the prominent effects on serotonin and D_1 by the new second-generation antipsychotics, suggest that the traditional dopamine hypothesis needs revision.

Understanding the projections of the dopamine system, as well as the differential localization of D_1 and D_2 receptors, clarifies some of the other effects of antipsychotic drugs. Some of these drugs have potent extrapyramidal side effects as a consequence of blocking D_2 receptors in the nigrostriatal pathway. Drugs that have a weak D_2 effect (of which

ular disorder of interest, such as bipolar disorder or schizophrenia. Thereafter, all available first-degree relatives (parents, siblings, children) are also evaluated using structured interviews and diagnostic criteria. The prevalence of the specific disorder under investigation is compared with the prevalence in a carefully selected control group. If an increased rate of the specific mental illness under study is observed in the first-degree relatives of the probands as compared with the first-degree relatives of the control subjects, then these results suggest that a disorder is familial and possibly genetic. These studies cannot exclude the possibility that the disorder has prominent nongenetic causes. Disorders can also run in families because of learned behavior, role modeling, or predisposing social environments. The following disorders have been found to "run in families": major depression, bipolar disorder, schizophrenia, panic disorder, social phobia, obsessive-compulsive disorder, antisocial personality disorder, borderline personality disorder, autistic disorder, and ADHD. Family studies have also led to the understanding that a spectrum of disorders is related to schizophrenia, including schizotypal personality disorder.

Twin Studies

Twin studies offer a better perspective on the extent to which a disorder is actually genetic. Twin studies typically compare the rate of a specific disorder in monozygotic (identical) versus dizygotic (nonidentical) twins. The rationale behind twin studies is that monozygotic twins have identical genetic material, whereas dizygotic twins theoretically share an average of 50% of their genetic material. The higher the rate of concordance in monozygotic twins, as compared with dizygotic twins, the greater the degree of genetic influence. Thus if a disorder were totally genetic and fully penetrant, the concordance rate in monozygotic twins would theoretically be 100%, whereas in dizygotic twins it would be 50%. In fact, actual rates for both groups are lower for most major mental illnesses. Table 3–1 shows the concordance rates for a variety of medical conditions that have been evaluated through twin studies. It is noteworthy that mental illnesses appear to be more highly genetic, as indicated by the twin method, than other medical disorders.

Although powerful, twin studies are not a perfect method for studying the genetics of major mental illnesses, because nongenetic psychological factors may play a significant role. Because twins are reared together, role modeling can be an influential factor. Furthermore, this factor is likely to be greater in monozygotic than in dizygotic twins because monozygotic twins are often treated as identical by their parents and peers, even being given the same toys and being dressed in the same clothing.

Candidate Gene Studies

Candidate gene studies provide an alternative approach. Typically, these studies begin with hypothesis-driven selection of a candidate gene. Candidate genes are chosen because they have single nucleotide polymorphisms (SNPs) and because they code for a protein that could have some effect leading to a specific mental illness. Examples of candidate genes include proteins regulating brain development such as brain-derived neurotrophic factor (*BDNF*), enzymes that affect neurotransmitter synthesis such as catechol-*O*-methyltransferase (*COMT*), or hormones that regulate brain activity such as neuropeptide Y. The strength of the candidate gene approach is that it directly permits investigators to determine whether a particular protein has any relevance to a specific mental illness. In the candidate gene approach, a group of patients with the specific disorder is usually compared with a group of normal control subjects to determine whether a specific allele occurs more frequently in the patients.

Candidate gene studies have some of the same limitations as the linkage studies. They may yield false-positive results, particularly if samples are not carefully chosen, and like linkage studies, their credibility depends on repeated replications. Despite these disclaimers, several candidate genes have been identified and replicated as potential vulnerability genes for schizophrenia. These include *BDNF, COMT,* dysbindin, Disrupted-in-Schizophrenia (*DISC*), and neuregulin 1. Several candidate genes that confer vulnerability to autism also have been identified, such as neurexin and ubiquitin, and the serotonin transporter gene has been implicated in mood disorders. In addition to examining disease association, investigators also have begun to do "deep phenotyping" of some genes using a variety of techniques such as animal models or neuroimaging. The *Met* allele in the *BDNF* promoter region is associated with schizophrenia, and individuals with this particular genotype also show decreased hippocampal activity during fMRI studies, smaller volume of frontal gray matter and hippocampus as measured with sMRI, progressive gray matter loss over the course of the disease, and poorer episodic memory than normal control subjects.

Copy Number Variants

Until relatively recently, it was assumed that all autosomal genes are present in two faithfully duplicated copies, with one allele inherited from each parent. We now know that large-scale variations in copy number are common and have the potential to confer disease liability. Copy number variants (CNVs) are mutations in DNA that are large

(1 kilobase or larger) and can include deletions, insertions, and duplications. It is estimated that there are an average of 12 CNVs per individual, that they cover approximately 12% of the human genome, and that at least half occur in protein-coding regions. This finding has launched a search for their possible relationship to a variety of diseases, including mental illnesses. They have now been found to be associated with rare disorders such as Prader-Willi and Angelman syndromes, but also with Alzheimer's disease and schizophrenia.

Genome-Wide Association Studies

Genome-wide association studies are another approach to finding genes for mental illnesses, made possible through advances such as the haplotype map of the entire human genome and the assembly of large databases containing DNA from thousands of individuals who suffer from specific disorders. To date, none of these genome-wide surveys has produced robust results. They have generated some evidence for genes on chromosomes 9, 10, and 12 for the dementias and chromosomes 1, 6, 8, 10, 11, 13, and 22 for the psychoses. However, evidence for linkage is often across a broad region, with different groups mapping to nonoverlapping areas of the same chromosome arm. Nonetheless, as statistical methods improve, and as haplotype map data are integrated with the method, genome-wide association studies may provide significant additional information about the location of the various genes over the next decade.

■ Self-Assessment Questions

1. Describe the functions performed by the prefrontal cortex.
2. Describe the locations and functions of the two major language regions in the brain.
3. Identify the anatomic components of the reward system and discuss its relationship to at least two psychiatric disorders.
4. Discuss the role of serotonin in modulating behavior and the ways that this role is associated with mental illnesses.
5. Describe the location and function of the dopamine system and discuss its relationship to at least two mental illnesses.
6. Describe the functions of glutamate and its possible relation to the symptoms of psychosis.

7. Describe the relative strengths of family studies, twin studies, and adoption studies as methods for determining the familiality of mental illnesses and the degree to which purely genetic factors play a causal role.

8. Discuss the possible interaction between genes and environmental factors in producing mental illness.

9. What are single nucleotide polymorphisms? Copy number variants? Genome-wide association studies? What have we learned from them about genetic mechanisms of mental illnesses?

TABLE 4–2. DSM-IV-TR diagnostic criteria for delirium due to a general medical condition

---

A. Disturbance of consciousness (i.e., reduced clarity of awareness of the environment) with reduced ability to focus, sustain, or shift attention.

B. A change in cognition (such as memory deficit, disorientation, language disturbance) or the development of a perceptual disturbance that is not better accounted for by a preexisting, established, or evolving dementia.

C. The disturbance develops over a short period of time (usually hours to days) and tends to fluctuate during the course of the day.

D. There is evidence from the history, physical examination, or laboratory findings that the disturbance is caused by the direct physiological consequences of a general medical condition.

Coding note: If delirium is superimposed on a preexisting Vascular Dementia, indicate the delirium by coding Vascular Dementia, With Delirium.

Coding note: Include the name of the general medical condition on Axis I, e.g., Delirium Due to Hepatic Encephalopathy; also code the general medical condition on Axis III (see Appendix G for codes).

Clinical Findings

The hallmark of delirium is the rapid development of disorientation, confusion, and global cognitive impairment. Characteristic features include a disturbance of consciousness evidenced by reduced clarity of awareness of the environment; difficulty focusing, sustaining, or shifting attention; impaired cognition; and perceptual disturbances (e.g., illusions). The patient may appear normal at one point and be disoriented and hallucinating at another. Other symptoms typical of delirium include sleep-wake cycle disturbances with worsening at night (sundowning); disorientation to place, date, or person; incoherence; restlessness; and agitation or excessive somnolence.

The following vignette illustrates a relatively typical case of delirium:

> An 84-year-old retired police chief was brought to the emergency department by his family because of a 4- to 5-day history of lassitude, lower-extremity weakness, bladder incontinence, and intermittent confusion and memory loss. The patient had fallen 4 weeks earlier and had sustained a scalp laceration that required suturing. He had no history of recent alcohol use.

The patient was cooperative but drowsy and easily distracted. He was oriented to person but was disoriented to date and situation. His memory for recent events was extremely poor, and he was unable to recall three objects either immediately or at 3 minutes. He thought that Franklin Roosevelt was the current president. Interestingly, the patient had known the paternal grandfather of one of the authors (D.W.B.) and was able to speak at length of this remote relationship.

A presumptive diagnosis of delirium was made, and a medical workup was begun. A computed tomography (CT) scan showed the presence of bilateral chronic subdural hematomas. The patient was transferred to the neurosurgery service, where burr hole evacuation was performed. The delirium cleared, but the patient had a residual dementia. He was transferred to a long-term nursing facility.

Etiology

Delirium most commonly occurs in persons who have a serious medical, surgical, or neurological illness or who are experiencing drug intoxication or withdrawal. The presence of a delirium should lead to an immediate search for a medical cause. Because delirium is a syndrome and not a disease, it is best seen as the final common pathway of many potential causes. These include metabolic disturbances, such as those caused by infection, febrile illness, hypoxia, hypoglycemia, drug intoxication or withdrawal states, or hepatic encephalopathy. Common causes of delirium that lie within the central nervous system (CNS) include brain abscesses, stroke, traumatic injuries, and postictal states. Other causes seen frequently in the elderly are new-onset arrhythmias (such as atrial fibrillation) and cardiac ischemia. Delirium can be influenced by environmental events, but these events do not cause delirium. For example, before delirium was well understood, patients who became delirious after surgery were thought to have an "ICU psychosis," presumably caused by the psychological reaction to the strange intensive care unit (ICU) environment.

Assessment

The medical evaluation should begin with a careful history and include a complete physical examination. Informants should be interviewed, because the patient may not be able to provide information. Close attention should be given to the presence of focal neurological signs, including weakness or sensory loss, papilledema, and frontal lobe release signs (e.g., suck, snout, palmomental, rooting reflexes) that indicate global deficit states. Laboratory tests should include routine blood and urine studies (e.g., complete blood count, urinalysis), chest X-ray, a CT scan or magnetic resonance imaging (MRI) scan of the brain, an electrocardiogram, lumbar puncture (in selected patients), toxicology screen, blood gases, and an electroencephalogram. Laboratory test results will vary depending on the underlying cause of the delirium. Serum urine toxicology is essential in patients presenting in emergency departments to evaluate for illicit drug use. Delirious patients frequently have temperature elevations that probably represent autonomic instability or an underlying infection. Generalized diffuse slowing is often found on the electroencephalogram.

The major problem in differential diagnosis is distinguishing delirium from a confusional state due to schizophrenia or a mood disorder. Delirious patients tend to have a more acute presentation, are globally confused, and have greater impairment in attention. Hallucinations, when present, are fragmentary and disorganized and tend to be visual or tactile as opposed to the auditory hallucinations seen in patients with psychotic disorders. Delirious patients are less likely to have a personal or family history of psychiatric illness. However, the presence of a prior psychiatric illness does not preclude the possibility of developing a delirium.

Clinical Management

First, the underlying medical condition must be corrected if possible. Measures taken to maintain the patient's health and safety should include constant observation, consistent nursing care, and frequent reassurance with repeated simple explanations. Restraints may be necessary in agitated patients. External stimulation should be minimized. Because shadows or darkness may be frightening, delirious patients tend to do better in quiet, well-lighted rooms. Unnecessary medication should be discontinued, including sedatives or hypnotics (e.g., benzodiazepines). Not only are delirious patients exquisitely sensitive to drug side effects, but the drugs may contribute to the delirium. Agitated patients may be calmed with low doses of high-potency antipsychotics (e.g., haloperidol, 1–2 mg every 2–4 hours as needed) or a second-generation antipsychotic (e.g., risperidone). Older drugs with significant anticholinergic effects (e.g., chlorpromazine, thioridazine) should be avoided because they can worsen or prolong the delirium. In fact, plasma anticholinergic levels correlate with delirium in surgical patients. When sedation is necessary, low doses of short-acting benzodiazepines (e.g., oxazepam, lorazepam) can be helpful. Unrecognized alcohol withdrawal can manifest as delirium, particularly in the post-surgical patient. This problem is common in hospitals, wherein a patient presents for surgery and fails to disclose a history of alcoholism; within days of the surgery, having had no alcohol, he or she becomes delirious. Benzodiazepines can be helpful in these cases because they will treat the withdrawal state. (See Chapter 9 for the treatment of alcohol withdrawal.)

Key points to remember about delirium

1. In the hospital, a quiet, restful setting that is well lighted is best for the confused patient.

2. Consistency of personnel is less likely to upset the delirious patient.

3. Reminders of day, date, time, place, and situation should be prominently displayed in the patient's room.

4. Medication for behavioral management should be limited to those cases in which behavioral interventions have failed.

    • Only essential drugs should be prescribed, and polypharmacy should be avoided.

    • Sedative-hypnotics and anxiolytics should be avoided; the exception is where the delirium is due to alcohol withdrawal.

    • Unmanageable behavior may require the use of antipsychotics or, alternatively, benzodiazepines with short half-lives (e.g., lorazepam).

■ Dementia

Dementia is a syndrome of impaired cognitive function accompanied by a decline in social and occupational functioning. Level of alertness (i.e., sensorium) is generally not disturbed. Cognitive impairment can involve the four *A*'s:

1. Aphasia (language disturbance)
2. Amnesia (memory disturbance)
3. Apraxia (inability to carry out complex motor activities)
4. Agnosia (failure to recognize or identify objects despite intact sensory function)

Dementias are acquired neurodegenerative disorders, unlike mental retardation, which is a neurodevelopmental source of cognitive impairment. The impairment created by dementia distinguishes it from the mild memory change that occurs during normal aging ("benign senescent forgetfulness"). A search for treatable causes is mandatory in the patient with dementia, even though most are irreversible. A small number of dementia cases are potentially reversible, but only 3% fully resolve.

Dementia is relatively uncommon in persons younger than 65 years. About 10% of persons between ages 65 and 75 have a dementia. Between ages 75 and 85, 25% or more have a dementia; by age 90, the rate is 50%. The rates of dementia are even higher among elderly hospitalized patients and physically ill persons. Because the growth in the United States population of those older than 65 is outstripping the growth in the general population, it is clear that the problem of dementia will be even greater in the future. Providing for the care of large numbers of dementia patients will be one of the major tasks that American society will need to address as the "baby boomers" age.

Clinical Findings

Dementia usually develops insidiously, and preliminary signs may be overlooked or misattributed to normal aging. (There are some forms of dementia that can develop fairly abruptly, such as a vascular dementia induced by a stroke.) In the earliest stages of dementia, the only symptom may be a subtle change in the patient's personality, a decrease in the range of the patient's interests, the development of apathy, or the development of labile or shallow emotions. Intellectual skills are gradually affected and may be noticed initially in work settings where high performance is required. At this point, the patient may be unaware of the loss of his or her intellectual sharpness or may deny the loss. Characteristics that help to separate delirium from dementia are highlighted in Table 4–3.

As the dementia advances, cognitive impairment becomes more pronounced, mood and personality changes become more exaggerated, and psychotic symptoms sometimes develop. Insight may be impaired such that the patient remains unconcerned even when the family has noticed substantial deficits. Because of the patient's poor insight, caregivers must intervene to restrict activities such as driving.

When the dementia is advanced, the patient may be unable to perform basic tasks such as self-feeding or caring for personal hygiene,

ability to read, write, and calculate. Thirty points are possible: a score of less than 25 is suggestive of impairment, and a score of less than 20 usually indicates definite impairment.

Laboratory testing is an important part of the evaluation to exclude irreversible medical sources of cognitive impairment. All patients with a new onset of dementia should have a complete blood count; liver, thyroid, and renal function tests; serologic tests for syphilis and HIV; urinalysis; electrocardiogram; and chest X-ray. Serum electrolytes, serum glucose, and vitamin B_{12} and folate levels should be measured. Most of the readily reversible metabolic, endocrine, vitamin deficiency, and infectious states, whether causal or complicating, will be uncovered with these simple tests when combined with the history and physical examination findings. Other laboratory tests are helpful in carefully selected patients; for example, a CT or an MRI structural brain scan is appropriate in the presence of a history suggestive of a mass lesion, focal neurological signs, or a very brief dementia. Electroencephalograms are appropriate for patients with altered consciousness or suspected seizures. Pulse oximetry is indicated when compromised respiratory function is evident. Although not widely available, single photon emission computed tomography or positron emission tomography (PET) imaging can help to distinguish Alzheimer's dementia from other forms of dementia. In fact, fluorodeoxyglucose PET imaging has been approved by Medicare as a diagnostic tool for distinguishing Alzheimer's from other dementias; in Alzheimer's dementia, there is characteristic temporal and parietal hypometabolism. The medical workup for dementia is summarized in Table 4–5.

Neuropsychological testing can be very helpful in the evaluation of dementia. Testing can be done to obtain baseline data by which to measure change both before and after treatment; can be helpful in evaluating highly educated individuals suspected of developing an early dementia when brain imaging or other test results are ambiguous; and also may help distinguish delirium from dementia and depression. These tests can be repeated serially to track changes in attention, memory, and cognition.

Mild cognitive impairment (MCI) is increasingly recognized as a prodromal state that may progress to dementia. It is currently defined as a condition in which the individual has no impairment in daily functioning but scores below age- and education-adjusted norms on memory tests. It has been estimated that approximately 12% of such persons progress to dementia each year.

Most patients with dementia can be evaluated on an outpatient basis. In practice, hospital admissions involving dementia patients are

TABLE 4–5.	**Medical workup for dementia**

1. Complete history
2. Thorough physical examination, including neurological examination
3. Mental status examination
4. Laboratory studies
    - Complete blood count, with differential
    - Serum electrolytes
    - Serum glucose
    - Blood urea nitrogen
    - Creatinine
    - Liver function tests
    - Serology for syphilis and HIV
    - Thyroid function tests
    - Serum vitamin B_{12}
    - Folate
    - Urinalysis and urine drug screen
    - Electrocardiogram
    - Chest X-ray
    - Pulse oximetry
    - Brain computed tomography or magnetic resonance imaging
5. Neuropsychological testing (e.g., attention, memory, cognitive function)
6. Optional tests
    - Functional neuroimaging (e.g., positron emission tomography, single-photon emission computed tomography)
    - Lumbar puncture

usually for the evaluation and treatment of behavioral and psychological complications such as aggression, violence, wandering, psychosis, or depression. Other reasons for hospitalization include suicidal threats or behaviors, rapid weight loss, or acute deterioration without an apparent cause.

Irreversible Causes of Dementia

Alzheimer's Disease

Alzheimer's disease is the most common cause of degenerative dementias and accounts for 50%–60% of all cases of dementia. It affects approximately 2.5 million Americans. In DSM-IV-TR, Alzheimer's dementia is divided into early (age 65 and younger) and late (older than 65 years) onset types. Most of the early-onset cases of Alzheimer's disease are classified as familial Alzheimer's disease. These patients often have an onset in the fifth decade, and the disorder has been linked to mutations on chromosomes 1, 14, and 21. The early-onset variant is relatively rare, however, and nearly all cases seen in the community are probably late (or sporadic) onset. (See Table 4–6 for the DSM-IV-TR diagnostic criteria for dementia of the Alzheimer's type.)

The onset is usually insidious, leading to death 8–10 years after symptoms are recognized. Estimates of the prevalence of Alzheimer's disease range from 5% at age 65 to 40% by age 90. Symptoms progressively worsen, eventually resulting in near collapse of cognitive functioning. Physical findings are generally absent, or they are present only in later stages: hyperactive deep tendon reflexes, Babinski's sign, and frontal lobe release signs. The presence of illusions, hallucinations, or delusions is associated with accelerated cognitive deterioration. Cortical atrophy and enlarged cerebral ventricles are typically seen on CT or MRI scans.

The case of composer Maurice Ravel illustrates the tragedy of dementia of the Alzheimer's type:

> Ravel, a leader of the French musical impressionist movement, excelled at piano composition and orchestration. At age 56, after completing his most famous work, Concerto in G Minor, he began to complain of fatigue and lassitude, symptoms that were in keeping with his chronic insomnia and lifelong hypochondriasis. His symptoms continued to progress, and his creative energy waned.
>
> The following year, after a minor automobile accident, Ravel's cognitive abilities began to erode. His capacity to remember names, to speak spontaneously, and to write became impaired. An eminent French neurologist noted that Ravel's ability to understand verbal speech was superior to his ability to speak or to write. Tragically, Ravel also developed *amusia*, the inability to comprehend musical sounds. His last public performance occurred shortly thereafter. He was no longer capable of the coordination, cognition, and speech necessary to lead an orchestra.
>
> Ravel's friends made futile attempts to help him, trying to stimulate him intellectually any way they could, but gradually his speech and intellectual functions declined further. Within 4 years of the onset of dementia, Ravel was mute and incapable of recognizing his own music.

Ravel died at age 62 after a neurosurgical procedure, the indications for which remain unclear. No autopsy was done, but his neurologist had suspected a cerebral degenerative disease. Syphilis, a common illness of the day, had been ruled out.

While new neuroimaging techniques are evolving rapidly toward the capability of an accurate diagnosis during life, the definitive diagnosis of Alzheimer's disease is largely still considered a histopathological diagnosis at autopsy. Two primary abnormalities characterize the histopathological features of Alzheimer's disease: amyloid plaques and neurofibrillary tangles. Amyloid plaques in the brain are generated from amyloid precursor protein (APP), which is cleaved by enzymes called secretases to form β-amyloid. The β-amyloid of the 42 amino acid type has been found to accumulate in excess in the brains of persons with Alzheimer's disease, and the β-amyloid-42 protein is known to aggregate into plaques that are associated with inflammation and neuronal death. The second characteristic histopathological feature is the presence of neurofibrillary tangles. These are comprised of hyperphosphorylated tau protein that folds within the intracellular cytoplasm of neurons and is also associated with cell death. In contrast to neuronal plaques, neurofibrillary tangles are seen more commonly in a variety of neurodegenerative diseases, such as frontotemporal dementia, as well as in persons with closed head injuries. To utilize these abnormalities as an in vivo marker, there has been research examining cerebrospinal fluid (CSF) levels of amyloid and tau proteins. Alzheimer's disease has been associated with a reduction in CSF amyloid levels compared with those in healthy subjects, which is thought to be due to sequestration of the amyloid within the neuronal plaques. Conversely, tau protein is elevated in the CSF of Alzheimer's patients compared to controls. This finding likely reflects that tau protein increases in the context of neuronal damage.

Risk factors for Alzheimer's disease include a history of head injury, Down syndrome, low educational and occupational level, and having a first-degree relative with Alzheimer's disease. In fact, up to 50% of the first-degree relatives of persons with dementia of the Alzheimer's type are affected with the disorder by age 90 years. A genetic polymorphism on chromosome 19, apolipoprotein E (*APOE*), has been found to influence the risk of Alzheimer's disease. The *APOE* ε4 allele increases risk and decreases age at onset of Alzheimer's disease, and the *APOE* ε2 allele has a protective effect. Alzheimer's disease susceptibility from *APOE* occurs worldwide.

TABLE 4–6. **DSM-IV-TR diagnostic criteria for dementia of the Alzheimer's type**

A. The development of multiple cognitive deficits manifested by both
  (1) memory impairment (impaired ability to learn new information or to recall previously learned information)
  (2) one (or more) of the following cognitive disturbances:
    (a) aphasia (language disturbance)
    (b) apraxia (impaired ability to carry out motor activities despite intact motor function)
    (c) agnosia (failure to recognize or identify objects despite intact sensory function)
    (d) disturbance in executive functioning (i.e., planning, organizing, sequencing, abstracting)
B. The cognitive deficits in Criteria A1 and A2 each cause significant impairment in social or occupational functioning and represent a significant decline from a previous level of functioning.
C. The course is characterized by gradual onset and continuing cognitive decline.
D. The cognitive deficits in Criteria A1 and A2 are not due to any of the following:
  (1) other central nervous system conditions that cause progressive deficits in memory and cognition (e.g., cerebrovascular disease, Parkinson's disease, Huntington's disease, subdural hematoma, normal-pressure hydrocephalus, brain tumor)
  (2) systemic conditions that are known to cause dementia (e.g., hypothyroidism, vitamin B_{12} or folic acid deficiency, niacin deficiency, hypercalcemia, neurosyphilis, HIV infection)
  (3) substance-induced conditions
E. The deficits do not occur exclusively during the course of a delirium.
F. The disturbance is not better accounted for by another Axis I disorder (e.g., Major Depressive Disorder, Schizophrenia).

Code based on presence or absence of a clinically significant behavioral disturbance:

> **Without Behavioral Disturbance:** if the cognitive disturbance is not accompanied by any clinically significant behavioral disturbance.

> **With Behavioral Disturbance:** if the cognitive disturbance is accompanied by a clinically significant behavioral disturbance (e.g., wandering, agitation).

TABLE 4–6.   DSM-IV-TR diagnostic criteria for dementia of the Alzheimer's type *(continued)*

Specify subtype:

With Early Onset: if onset is at age 65 years or below

With Late Onset: if onset is after age 65 years

Coding note: Also code Alzheimer's disease on Axis III. Indicate other prominent clinical features related to the Alzheimer's disease on Axis I (e.g., Mood Disorder Due to Alzheimer's Disease, With Depressive Features, and Personality Change Due to Alzheimer's Disease, Aggressive Type).

Dementia With Lewy Bodies

Dementia with Lewy bodies may account for up to 25% of dementia cases and is progressive and irreversible, with clinical features similar to those of Alzheimer's disease. Prominent visual hallucinations and parkinsonian features tend to occur early in the illness. The course is often slightly more rapid than in Alzheimer's disease. In addition to changes in the brain parenchyma typical for Alzheimer's disease, Lewy bodies—eosinophilic inclusion bodies—are seen in the cerebral cortex and brainstem. Patients with this form of dementia are very sensitive to extrapyramidal side effects of conventional antipsychotics. Second-generation antipsychotics are better tolerated if medication is needed for behavioral management.

Frontotemporal Dementia

Frontotemporal dementia is increasingly recognized as a major source of dementia. The original concept of Pick's disease has broadened to the more inclusive term of *frontotemporal dementia* because the disorder is now known to have a fairly heterogeneous histopathology. In general, this dementia is characterized by tau-positive inclusions and a subgroup of cases with parkinsonian features linked to chromosome 17. There are two main clinical syndromes; one is characterized by disinhibition and shallow affect, the other by early and progressive loss of expressive language, with severe naming difficulties.

Huntington's Disease

Huntington's disease is a neuropsychiatric disorder with autosomal-dominant inheritance. Its gene has been located on the short arm of chromosome 4. Psychiatric manifestations range from mild depression, anxiety, and irritability to frank hallucinations and delusions, all of which may precede the onset of choreiform movements. Dementia occurs in the terminal phase of the illness and is characterized by impaired cognition without a language disorder.

Creutzfeldt-Jakob Disease

Creutzfeldt-Jakob disease is a virulent and irreversible cause of dementia. It is caused by prions, which are small proteinaceous particles that cause spongiform changes in the brain. In the past, Creutzfeldt-Jakob disease and other spongiform encephalopathies were thought to be due to "slow viruses." Creutzfeldt-Jakob disease is rare, has a peak incidence between 50 and 70 years, and is characterized by a rapidly progressive dementing illness that causes death, usually within a few months. The incubation period can be months to years. Severe cerebellar and/or extrapyramidal signs, along with myoclonus, are present. Akinetic mutism and cortical blindness sometimes occur. Triphasic complexes are found on electroencephalograms in about 80% of the cases. Histopathology shows spongiform changes, which consist of fine vacuolation of the neuropil of the gray matter, associated with astrocytosis and neuronal loss. Creutzfeldt-Jakob disease occurs sporadically and may be inherited or transmitted by intracerebral electrodes, grafts of dura mater, corneal transplants, and human-derived growth hormone and gonadotropin. The disease is invariably fatal, and there are no known treatments. A new variant recently has been described that has an earlier onset (average age of 27 years vs. 60 years), more psychiatric symptoms, a longer course (14 months vs. 4 months), and an absence of triphasic complexes on electroencephalography.

Other Irreversible Causes of Dementia

Other irreversible forms of dementia include diseases of the basal ganglia (Parkinson's disease), cerebellum (cerebellar, spinocerebellar, and olivopontocerebellar degeneration), and motor neurons (amyotrophic lateral sclerosis); the parkinsonism-dementia complex of Guam; herpes simplex encephalitis; and the dementia of multiple sclerosis. Numerous hereditary metabolic diseases are associated with irreversible dementia, including Wilson's disease (hepatolenticular degeneration), metachromatic leukodystrophy, the adrenoleukodystrophies, and the neuronal storage diseases (e.g., Tay-Sachs disease).

TABLE 4–7. Cognitive enhancement medications

Drug	Trade name	Dosage range (mg/day)
Donepezil	Aricept	5–10
Galantamine	Reminyl	8–24
Memantine	Namenda	10–20
Rivastigmine	Exelon	1.5–6
Tacrine	Cognex	40–160

Clinical Management

Cholinergic therapies address the well-known deficit of acetylcholine in Alzheimer's disease. Three cholinesterase inhibitor drugs are commonly used: donepezil, rivastigmine, and galantamine. These drugs are equally effective and work to slow the rate of cognitive decline. Another drug, tacrine, is also U.S. Food and Drug Administration (FDA) approved but is used infrequently because of poor tolerability and the need to monitor liver enzymes. There is a marked variation in response—some patients show tremendous improvement, whereas others show very little improvement. These drugs do not alter the course of the disease and work best in persons in the earliest stages of the disease. Side effects across this class of drugs include nausea, emesis, diarrhea, anorexia, and weight loss, all of which tend to be mild and temporary. Dosages are titrated slowly to the target.

Memantine is the first of a new generation of cognitive enhancers, and it blocks the *N*-methyl-D-aspartate (NMDA) receptor, one of two receptors that normally bind glutamate. This receptor is thought to mediate certain aspects of learning and memory. The drug is approved by the FDA to treat moderate to severe Alzheimer's disease. Like the cholinesterase inhibitors, the main benefit of the drug is to slow the inevitable decline in cognitive functioning. (See Table 4–7 for a list of the cognitive enhancers.)

Other medications are used for the symptomatic treatment of associated anxiety, psychosis, or depression, including the anxiolytics, antipsychotics, and antidepressants, respectively. The physician must find the lowest effective dosage, because patients with dementia often poorly tolerate drug side effects. In treating depression in patients with dementia, physicians should avoid tricyclic antidepressants and use the

TABLE 4–8.   Examples of preventable or treatable causes of dementia

Vascular
  Multiple infarcts
  Subacute bacterial endocarditis
  Myocardial infarction, heart failure

Metabolic and endocrine
  Hypothyroidism
  Hyperparathyroidism
  Pituitary insufficiency
  Uremia
  Hepatic encephalopathy

Nutrition
  Pernicious anemia
  Alcoholism and thiamine deficiency
  Pellagra

Toxicity
  Bromides
  Mercury
  Lead

Infections
  Cryptococcal meningitis
  Encephalitis
  Sarcoidosis
  Postinfectious encephalomyelitis

Mass effect
  Intracranial tumor (e.g., subfrontal meningioma)
  Subdural hematoma
  Subclinical seizures
  Demyelinating disease
  Normal-pressure hydrocephalus

few hours earlier. This disorder can be caused by trauma, tumor, infection, infarction, seizures, or drugs, but the most common cause is severe alcohol abuse. Alcohol-related amnesia is probably caused by chronic thiamine deficiency. This syndrome may occur in association with *Wernicke's encephalopathy,* characterized by ophthalmoplegia, ataxic gait, nystagmus, and mental confusion, and requires emergency treatment with thiamine. This condition may not improve despite abstinence from alcohol and maintenance on thiamine. The term *Wernicke-Korsakoff syndrome* is used when cognitive and memory impairment endures. Autopsies of patients with this condition show hemorrhage and sclerosis of the hypothalamic mamillary bodies and nuclei of the thalamus as well as more diffuse lesions in the brainstem, cerebellum, and limbic system.

■ Self-Assessment Questions

1. What are the differences between delirium and dementia? How are they alike?

2. What does the medical workup for delirium and dementia involve?

3. Describe Alzheimer's disease. What are its histopathological findings?

4. What are the two clinical syndromes seen in frontotemporal dementia?

5. What does the "symptom triad" in normal-pressure hydrocephalus consist of?

6. List some of the different causes of dementia.

7. What is pseudodementia? What are its signs and symptoms?

8. How are dementia patients clinically managed? What is the proposed mechanism of action for the cognitive enhancers?

9. What is Wernicke's encephalopathy and what is its relationship to the Wernicke-Korsakoff syndrome? What is its cause?

CHAPTER 5

Schizophrenia and Other Psychotic Disorders

I felt a Cleaving in my Mind—
As if my Brain had split—
I tried to match it—Seam by Seam—
But could not make them fit.

Emily Dickinson

SCHIZOPHRENIA IS not a "split personality," as many people assume, based on its name. The illness is called "schizo" (fragmented or split apart) "phrenia" (mind) because it causes its victims to experience profound disabilities in their capacity to think clearly and to feel normal emotions. It is probably the most devastating illness that psychiatrists treat. Schizophrenia strikes people just when they are preparing to enter the phase of their lives in which they can achieve their highest growth and productivity—typically in the teens or early 20s—leaving most of them unable to return to normal young adult lives: to go to school, to find a job, or to marry and have children. According to *The Global Burden of Disease,* a World Health Organization–sponsored study of the cost of medical illnesses worldwide, schizophrenia is among the 10 leading causes of disability in the world among people in the 15–44 age range.

Although schizophrenia is arguably the most important of the psychotic disorders, several other less common psychotic disorders are also reviewed in this chapter. These include delusional disorder, schizoaffective disorder, schizophreniform disorder, brief psychotic disorder, and shared psychotic disorder. A residual category, *psychotic disorder not otherwise specified,* is used for individuals who do not fit into any of the better-defined categories.

■ Schizophrenia

Definition

One of the greatest challenges to the student of schizophrenia is to understand the multiplicity of signs and symptoms that arise from its underlying cognitive and emotional impairments. The characteristic symptoms include dysfunctions in nearly every capacity of which the human brain is capable—perception, inferential thinking, language, memory, and executive functions. The symptoms are sometimes divided into two groups: positive and negative. Positive symptoms (e.g., hearing voices) are characterized by the presence of something that should be absent. Negative symptoms (e.g., avolition), on the other hand, are characterized by the absence of something that should be present.

In DSM-IV-TR, schizophrenia is defined by a group of characteristic symptoms, such as hallucinations, delusions, or negative symptoms (i.e., affective flattening, alogia, avolition); deterioration in social, occupational, or interpersonal relationships; and continuous signs of the disturbance for at least 6 months. (See Table 5–1 for the complete DSM-IV-TR diagnostic criteria for schizophrenia.)

Epidemiology

The worldwide prevalence of schizophrenia has been estimated at between 0.5% and 1%. Schizophrenia can develop at any age, but the age at first psychotic episode is typically 18–25 years for men and 21–30 years for women. Age at onset is probably under both genetic and environmental control, but it is unknown why women develop the illness later than men. Patients with schizophrenia tend not to marry and are less likely to have children than persons in the general population.

People with schizophrenia are at high risk for suicidal behavior. About one-third will attempt suicide, and 1 in 10 will eventually kill themselves.

Risk factors for suicide include male gender, age less than 30 years, unemployment, chronic course, prior depression, past treatment for depression, history of substance abuse, and recent hospital discharge.

Clinical Findings

Because schizophrenia is characterized by so many different types of symptoms, clinical investigators have tried to simplify the conceptualization of the disorder. Using factor analysis, research has repeatedly identified three dimensions (or groups of related symptoms) in schizophrenia: psychoticism, disorganization, and negative symptoms. (The many symptoms of schizophrenia, and their frequencies, are summarized in Table 5–2.)

The Psychotic Dimension

The *psychotic dimension* refers to hallucinations and delusions, two classic "psychotic" symptoms that reflect a patient's confusion about the loss of boundaries between him- or herself and the external world. *Hallucinations* are perceptions experienced without an external stimulus to the sense organs and have a quality similar to a true perception. Patients with schizophrenia commonly report auditory, visual, tactile, gustatory, or olfactory hallucinations or a combination of these. Auditory hallucinations are the most frequent; they are typically experienced as speech ("voices"). The voices may be mumbled or heard clearly, and they may speak words, phrases, or sentences. Visual hallucinations may be simple or complex and include flashes of light, persons, animals, or objects. Olfactory and gustatory hallucinations are often experienced together, especially as unpleasant tastes or odors. Tactile hallucinations may be experienced as sensations of being touched or pricked, electrical sensations, or the sensation of insects crawling under the skin, which is called *formication.*

Delusions involve disturbance in thought rather than perception; they are firmly held beliefs that are untrue as well as contrary to a person's educational and cultural background. Delusions occurring in schizophrenic patients may have somatic, grandiose, religious, nihilistic, sexual, or persecutory themes (Table 5–3). The type and frequency of the delusions tend to differ according to the patient's culture. For example, in the United States, a patient might worry about being spied on by the FBI or CIA; in sub-Saharan Africa, a Bantu or Zulu patient would more likely worry about persecution by demons or spirits.

TABLE 5–1.   DSM-IV-TR diagnostic criteria for schizophrenia

A. *Characteristic symptoms:*   Two (or more) of the following, each present for a significant portion of time during a 1-month period (or less if successfully treated):
   (1) delusions
   (2) hallucinations
   (3) disorganized speech (e.g., frequent derailment or incoherence)
   (4) grossly disorganized or catatonic behavior
   (5) negative symptoms, i.e., affective flattening, alogia, or avolition
   Note: Only one Criterion A symptom is required if delusions are bizarre or hallucinations consist of a voice keeping up a running commentary on the person's behavior or thoughts, or two or more voices conversing with each other.

.B. *Social/occupational dysfunction:*   For a significant portion of the time since the onset of the disturbance, one or more major areas of functioning such as work, interpersonal relations, or self-care are markedly below the level achieved prior to the onset (or when the onset is in childhood or adolescence, failure to achieve expected level of interpersonal, academic, or occupational achievement).

C. *Duration:*   Continuous signs of the disturbance persist for at least 6 months. This 6-month period must include at least 1 month of symptoms (or less if successfully treated) that meet Criterion A (i.e., active-phase symptoms) and may include periods of prodromal or residual symptoms. During these prodromal or residual periods, the signs of the disturbance may be manifested by only negative symptoms or two or more symptoms listed in Criterion A present in an attenuated form (e.g., odd beliefs, unusual perceptual experiences).

D. *Schizoaffective and Mood Disorder exclusion:*   Schizoaffective Disorder and Mood Disorder With Psychotic Features have been ruled out because either (1) no Major Depressive, Manic, or Mixed Episodes have occurred concurrently with the active-phase symptoms; or (2) if mood episodes have occurred during active-phase symptoms, their total duration has been brief relative to the duration of the active and residual periods.

E. *Substance/general medical condition exclusion:*   The disturbance is not due to the direct physiological effects of a substance (e.g., a drug of abuse, a medication) or a general medical condition.

TABLE 5–1.   DSM-IV-TR diagnostic criteria for schizophrenia *(continued)*

F. *Relationship to a Pervasive Developmental Disorder:*   If there is a history of Autistic Disorder or another Pervasive Developmental Disorder, the additional diagnosis of Schizophrenia is made only if prominent delusions or hallucinations are also present for at least a month (or less if successfully treated).

Classification of longitudinal course (can be applied only after at least 1 year has elapsed since the initial onset of active-phase symptoms):

  Episodic With Interepisode Residual Symptoms (episodes are defined by the reemergence of prominent psychotic symptoms); *also specify if:*   **With Prominent Negative Symptoms**

  Episodic With No Interepisode Residual Symptoms

  Continuous (prominent psychotic symptoms are present throughout the period of observation); *also specify if:*   **With Prominent Negative Symptoms**

  Single Episode in Partial Remission; *also specify if:*   **With Prominent Negative Symptoms**

  Single Episode in Full Remission

  Other or Unspecified Pattern

Although delusions and hallucinations are most common in schizophrenia, they also occur in other disorders such as the dementias or the mood disorders. However, a German psychiatrist working in the early twentieth century, Kurt Schneider, argued that certain types of hallucinations and delusions were of the "first rank," meaning that they are especially characteristic of schizophrenia. Examples include delusions of being forced to do things against one's will or that thoughts are being withdrawn from or inserted into one's mind. These symptoms all reflect a patient's confusion about the loss of boundaries between him- or herself and the external world.

The following case is of a patient evaluated in our hospital and illustrates symptoms characteristic of the paranoid subtype of schizophrenia:

> Jane, a 55-year-old woman, was admitted to the hospital for evaluation of agitation and paranoia. A former schoolteacher, she had lived in a series of rooming houses and had held only temporary jobs in the past 10 years. She was socially isolated and interacted with others only at her church.

The Negative Dimension

DSM-IV-TR lists three negative symptoms as characteristic of schizophrenia: alogia, affective blunting, and avolition. Another negative symptom common in schizophrenia is anhedonia. These are described below:

- *Alogia* is characterized by a diminution in the amount of spontaneous speech or a tendency to produce speech that is empty or impoverished in content when the amount is adequate.
- *Affective flattening or blunting* is a reduced intensity of emotional expression and response. It is manifested by unchanging facial expression, decreased spontaneous movements, poverty of expressive gestures, poor eye contact, lack of voice inflections, and slowed speech.
- *Avolition* is a loss of the ability to initiate goal-directed behavior and to carry it through to completion. Patients seem to have lost their will or drive.
- *Anhedonia* is the inability to experience pleasure. Many patients describe themselves as feeling emotionally empty. They are no longer able to enjoy activities that previously gave them pleasure, such as playing sports or seeing family or friends.

Other Symptoms

Lack of insight is common in schizophrenia. A patient may not believe that he or she is ill or abnormal in any way. Orientation and memory usually are normal, unless they are impaired by the patient's psychotic symptoms, inattention, or distractibility.

Nonlocalizing neurological soft signs occur in some patients and include abnormalities in stereognosis, graphesthesia, balance, and proprioception. Some patients have disturbances of sleep, sexual interest, and other bodily functions. Many schizophrenic patients have inactive sex drives and avoid sexual intimacy.

Alcohol and drug abuse are common in patients with schizophrenia. Drug-using patients tend to be young, male, and poorly adherent with treatment; they also tend to have frequent hospitalizations. It is believed that many abuse drugs in an attempt to treat their depression or their medication side effects (e.g., akinesia) or to reduce their lack of motivation and pleasure.

Subtypes of Schizophrenia

Five subtypes of schizophrenia are recognized in DSM-IV-TR: paranoid, disorganized, catatonic, undifferentiated, and residual. Their usefulness is primarily descriptive because their reliability and validity are not established. As a practical matter, many patients seem to fit several of these subtypes during the course of their illness:

- *Paranoid:* This subtype involves preoccupation with one or more systematized delusions or frequently auditory hallucinations; disorganized speech and behavior, catatonic behavior, and flat or inappropriate affect are not prominent. Compared with patients with the disorganized subtype, paranoid patients tend to have an older age at onset and are more likely to be married, to have children, and to be employed; both their premorbid functioning and their outcome tend to be better.
- *Disorganized:* This subtype is characterized by disorganized speech and behavior and flat or inappropriate affect. Delusions and hallucinations, when present, tend to be fragmentary, unlike the often well-systematized delusions of the paranoid schizophrenic patient. Onset occurs at an early age with the development of negative symptoms such as avolition, flat affect, and cognitive impairment. These patients often seem silly and childlike and occasionally grimace, giggle inappropriately, and appear self-absorbed.
- *Catatonic:* This subtype is dominated by at least two of the following: motoric immobility (e.g., catalepsy, stupor), excessive motor activity, extreme negativism, peculiarities of voluntary movement (e.g., stereotypies, mannerisms, grimacing), and echolalia or echopraxia. This subtype is less common than it was in the past, but isolated catatonic symptoms do occur from time to time.
- *Undifferentiated:* This subtype is a residual category for patients meeting criteria for schizophrenia but not for the paranoid, disorganized, or catatonic subtypes.
- *Residual:* Residual schizophrenia is a diagnosis for patients who no longer have prominent psychotic symptoms but who once met criteria for schizophrenia and have ongoing evidence of illness such as blunted affect or eccentric behavior.

Course of Illness

Schizophrenia typically begins with a prodromal phase in the mid to late teens that is characterized by subtle changes in emotional, cognitive, and social functioning. This is followed by an active phase, during which psychotic symptoms develop. The person usually does not disclose these symptoms to others right away, and many patients go for as long as 2 years before symptoms become so troubling that a psychiatrist is consulted. The

TABLE 5–4. Typical stages of schizophrenia

Stage	Typical features
Prodromal phase	Insidious onset occurs over months or years; subtle behavior changes include social withdrawal, work impairment, blunting of emotion, avolition, and odd ideas and behavior.
Active phase	Psychotic symptoms develop, including hallucinations, delusions, or disorganized speech and behavior. These symptoms eventually lead to medical intervention.
Residual phase	Active-phase symptoms are absent or no longer prominent. There is often role impairment, negative symptoms, or attenuated positive symptoms. Acute-phase symptoms may reemerge during the residual phase ("acute exacerbation").

psychotic symptoms usually respond relatively well to antipsychotic treatment, but ongoing problems such as blunted emotions or odd behavior tend to persist as the person passes into a residual phase. Acute exacerbations tend to occur from time to time, even when the patient continues to take medication. Typical stages of schizophrenia are outlined in Table 5–4.

Because schizophrenia is such a serious illness, it can be difficult to "break the news" about the diagnosis to the patient and his or her family. The first question that they will ask is "What does the future hold?" For many years, two different kinds of messages were taught to clinicians. The most common teaching has been that schizophrenia is a severe chronic illness with a poor outcome. Alternatively, clinicians were sometimes taught the "rule of thirds": about one-third of patients first diagnosed with schizophrenia will have a relatively good outcome, with minimal symptoms and mild impairments in cognition and social functioning; one-third will have a poor outcome, with persistence of psychotic symptoms, prominent negative symptoms, and significant psychosocial impairment; and one-third will have an outcome somewhere in the middle. As originally formulated, the rule of thirds was based on relatively limited clinical observation rather than rigorous scientific studies. Nonetheless, these limited studies stressed an important fact: schizophrenia has a heterogeneous outcome. Several well-designed longitudinal studies conducted during recent years have in-

TABLE 5–5. Features associated with good and poor outcome in schizophrenia

Feature	Good outcome	Poor outcome
Onset	Acute	Insidious
Duration of prodrome	Short	Since childhood
Age at onset	Late 20s to 30s	Early teens
Mood symptoms	Present	Absent
Psychotic or negative symptoms	Mild to moderate	Severe
Obsessions/compulsions	Absent	Present
Gender	More common in females	More common in males
Premorbid functioning	Good	Poor
Marital status	Married	Never married
Psychosexual functioning	Good	Poor
Neurological functioning	Normal	Soft signs present
Structural brain abnormalities	None	Present
Intelligence level	High	Low
Family history of schizophrenia	Negative	Positive

corporated cognitive measures and quantitative structural brain imaging measures obtained from magnetic resonance imaging (MRI) scans. Although it is difficult to definitively predict outcome for a specific patient based on these studies, a variety of features have been identified that are associated with good and poor outcome. These are summarized in Table 5–5. Among these, IQ is the strongest predictor of outcome, with age at onset, gender, severity and type of initial symptoms, and structural brain abnormalities also having some predictive value.

Additionally, cross-cultural studies have shown that patients in less developed countries tend to have better outcomes than those in more developed countries. It may be that the schizophrenic patient is better accepted in less developed societies, has fewer external demands, and is more likely to be taken care of by family members. Women, in general, tend to have a better outcomes than men.

Differential Diagnosis

Schizophrenia should be thought of as a diagnosis of exclusion because the consequences of the diagnosis are severe and limit therapeutic options. First, a thorough physical examination and history should be performed to help rule out medical causes of schizophrenic symptoms. Psychotic symptoms are found in many other illnesses, including substance abuse (e.g., hallucinogens, phencyclidine, amphetamines, cocaine, alcohol), intoxication due to commonly prescribed medications (e.g., corticosteroids, anticholinergics, levodopa), infections, metabolic and endocrine disorders, tumors and mass lesions, and temporal lobe epilepsy. Routine laboratory tests may be helpful in ruling out medical etiologies. Testing may include a complete blood count, urinalysis, liver enzymes, serum creatinine, blood urea nitrogen, thyroid function tests, and serologic tests for evidence of an infection with syphilis or HIV. MRI may be useful in selected patients to rule out focal brain disorder (e.g., tumors, strokes) during the initial workup for new-onset cases.

The major differential diagnosis involves separating schizophrenia from schizoaffective disorder, mood disorder, delusional disorder, and personality disorders (Table 5–6). The chief distinction from schizoaffective disorder and psychotic mood disorders is that in schizophrenia, a full depressive or manic syndrome either is absent, develops after the psychotic symptoms, or is brief relative to the duration of psychotic symptoms. Unlike delusional disorder, schizophrenia is often characterized by bizarre delusions, and hallucinations are common. Patients with personality disorders, particularly those disorders within the eccentric cluster (e.g., schizoid, schizotypal, and paranoid), may be indifferent to social relationships and have a restricted affect, bizarre ideation, or odd speech, but they are not psychotic.

Other psychiatric disorders also must be ruled out, including schizophreniform disorder, brief psychotic disorder, factitious disorder with psychological symptoms, and malingering.

Etiology and Pathophysiology

Schizophrenia is best conceptualized as a "multiple-hit" illness similar to cancer, diabetes, and cardiovascular disease. Individuals may carry a genetic predisposition, but this vulnerability is not "released" unless other factors also intervene. Although most of these factors are considered environmental, in the sense that they are not encoded in DNA and could potentially produce mutations or influence gene expression, most are

TABLE 5–6. Differential diagnosis of schizophrenia

Psychiatric illness	Other medical illness
Bipolar disorder with psychotic features	Temporal lobe epilepsy
	Tumor, stroke, brain trauma
Major depression with psychotic features	Endocrine/metabolic disorders (e.g., porphyria)
Schizoaffective disorder	Vitamin deficiency (e.g., B_{12})
Brief psychotic disorder	Infectious disease (e.g.,
Schizophreniform disorder	neurosyphilis)
Delusional disorder	Autoimmune disorder (e.g.,
Shared psychotic disorder	systemic lupus erythematosus)
Panic disorder	Toxic illness (e.g., heavy metal
Depersonalization disorder	poisoning)
Obsessive-compulsive disorder	**Drugs**
Personality disorders (e.g., "eccentric cluster")	Stimulants (e.g., amphetamine, cocaine)
	Hallucinogens
	Anticholinergics (e.g., belladonna alkaloids)
	Alcohol withdrawal
	Barbiturate withdrawal

also biological rather than psychological and include factors such as birth injuries, poor maternal nutrition, or maternal substance abuse. Current studies of the neurobiology of schizophrenia examine a multiplicity of factors, including genetics, anatomy (primarily through structural neuroimaging), functional circuitry (through functional neuroimaging), neuropathology, electrophysiology, neurochemistry and neuropharmacology, and neurodevelopment.

Genetics

There is substantial evidence that schizophrenia has a strong genetic component. Summaries of family studies have shown that siblings of schizophrenic patients have about a 10% chance of developing schizophrenia, whereas children who have one parent with schizophrenia have a 5%–6% chance. The risk of family members developing schizophrenia increases markedly when two or more family members have the illness. The risk of developing schizophrenia is 17% for persons with one sibling and one parent with schizophrenia and 46% for the children

and second-generation antipsychotics (e.g., risperidone, olanzapine) are considered first-line treatments for schizophrenia. Although the second-generation antipsychotics are generally better tolerated because they have less potential to cause extrapyramidal side effects, they can cause weight gain, glucose intolerance, and lipid dysregulation. Clozapine is a second-line choice because of its propensity to cause agranulocytosis. Nonetheless, it is associated with a reduction in suicidal behavior and may be particularly useful in patients with schizophrenia at high risk for suicide. The use of these drugs is further described in Chapter 20.

Maintenance Therapy

Patients benefiting from short-term treatment with antipsychotic medications are candidates for long-term maintenance treatment, which has as its goal the sustained control of psychotic symptoms. At least 1–2 years of treatment are recommended after the initial psychotic episode because of the high risk of relapse and the possibility of social deterioration from further relapses. At least 5 years of treatment for multiple episodes is recommended because a high risk of relapse remains. Beyond this, data are incomplete, but indefinite (perhaps lifelong) treatment is likely to be needed by most patients. Long-acting injectable formulations (e.g., haloperidol decanoate, risperidone) may be used for patient convenience and to improve adherence.

Adjunctive Treatments

Adjunctive psychotropic medications are sometimes useful in the schizophrenic patient, but their role has not been clearly defined. Many patients benefit from anxiolytics (e.g., benzodiazepines) when anxiety is prominent. Lithium carbonate, valproate, and carbamazepine can be used to reduce impulsive and aggressive behaviors, hyperactivity, or mood swings, although their effectiveness in patients with schizophrenia has not been adequately determined. Antidepressants are sometimes used to treat depression in schizophrenic patients and appear to be effective.

Psychosocial Interventions

As hospitalizations have become briefer, the locus of treatment has shifted to outpatient settings and to the community. Hospitalization now is reserved for patients who pose a danger to themselves or others; who are unable to properly care for themselves (e.g., refuse food or fluids); or

---

TABLE 5–7.   Reasons to hospitalize patients with schizophrenia

---

1. When the illness is new, to rule out alternative diagnoses and to stabilize the dosage of antipsychotic medication
2. For special medical procedures such as electroconvulsive therapy
3. When aggressive or assaultive behavior presents a danger to the patient or others
4. When the patient becomes suicidal
5. When the patient is unable to properly care for himself or herself (e.g., refuses to eat or take fluids)
6. When medication side effects become disabling or potentially life threatening (e.g., severe pseudoparkinsonism, neuroleptic malignant syndrome)

---

who require special medical observation, tests, or treatments. (See Table 5–7 for the reasons to hospitalize patients with schizophrenia).

Patients with schizophrenia who do not need to be hospitalized may benefit from partial hospital or day treatment programs, especially patients with substantial symptoms that have not responded adequately to medication. These programs generally operate on weekdays, and patients return home in the evenings and on weekends. Pharmacological management is provided along with psychosocial rehabilitation. In these programs, the services provided and frequency of attendance will be individualized to fit the needs of the patient.

The outpatient clinic will be the best setting in which to coordinate care for most schizophrenic patients. A well-equipped clinic should be able to provide medication management and a variety of adjunctive behavioral and cognitive treatments.

Assertive community treatment (ACT) programs are available in some areas. They employ careful monitoring of patients through mobile mental health teams and individually tailored programming. ACT programs have staff available 24 hours a day and have been shown to reduce hospital admission rates and to improve the quality of life for many patients with schizophrenia. ACT involves teaching patients basic living skills, helping patients work with community agencies, and helping patients develop a social support network. Voluntary job placement and supported work settings (i.e., sheltered workshops) are an important part of the program.

Family Therapy

Family therapy, combined with antipsychotic medication, has been shown to reduce relapse rates in schizophrenia. Families often want to learn more about the nature of the illness. They need realistic and accurate information about the cause of illness, prognostic indicators, and available treatments. They also will benefit from learning how to improve communications with their schizophrenic relative and how to provide constructive support.

Cognitive Rehabilitation

Cognitive rehabilitation therapy has as its goal the remediation of abnormal thought processes known to occur in schizophrenia and uses techniques pioneered in the treatment of brain-injured persons. Work with schizophrenic patients is focused on improving information-processing skills such as attention, memory, vigilance, and conceptual abilities. Patients may also learn various coping strategies such as listening to music to mask auditory hallucinations or reality testing of delusional beliefs.

Social Skills Training

Social skills training aims to help patients develop more appropriate behavior. This training is accompanied by modeling and social reinforcement and by providing opportunities, both individual and group, to practice the new behaviors. This could be as simple as helping the patient learn to maintain eye contact or as complicated as helping him or her learn better conversational skills.

Psychosocial Rehabilitation

The goal of psychosocial rehabilitation is to integrate the patient back into his or her community rather than segregating the patient in separate facilities, as has occurred in the past. In some locations, patient clubhouses are available to promote psychosocial rehabilitation, such as Fountain House, a program in New York that patients help to manage. Appropriate and affordable housing is a major concern for many patients, and depending on the community, options may range from supervised shelters and group homes (halfway houses) to boarding homes to supervised apartment living. Group homes provide peer support and companionship, along with on-site staff supervision. Supervised apartments provide greater independence and offer the availability and backup of trained staff.

Vocational interventions can help patients find and maintain paid jobs. Vocational rehabilitation may involve supported employment, competitive work in integrated settings, and more formal job training programs. A simple, repetitive job environment offering both interpersonal distance and on-site supervision may be the best initial setting, such as that found in a sheltered workshop. Although some patients will not be employable in any setting because of apathy, amotivation, or chronic psychosis, employment should be encouraged in able patients. A job will serve to improve self-esteem, provide additional income, and provide a social outlet for the patient. With the aid of modern treatments, some patients are able to achieve regular paid employment that improves their integration into society.

Key points to remember about schizophrenia

1. Psychotic symptoms should be treated aggressively with medication.

    • Both high-potency conventional antipsychotics and second-generation antipsychotics are considered first-line therapy because they are effective and well tolerated.

    • Intramuscular medication is useful in noncompliant patients or those who prefer the convenience of bimonthly or monthly injections.

2. The clinician should engage the patient in an empathic relationship.

    • This task may at times be challenging because some patients are unemotional, aloof, and withdrawn.

    • The clinician should be practical and help the patient with problems that matter to him or her, such as finding adequate housing.

3. The clinician should help the patient find a daily routine that he or she can manage, to help improve socialization and reduce boredom.

    • Partial hospitalization or day treatment programs are available in many areas.

    • Sheltered workshops that provide simple, repetitive chores may be helpful.

4. The clinician should develop a close working relationship with local social services.

    • Patients tend to be poor and disabled; finding adequate housing and food takes the skills of a social worker.

    • The clinician should help the patient obtain disability benefits.

> **Key points to remember about schizophrenia** *(continued)*
>
> 5. Family therapy is important for the patient who lives at home or who still has close family ties.
>   - As a result of the illness, many patients will have broken their family ties.
>   - Families desperately need education about schizophrenia.
>   - The clinician should help family members find a support group through referral to a local chapter of the National Alliance on Mental Illness (NAMI).

■ Delusional Disorder

Delusional disorder is an important but relatively rare psychotic disorder. It is characterized by the presence of well-systematized, nonbizarre delusions accompanied by affect appropriate to the delusion and occurring in the presence of a relatively well-preserved personality. The delusions will have lasted at least 1 month; behavior is generally not odd or bizarre apart from the delusion or its ramifications; active-phase symptoms that may occur in schizophrenia (e.g., hallucinations, disorganized speech) are absent; and the disorder is not due to a mood disorder, is not substance induced, and is not due to a medical condition (see Table 5–8).

The core feature of delusional disorder is the presence of a well-systematized, encapsulated, nonbizarre delusion. Nonbizarre delusions are ones that, although technically possible, are improbable nonetheless. (An example of an impossible delusion is the belief that one is controlled by green Martians.) The term *systematized* indicates that the delusion and its ramifications fit into a complex, all-encompassing scheme that makes logical sense to the patient. The term *encapsulated* indicates that apart from the delusion or its ramifications, the patient generally behaves normally, or at least is not obviously odd or bizarre.

Epidemiology, Etiology, and Course

Delusional disorder is relatively rare, with an estimated prevalence of between 24 and 30 per 100,000 persons. Considered a disorder of middle to late adult life, it affects more women than men. Most delusional disorder patients marry, but they tend to be poorly educated and from lower income groups.

TABLE 5–8.   DSM-IV-TR diagnostic criteria for delusional disorder

A. Nonbizarre delusions (i.e., involving situations that occur in real life, such as being followed, poisoned, infected, loved at a distance, or deceived by spouse or lover, or having a disease) of at least 1 month's duration.

B. Criterion A for Schizophrenia has never been met.   **Note:** Tactile and olfactory hallucinations may be present in Delusional Disorder if they are related to the delusional theme.

C. Apart from the impact of the delusion(s) or its ramifications, functioning is not markedly impaired and behavior is not obviously odd or bizarre.

D. If mood episodes have occurred concurrently with delusions, their total duration has been brief relative to the duration of the delusional periods.

E. The disturbance is not due to the direct physiological effects of a substance (e.g., a drug of abuse, a medication) or a general medical condition.

Specify type (the following types are assigned based on the predominant delusional theme):

> **Erotomanic Type:**   delusions that another person, usually of higher status, is in love with the individual
>
> **Grandiose Type:**   delusions of inflated worth, power, knowledge, identity, or special relationship to a deity or famous person
>
> **Jealous Type:**   delusions that the individual's sexual partner is unfaithful
>
> **Persecutory Type:**   delusions that the person (or someone to whom the person is close) is being malevolently treated in some way
>
> **Somatic Type:**   delusions that the person has some physical defect or general medical condition
>
> **Mixed Type:**   delusions characteristic of more than one of the above types but no one theme predominates
>
> **Unspecified Type**

There is no known cause of delusional disorder. Paranoid personality traits (e.g., suspiciousness, jealousy) have been found in relatives of delusional disorder probands, suggesting that the disorder may have a hereditary basis.

Stressful situations were long thought to cause delusional disorder in some persons. For example, people migrating from one country to another were long noted to be at greater risk of developing persecutory delusions ("migration psychosis"). Solitary confinement in prison is another example of a stressor thought to induce a delusional disorder in some persons.

Delusional disorder tends to be chronic and lifelong. Yet unlike the person with schizophrenia, people with delusional disorder are generally employed and self-supporting.

Clinical Findings

Patients with delusional disorder tend to be socially isolated and chronically suspicious. Those with persecutory or jealous delusions sometimes become angry and hostile, emotions that can lead to violent outbursts. Many will become litigious and end up as lawyers' clients rather than as psychiatrists' patients. Sexual disorders and depressive symptoms are common. Patients may become overtalkative and circumstantial, particularly when discussing their delusions.

The following DSM-IV-TR subtypes are based on the predominant delusional theme:

- *Persecutory type*: The belief that one is being treated badly in some way
- *Erotomanic type* (de Clerambault's syndrome): The belief that a person, usually of higher status, is in love with the patient
- *Grandiose type*: The belief that one is of inflated worth, power, knowledge, or identity or that one has a special relationship to a deity or famous person
- *Jealous type*: The belief that one's sexual partner is unfaithful
- *Somatic type*: The belief that one has some physical defect, disorder, or disease, such as AIDS

The residual category *unspecified type* is for patients who do not fit the previous categories (e.g., those who have been ill less than 1 month). The category *mixed type* is used for those with delusions characteristic of more than one subtype but without any single theme predominating.

The following patient seen in our hospital illustrates the erotomanic subtype:

Doug, a 33-year-old restaurant manager, was brought to the hospital under court order. He allegedly had harassed and threatened a young woman. The following story gradually unfolded.

Doug was convinced that an attractive young woman who worked in a local bookstore was in love with him, even though they had never met. He took as evidence of her affection glances and smiles they had exchanged when crossing paths in their small town. After learning her name and address, he sent her a "sexual business letter." Doug continued to send additional love letters over the next few years and carefully tracked her whereabouts. There were no other communications, but the letters indicated his belief that she was infatuated with him.

The young woman reported her concerns to the police; they warned Doug not to call or write her, but this had little effect. (Interestingly, Doug himself complained to the police about his imagined harassment by her.) Eventually a court order was sought when Doug's letters took a more threatening tone, and a "no contact" order failed to keep him away from the bookshop where she worked.

Doug was indignant about his hospitalization. Although he was circumstantial in describing his fantasy relationship, there was no evidence of a mood disorder, hallucinations, or bizarre delusions. He reported a history of a similar relationship 10 years earlier, consisting mostly of letters, which ended only when the girl moved out of town. Doug was a loner with few friends but functioned well in his position at work and was active in several community organizations.

At his mental health hearing, Doug denied that his behavior was inappropriate, but he agreed to undergo outpatient psychiatric treatment. The young woman eventually moved out of town.

Differential Diagnosis

The major differential diagnosis involves separating delusional disorder from mood disorders with psychotic features, schizophrenia, and paranoid personality. The chief distinction from psychotic mood disorders is that in delusional disorder, a depressive or manic syndrome is absent, develops after the psychotic symptoms, or is brief in relation to the psychotic symptoms. Unlike schizophrenia, delusional disorders are characterized by nonbizarre delusions and generally either no hallucinations or hallucinations that are not prominent or are very brief. (Tactile and olfactory hallucinations may be present when they are related to the delusional theme.) Furthermore, patients with delusional disorders do not develop other symptoms typically associated with schizophrenia, such as incoherence or grossly disorganized behavior, and personality is generally preserved. Persons with paranoid personality may be suspicious and hypervigilant, but they are not delusional.

Clinical Management

Because delusional disorder is so uncommon, treatment recommendations are based on clinical observation and not careful research. Clinical experience suggests that response to antipsychotics is poor and that although they may help relieve agitation and anxiety, they may leave the core delusion intact. Any of the antipsychotics can be used, including one of the high-potency conventional antipsychotics (e.g., haloperidol 5–10 mg/day) or a second-generation antipsychotic (e.g., risperidone 2–6 mg/day). *Monohypochondriacal paranoia* (i.e., delusional disorder, somatic subtype) has been specifically reported to respond to the antipsychotic pimozide at dosages of 4–8 mg/day. Selective serotonin reuptake inhibitors (e.g., fluoxetine, paroxetine) also have been reported to be helpful in reducing delusional beliefs in some patients.

The physician should make an effort to develop a trusting relationship with the patient, after which he or she may gently challenge the patient's beliefs by showing how they interfere with the patient's life. The patient should be assured of the confidential nature of the doctor–patient relationship. Tact and skill are necessary to persuade a patient to accept treatment, and the physician must neither condemn nor collude in the beliefs. Group therapy is not recommended because patients with delusional disorder tend to be suspicious and hypervigilant and are prone to misinterpret situations that may arise in the course of the therapy.

Key points to remember about delusional disorder

1. Because the patient with delusional disorder is so suspicious, it may be very difficult to establish a therapeutic relationship.
   - Building a relationship will take time and patience.
   - The therapist must neither condemn nor collude in the delusional beliefs of the patient.
   - The patient must be assured of complete confidentiality.

2. Once rapport is established, the patient's delusional beliefs may be gently challenged by pointing out how they interfere with his or her functioning.
   - Tact and skill are needed to convince the patient to accept treatment.

3. A patient with delusional disorder may be more accepting of medication if it is explained as a treatment for the anxiety, dysphoria, and stress that the patient invariably experiences as a result of his or her delusions.

> **Key points to remember about delusional disorder** *(continued)*
>
> - Antipsychotic medication should be tried, although results are unpredictable.
> - Patients with the somatic subtype may preferentially respond to pimozide.

■ Schizoaffective Disorder

The term *schizoaffective* was first used in 1933 by Jacob Kasanin to describe a small group of patients who had a mixture of psychotic and mood symptoms and who were severely ill. In DSM-IV-TR, its hallmark is the presence of either a depressive or a manic episode concurrent with symptoms characteristic of schizophrenia, such as bizarre delusions (see Table 5–9). During the illness, hallucinations or delusions must be present for 2 weeks or more in the absence of prominent mood symptoms, but mood symptoms must be present for a substantial portion of the total duration of the illness. (Some experts consider a "substantial portion" to constitute 30% or more of the total duration.) Finally, the effects of medical illness and drugs must have been excluded as having caused the symptoms. There are two subtypes: the bipolar type, marked by a current or previous manic syndrome, and the depressive type, marked by the absence of any manic syndromes.

Schizoaffective disorder is thought to have a prevalence of less than 1% and to occur more often in women. The diagnosis is common in psychiatric hospitals and clinics but is primarily a diagnosis of exclusion. The differential diagnosis for schizoaffective disorder consists primarily of schizophrenia, psychotic mood disorders, and disorders induced by medical illness or drugs. In schizophrenia, the duration of all episodes of a mood syndrome is brief relative to the total duration of the psychotic disturbance. Although psychotic symptoms may occur in persons with mood disorders, they are generally not present in the absence of depression or mania, helping to set the boundary between schizoaffective disorder and psychotic mania or depression. It is usually clear from the history, physical examination, or laboratory tests when a drug or medical illness has initiated and maintained the disorder.

Family studies have shown an increased prevalence of both schizophrenia and mood disorders in relatives of patients with schizophrenia. In general, schizoaffective patients have higher rates of schizophrenia

---

TABLE 5–9.   DSM-IV-TR diagnostic criteria for schizoaffective disorder

---

A. An uninterrupted period of illness during which, at some time, there is either a Major Depressive Episode, a Manic Episode, or a Mixed Episode concurrent with symptoms that meet Criterion A for Schizophrenia.
   Note: The Major Depressive Episode must include Criterion A1: depressed mood.
B. During the same period of illness, there have been delusions or hallucinations for at least 2 weeks in the absence of prominent mood symptoms.
C. Symptoms that meet criteria for a mood episode are present for a substantial portion of the total duration of the active and residual periods of the illness.
D. The disturbance is not due to the direct physiological effects of a substance (e.g., a drug of abuse, a medication) or a general medical condition.

Specify type:
   Bipolar Type: if the disturbance includes a Manic or a Mixed Episode (or a Manic or a Mixed Episode and Major Depressive Episodes)
   Depressive Type: if the disturbance only includes Major Depressive Episodes

---

and lower rates of mood disorders in their relatives than do patients with mood disorder but higher rates of mood disorder and lower rates of schizophrenia in their relatives than do patients with schizophrenia. Other research also suggests that patients with schizoaffective disorder are a mixture of patients with schizophrenia with severe mood symptoms and mood disorder patients with severe psychoses.

The signs and symptoms of schizoaffective disorder include those seen in schizophrenia and the mood disorders. The symptoms may present together or in an alternating fashion, and psychotic symptoms may be mood congruent or mood incongruent. The course of schizoaffective disorder is variable but represents a middle ground between that of schizophrenia and the mood disorders. A worse outcome is associated with poor premorbid adjustment, insidious onset, lack of a precipitating stressor, predominance of psychotic symptoms, early onset, unremitting course, and a family history of schizophrenia.

The treatment of schizoaffective disorder should target both psychotic and mood symptoms. With second-generation antipsychotics, a single drug may adequately target both psychotic and mood symptoms, so these drugs may represent an ideal first-line treatment. In fact, paliperidone was recently approved as monotherapy by the U.S. Food and Drug Administration for the treatment of schizoaffective disorder. Some patients may benefit from the addition of a mood stabilizer (e.g., lithium, valproate) or an antidepressant. Patients not responding to medication may respond to electroconvulsive therapy, although medication is typically reinstituted for long-term maintenance. Schizoaffective patients who are a danger to themselves or others or who are unable to properly care for themselves should be hospitalized.

■ Schizophreniform Disorder

The diagnosis of schizophreniform disorder is used for patients who present with typical schizophrenia symptoms but who have been ill for less than 6 months. In DSM-IV-TR, the definition of *schizophreniform disorder* requires that the following features be present: 1) the patient has psychotic symptoms characteristic of schizophrenia, 2) the symptoms are not due to a substance or general medical condition, 3) schizoaffective disorder and mood disorder with psychotic features have been ruled out, and 4) the duration is at least 1 month but less than 6 months.

The diagnosis changes to schizophrenia once the symptoms have extended past 6 months, even if the only symptoms remaining are residual ones, such as blunted affect. The diagnosis is considered provisional in patients who have not recovered, because many persons who meet criteria for schizophreniform disorder will eventually meet criteria for schizophrenia.

Research has not supported the validity of schizophreniform disorder as a distinct diagnosis. The diagnosis appears to identify a widely varying group of patients, most of whom eventually develop either schizophrenia, a mood disorder, or schizoaffective disorder.

Clearly, the proper boundaries of this disorder remain in question. Its main use is to guard against premature diagnosis of schizophrenia. Treatment of schizophreniform disorder has not been systematically evaluated. The principles for its management are similar to those for an acute exacerbation of schizophrenia.

■ Brief Psychotic Disorder

Patients with a brief psychotic disorder have psychotic symptoms that last at least 1 day but no more than 1 month, with gradual recovery. Psychotic mood disorders, schizophrenia, and the effects of drugs or medical illness have been ruled out as causing the symptoms. Signs and symptoms are similar to those seen in schizophrenia, including hallucinations, delusions, and grossly disorganized behavior. The three subtypes are 1) with marked stressor(s), 2) without marked stressor(s), and 3) with postpartum onset. In the past, patients with marked stressors would have received a diagnosis of a reactive, hysterical, or psychogenic psychosis. This disorder is similar to what Scandinavian psychiatrists regard as *reactive psychoses,* conditions that arise in psychologically vulnerable persons subjected to stressful situations.

Patients with postpartum onset generally develop symptoms within 1–2 weeks after delivery. Symptoms include disorganized speech, misperceptions, labile mood, confusion, and hallucinations. *Postpartum psychosis,* as it is often called, tends to arise in otherwise normal individuals and resolves within 2–3 months. The disorder should be distinguished from *postpartum blues,* which occurs in up to 80% of new mothers, lasts for a few days after delivery, and is considered normal.

The prevalence and gender ratio of brief psychotic disorder are unknown. The disorder is thought to occur more commonly in lower income groups and among individuals with personality disorders, especially the borderline and schizotypal types.

As with any acute psychosis, hospitalization may be necessary for the safety of the patient or others. Because a brief psychotic disorder is probably self-limiting, no specific treatment is indicated, and the hospital milieu itself may be sufficient to help the patient recover. Antipsychotics may be helpful early on, especially when the patient is highly agitated or experiencing great emotional turmoil. After the patient has sufficiently recovered, the clinician can help him or her explore the meaning of the psychotic reaction and of the triggering stressor. Supportive psychotherapy may help restore morale and self-esteem.

■ Shared Psychotic Disorder

The essence of shared psychotic disorder is the transmission of delusional beliefs from one person to another. In DSM-IV-TR, a shared psychotic disorder involves the presence of a delusion that develops in the context of a close relationship with another person, who already has an established delusion. In the past, these rare cases were called *folie à deux*, a French term meaning "double insanity."

Most cases of shared psychotic disorder involve two members of the same family, most commonly siblings, a parent and child, or a husband and wife. Its development requires the presence of a dominant person with an established delusion and a more submissive and suggestible person who gains the acceptance of the more dominant individual by adopting his or her delusional beliefs. Clinical observation suggests that separation may result in rapid improvement of the submissive person.

■ Self-Assessment Questions

1. How is schizophrenia diagnosed? What is its differential diagnosis?

2. What are typical signs and symptoms of schizophrenia?

3. What are the subtypes of schizophrenia?

4. What evidence supports a neurobiological basis for schizophrenia?

5. What is the natural history of schizophrenia?

6. How is schizophrenia managed, both pharmacologically and psychosocially?

7. How does delusional disorder differ from schizophrenia?

8. What are the subtypes of delusional disorder?

9. How does schizoaffective disorder differ diagnostically from both schizophrenia and psychotic mood disorders?

10. What is the differential diagnosis of a brief psychotic disorder?

11. What is the commonly accepted treatment in shared psychotic disorder for the patient who develops a delusion in the context of a close relationship with another person?

CHAPTER 6

Mood Disorders

I see the lost are like this, and their curse
To be, as I am mine, their sweating selves. But worse.

Gerard Manley Hopkins

MOOD DISORDERS have a high prevalence, a high morbidity, and a high mortality rate. Masked as complaints about insomnia, fatigue, or unexplained pain, mood disorders often lead people to seek medical care in primary care settings. Many patients receive treatment there, but some are referred on to specialists (and potentially to the wrong specialist if the diagnosis of depression is missed). Therefore, all physicians who have direct personal contact with patients need to learn the fundamentals about diagnosing and treating mood disorders. Mood disorders can be costly and disabling if not correctly diagnosed and treated. For people ages 15–45 years, depression accounts for an astonishing 10.3% of all costs of biomedical illnesses worldwide. Furthermore, bipolar disorder (manic-depressive illness), the severe form of mood disorder characterized by extreme mood swings, ranks sixth among the world's most disabling illnesses. Yet these substantial costs to society from disability due to mood disorders, documented in *The Global Burden of Disease,* may be unnecessary. When correctly diagnosed and treated, mood disorders usually respond well.

■ Major Depressive Episode

The DSM-IV-TR criteria for an episode of major depression specify that the patient must have at least five of nine symptoms of depression (and one of them must be depressed mood or loss of interest or pleasure). These characteristic symptoms define major depression, and they must be present for at least 2 weeks to rule out transient mood fluctuations. Criteria B, D, and E serve to rule out other conditions, such as a bipolar disorder (e.g., presence of a mixed episode), abnormalities in mood due to abuse of a substance (e.g., amphetamines) or to a general medical condition (e.g., myxedema), or a disturbance in mood due to bereavement. Criterion C specifies that the symptoms must cause distress or impairment in order to differentiate a disorder from normal fluctuations in mood (Table 6–1).

Because major depression is the most common psychiatric illness that clinicians in any branch of medicine are likely to encounter, it is worthwhile to commit the nine characteristic symptoms to memory. When interviewing patients to determine whether they are depressed, the clinician must mentally run through this list of symptoms. Consequently, it is convenient to have it stored in an accessible memory bank so that the evaluation can be done fluently and smoothly. This can be facilitated through the use of a simple mnemonic: "Depression Is Worth Studiously Memorizing Extremely Grueling Criteria. Sorry." (DIWSMEGCS). The initials stand for Depressed mood, Interest, Weight, Sleep, Motor activity, Energy, Guilt, Concentration, Suicide.

Clinical Findings

The basic abnormality in depression is an alteration in mood: a person who is depressed feels sad, despondent, down in the dumps, or full of despair. Occasional patients will complain of feeling tense or irritable, with only a small component of sadness, or of having lost their ability to feel pleasure or to experience interest in things they normally enjoy.

The depressive syndrome is frequently accompanied by a group of *vegetative symptoms* (also known as *somatic symptoms*), such as decreased appetite or insomnia. Decreased appetite often leads to some weight loss, although some depressed persons will force themselves to eat despite decreased appetite, or they may be urged to eat by a parent or spouse. Less frequently, depression expresses itself as a desire to eat excessively and is accompanied by weight gain.

Insomnia may be initial, middle, or terminal. *Initial insomnia* means that the patient has difficulty falling asleep, often tossing or turning for several

TABLE 6–1. DSM-IV-TR diagnostic criteria for major depressive episode

A. Five (or more) of the following symptoms have been present during the same 2-week period and represent a change from previous functioning; at least one of the symptoms is either (1) depressed mood or (2) loss of interest or pleasure.
   Note: Do not include symptoms that are clearly due to a general medical condition, or mood-incongruent delusions or hallucinations.
   (1) depressed mood most of the day, nearly every day, as indicated by either subjective report (e.g., feels sad or empty) or observation made by others (e.g., appears tearful). **Note:** In children and adolescents, can be irritable mood.
   (2) markedly diminished interest or pleasure in all, or almost all, activities most of the day, nearly every day (as indicated by either subjective account or observation made by others)
   (3) significant weight loss when not dieting or weight gain (e.g., a change of more than 5% of body weight in a month), or decrease or increase in appetite nearly every day. **Note:** In children, consider failure to make expected weight gains.
   (4) insomnia or hypersomnia nearly every day
   (5) psychomotor agitation or retardation nearly every day (observable by others, not merely subjective feelings of restlessness or being slowed down)
   (6) fatigue or loss of energy nearly every day
   (7) feelings of worthlessness or excessive or inappropriate guilt (which may be delusional) nearly every day (not merely self-reproach or guilt about being sick)
   (8) diminished ability to think or concentrate, or indecisiveness, nearly every day (either by subjective account or as observed by others)
   (9) recurrent thoughts of death (not just fear of dying), recurrent suicidal ideation without a specific plan, or a suicide attempt or a specific plan for committing suicide
B. The symptoms do not meet criteria for a Mixed Episode.
C. The symptoms cause clinically significant distress or impairment in social, occupational, or other important areas of functioning.
D. The symptoms are not due to the direct physiological effects of a substance (e.g., a drug of abuse, a medication) or a general medical condition (e.g., hypothyroidism).
E. The symptoms are not better accounted for by Bereavement, i.e., after the loss of a loved one, the symptoms persist for longer than 2 months or are characterized by marked functional impairment, morbid preoccupation with worthlessness, suicidal ideation, psychotic symptoms, or psychomotor retardation.

hours before dozing off. *Middle insomnia* refers to awakening in the middle of the night, remaining awake for an hour or two, and finally falling asleep again. *Terminal insomnia* refers to awakening early in the morning and being unable to return to sleep. Patients with insomnia will often worry and ruminate while they are lying awake. Patients who have terminal insomnia may have more severe depressive syndromes. Occasionally, the sleep difficulty may involve a need to sleep excessively: the patient may complain of feeling chronically tired and needing to spend 10–14 hours in bed each day.

Motor activity is often altered in depression. Patients with *psychomotor retardation* may sit quietly in a chair for hours without speaking to anyone, simply staring into space. When these patients get up and move about, they walk at a snail's pace, their speech is slow, and their replies are brief and laconic. If asked about their thinking, they may complain that it is markedly slowed down. Conversely, patients with *psychomotor agitation* are restless and seem extremely nervous. Agitated patients may complain more of irritability or tenseness than of depression. They are unable to sit in a chair and frequently pace about. They may wring their hands or perform repetitive gestures such as drumming their fingers on a table or pulling on their hair or clothing.

Depressed patients also complain frequently of fatiguing too easily or lacking energy. In a general medical setting, this may be one of the most common presenting complaints of depression.

Feelings of worthlessness and guilt are also very common. Depressed persons may lose confidence in themselves so that they are fearful of going to work, taking examinations, or assuming responsibility for household tasks. They may not answer the telephone or return telephone calls to avoid responsibilities or social relationships that they feel unable to handle. They may become completely hopeless and full of despair, believing that their situation can never be improved or even that they do not deserve to feel better. Depressed patients may feel quite guilty over actual or fantasized misdeeds they have committed in the past. Usually the misdeed is seen as more terrible than it actually was, so that depressed persons believe that they should be social pariahs because of a lie told as a child or sent to prison for a long term because of a questionable deduction taken on an income tax return.

Complaints of difficulty in concentrating or thinking clearly are also common in depression. Depressed patients feel that they function less well at work, are unable to study, or in severe cases are even unable to perform simple cognitive tasks such as watching a football game on television or reading.

Depressed patients may think a great deal about death or suicide. This may be seen either as an escape from their suffering or as a deserved punishment for their various misdeeds. The suicidal patient often expresses the notion that "everyone would be better off without me." Suicide risk is high in depressed patients and should always be assessed carefully. (See Chapter 15 for more detail on evaluation and management of the suicidal patient.)

In addition to the nine core symptoms summarized in the diagnostic criteria, other symptoms may occur in patients with depression. *Diurnal variation* is a fluctuation in mood during the course of a 24-hour day. Most typically, patients state that their mood is worse in the morning but that it improves as the day progresses, so that they feel best in the evening.

Sex drive may decrease markedly, so that the patient has no interest in sex or even begins to experience impotence or anorgasmia. The depressed patient also may complain of other physical symptoms such as constipation or dry mouth.

Occasionally, patients experience *masked depression*. This term means that the full depressive syndrome is not immediately obvious because the patient does not report a depressed mood. Masked depression may be especially important in primary care settings. For example, an older person may come in complaining primarily of somatic symptoms (e.g., insomnia, loss of energy and appetite) so troubling that he or she is unable to concentrate, work, and sleep. Although a careful medical workup reveals no physical abnormalities, the patient continues to insist on the troubling nature of the various somatic and depressive symptoms. When the masked depression is diagnosed and remits with appropriate treatment, however, the physical complaints tend to disappear, making it clear that they were related to a depressive syndrome.

About one-fifth of severely depressed patients may experience *psychotic symptoms* such as delusions or hallucinations. These are usually congruent with the depressed mood. For example, people who are depressed may hear the voice of the Devil telling them that they have fallen from God's ways and that they will be tormented in Hell. They may think that a fatal disease is consuming their bodies and rotting away their internal organs. Less frequently, the delusions will not be consistent with depressed mood. For example, patients may report that they are being spied on because they are on the verge of developing some great invention that others are attempting to steal—a persecutory delusion that is not directly related to depressed mood.

The following case is that of a patient with major depressive episode:

Wilma, a 41-year-old woman, was brought to the hospital at the request of her family. She described herself as being despondent and demoralized because her husband, Bill, was having an affair with Lydia, a woman who had been his office assistant. Her husband adamantly denied having an affair.

Wilma admitted to having a depressed mood plus a full constellation of depressive symptoms, including feelings of worthlessness, suicidal thoughts, hypersomnia, increased appetite and weight gain, and decreased interest in and enjoyment of activities she normally found pleasurable (such as following the many activities of her four teenage children). Wilma had had one prior episode of depression that had been successfully treated with antidepressants approximately 5 years earlier.

Wilma attributed most of her depressive symptoms to this situation, which she believed had been going on for at least 6 months (as had her depression). She had no conclusive evidence to support the occurrence of the affair, but she said that her husband had been away more in the evenings, had a marked decrease in sexual interest, and had talked frequently about Lydia's administrative skills until Wilma became jealous and angry. Because of pressure from Wilma, her husband eventually urged Lydia to seek another position, but Wilma believed that her husband was continuing to see Lydia secretly.

Depression was diagnosed, and Wilma was given imipramine, with the dosage gradually increased to 150 mg/day. She showed some improvement on this medication, and both Bill and Wilma also were seen for marital counseling. Their relationship improved somewhat, but Wilma continued to be suspicious.

After 3 months of psychotherapy, she came in one day with a new firmness of step and her eyes flashing with anger. While cleaning out the pockets of one of her husband's suits in preparation for sending it to the cleaners, she had found a love letter from Lydia. She did not confront Bill immediately but instead followed him the next night when he indicated that he was going back to the office to get caught up on some work. Ten minutes after his departure, Wilma left, drove past Lydia's house, and found Bill's car parked in her garage. She confronted him, and he finally confessed to an affair that had been going on for nearly 2 years.

The direction of marital counseling changed sharply, and Bill was urged to seek individual psychotherapy himself. Wilma continued to take antidepressant medication for another 6 months, and she gradually came to terms with the fact of her husband's infidelity (which was actually more painful than having her suspicions discounted by both her husband and the medical community). Eventually, however, the couple was able to work through this situation, to remain married, and eventually to establish a reasonably good relationship with each other.

Course and Outcome

A depressive episode may begin either suddenly or gradually. The duration of an untreated episode may range from a few weeks to months or even years, although most depressive episodes clear spontaneously within approximately 6 months. The prognosis for any single depressive episode is quite good, particularly in view of the efficacy of the available antidepressant medications. Unfortunately, a substantial number of patients will have a recurrence of depression at some time in their lives, and about 20% will develop a chronic form of depression.

Suicide is the most serious complication of depression. Approximately 10%–15% of all patients hospitalized with depression will eventually take their own lives. Several factors suggest an increase in suicidal risk: being divorced or living alone, having a history of alcohol or drug abuse, being older than 40, having a history of a prior suicide attempt, and expressing suicidal ideation (particularly when detailed plans have been formulated). Suicidal risks always should be carefully evaluated in any patient with depression, beginning with a direct inquiry as to whether the patient has considered taking his or her life. A patient considered at risk for suicide usually should be treated as an inpatient rather than as an outpatient to minimize the risk. Suicide is discussed in more detail in Chapter 15.

A broad range of other social and personal complications also may occur. Decreased energy, poor concentration, and lack of interest may cause poor performance at school or work. Apathy and decreased sexual interest may lead to marital discord. Patients may attempt to treat depressive symptoms themselves with sedatives, alcohol, or stimulants, thereby initiating problems with drug and alcohol abuse.

■ Manic Episode

The DSM-IV-TR criteria for a manic episode require the presence of an abnormally elevated, expansive, or irritable mood lasting at least 1 week plus three of seven characteristic symptoms (Table 6–2). The criteria are similar to those used to define depression, in that the mood disturbance must be sufficiently severe to cause marked impairment or to require hospitalization. As in the case of depression, the symptoms cannot be due to the physiological effects of drugs of abuse, medications, or a general medical condition.

Clinical Findings

The manic patient's mood is typically cheerful, enthusiastic, and expansive. The cheerfulness often has an infectious quality, making interviewing an enjoyable and sometimes amusing experience. Sometimes,

TABLE 6–2.   DSM-IV-TR diagnostic criteria for manic episode

A. A distinct period of abnormally and persistently elevated, expansive, or irritable mood, lasting at least 1 week (or any duration if hospitalization is necessary).
B. During the period of mood disturbance, three (or more) of the following symptoms have persisted (four if the mood is only irritable) and have been present to a significant degree:
    (1) inflated self-esteem or grandiosity
    (2) decreased need for sleep (e.g., feels rested after only 3 hours of sleep)
    (3) more talkative than usual or pressure to keep talking
    (4) flight of ideas or subjective experience that thoughts are racing
    (5) distractibility (i.e., attention too easily drawn to unimportant or irrelevant external stimuli)
    (6) increase in goal-directed activity (either socially, at work or school, or sexually) or psychomotor agitation
    (7) excessive involvement in pleasurable activities that have a high potential for painful consequences (e.g., engaging in unrestrained buying sprees, sexual indiscretions, or foolish business investments)
C. The symptoms do not meet criteria for a Mixed Episode.
D. The mood disturbance is sufficiently severe to cause marked impairment in occupational functioning or in usual social activities or relationships with others, or to necessitate hospitalization to prevent harm to self or others, or there are psychotic features.
E. The symptoms are not due to the direct physiological effects of a substance (e.g., a drug of abuse, a medication, or other treatment) or a general medical condition (e.g., hyperthyroidism).
    Note: Manic-like episodes that are clearly caused by somatic antidepressant treatment (e.g., medication, electroconvulsive therapy, light therapy) should not count toward a diagnosis of Bipolar I Disorder.

however, the patient's mood is simply irritable, particularly if the person feels thwarted, and such irritable manic patients can be quite difficult to manage. Because of their euphoria, manic patients usually have very little insight into their problems. In fact, they may deny that anything is wrong with them and instead blame friends or family for attributing an abnormality to them that is not actually present.

Manic patients typically have inflated self-esteem and grandiosity, which may reach delusional proportions. Manic patients may believe that they have special abilities or powers that clearly are outside the normal range for their educational background or intellectual achievement. They may develop plans to write books, record compact discs, lead religious movements, or undertake expansive business ventures. When the grandiosity reaches delusional proportions, patients may report that they are rock stars, famous athletes or politicians, or even religious figures such as the Messiah.

The euphoria and grandiosity are typically accompanied by increased energy, activity levels, and cognitive speed. Patients with mania usually require less sleep than usual, often getting by on only 2 or 3 hours per night. Patients may become more social and gregarious, going to bars, planning parties, or calling friends at all hours of the night. Interest in sex is often increased, leading the manic patient to exhaust his or her partner or to make inappropriate overtures to casual acquaintances or strangers. Patients with mania are usually physically restless and unable to sit still. The increased level of activity is often accompanied by poor judgment. Patients with mania tend to overextend themselves in ways that lead them into serious trouble after the manic episode is over. They spend money excessively, commit themselves to projects that they are unable to complete, become involved in extramarital affairs, or engage in quarrels with business associates or family members who disagree with them or try to slow them down.

Manic patients tend to talk excessively and to manifest *pressured speech*. Thus, they answer questions at great length, continue to talk even when interrupted, and sometimes talk when no one is listening. Their speech usually is rapid, loud, and emphatic. Underlying the pressured speech is probably a rapid flow of thought, sometimes referred to as *flight of ideas*. This increased speed in cognitive functioning is inferred by listening to the patient's speech, which manifests derailment, incoherence, and distractibility. Manic patients tend to skip from one topic to another as they describe their experiences, ideas, or symptoms. Distractibility is observed in both their speech and their social behavior. While speaking, they may shift their topic in response to some stimulus in the environment, and they manifest the same pattern of distractibility when trying to perform tasks or complete activities.

Approximately one-half of manic patients have psychotic symptoms, which may include either delusions or hallucinations that typically express themes consistent with the mood, such as delusions about special abilities or powers. Less commonly, the delusions may be mood incongruent and express themes that are not related to the patient's euphoric and grandiose mood.

The following case illustrates a manic episode:

> Charles, a 43-year-old man, was brought to the emergency room by the local police after he had jumped from his seat in the middle of a perfor-

mance of *Les Misérables*, run onto the stage, and begun yelling that the injustices of the Bush administration were as extensive and profound as those portrayed in the performance. He had begun conversing with Jean Valjean, urging him to leave the performance, to join the Democratic Party, and to assist in the effort to place a Democrat in the White House. This speech was accompanied by an extensive speech on the injustice of packing the Supreme Court with a group of extreme conservatives.

In the emergency room, Charles indicated that he did not live in Iowa City but had come from Des Moines (100 miles away) to attend the performance and to consult with friends and colleagues at the law school. He described himself as a prominent lawyer, a graduate of Harvard Law School who had edited the *Law Review*, a close friend of the Clinton family and other prominent Democrats, and a dedicated crusader against social injustice. He described the Bush administration as a rerun of the industrial-totalitarian axis that had been created in Nazi Germany, complained about a conspiracy that he believed was under way to destroy the Democratic party by either persecution or assassination of key figures, and indicated that one of the purposes of his trip to Iowa City was to warn his colleagues at the law school about these dangerous circumstances.

His appearance was somewhat unkempt and disheveled, inconsistent with his description of his prominent status. Although he was attired in an expensive-appearing pinstripe suit, his hair was uncombed, his eyes were red, and he was unshaven. Charles spoke excitedly in a rapid manner, and his voice rose to a shout at times. His speech was disjointed and difficult to follow, as his topic changed from his own special importance and abilities to the various conspiracies that he thought were under way in the Bush government.

When admission to the hospital was proposed, he became physically agitated and tried to run away. He became physically combative at attempts to restrain him. A decision was made to obtain an emergency hospitalization order. His claims of special importance and abilities were discounted and attributed to his manic state. Later, as more history was obtained, it became evident that Charles was indeed a prominent attorney with many important national connections. The conspiracy against the Democratic party, although potentially bearing some credence, contained enough implausible elaborations to qualify as delusional thinking. Interviews with his family members revealed that he had had one prior hospitalization for mania and had been treated for depression as an outpatient. He had been taking maintenance lithium but had decided to discontinue it abruptly approximately 3 days earlier.

Charles was given a therapeutic dose of lithium, and his symptoms cleared rapidly over the course of 5–7 days. He was able to leave the hospital and to return to work within 1 week.

Course and Outcome

The onset of mania is frequently abrupt, although it may begin gradually over the course of a few weeks. The episodes usually last from a few days to months. They tend to be briefer and to have a more abrupt termination than depressive episodes. Although the prognosis for any particular episode is reasonably good, especially with the availability of effective treatments such as lithium and antipsychotics, the risk for recurrence is significant. Not uncommonly, an episode of mania is followed by an episode of depression. Some patients with bipolar disorder recover relatively fully, but a substantial subset continue to have chronic mild instability of mood, particularly recurrent episodes of mild depression.

The complications of mania are primarily social: marital discord, divorce, business difficulties, financial extravagance, and sexual indiscretions. Drug or alcohol abuse may occur during a manic episode. When mania is relatively severe, the patient may be almost completely incapacitated and require protection from the consequences of poor judgment or hyperactivity. The excessive activity level continues to be a significant risk in patients with cardiac problems. A manic syndrome can switch rapidly to depression, and the risk for suicide is heightened when the patient becomes remorsefully aware of inappropriate behavior that occurred during the manic episode.

■ Mixed and Hypomanic Episodes

A small number of patients present with a mixture of both manic and depressive symptoms within a single episode of illness. When this occurs, it is referred to as a *mixed episode.* The clinical presentation of mixed episodes can be quite confusing because the patient's mood and symptom picture tend to alternate rapidly. At one moment, the patient will be talkative, energetic, and expansive and minutes later may burst into tears and complain of feeling hopeless and suicidal. DSM-IV-TR requires that full criteria for both a manic and a depressive episode be met within a 1-week period to diagnose the presence of a mixed episode. Clinicians sometimes apply the term "mixed" more broadly than defined in DSM-IV-TR to include admixtures of depressive and manic symptoms that don't meet full criteria. Patients with a mixed episode are difficult to treat because medications must target both poles of mood disorder.

Hypomania is another important form of mood disorder. The syndrome is similar to mania, but it is milder and briefer. During a hypomanic episode, the patient experiences the elevated mood and other classic symptoms that define mania, but they are not accompanied by delusional beliefs or hallucinations, and they are not severe enough to require hospitalization or to markedly impair social and occupational functioning. Many patients with hypomania also have chronic mild depression, so it can sometimes be difficult to determine whether they are "back to their usual selves" or "just feeling good for a change." Obtaining information from family and friends usually is helpful in determining whether the presence of a good mood is indeed pathological rather than a patch of normal happiness in the midst of feeling chronically blue. Course of illness may also be informative because like manic episodes, hypomanic episodes are often followed by a crash into a depressive episode.

■ Dysthymia and Cyclothymia

DSM-IV-TR also recognizes additional forms of mood disorder: *dysthymic disorder* and *cyclothymic disorder.*

Dysthymic disorder (sometimes referred to as *depressive neurosis*) is a chronic and persistent disturbance in mood that has been present for at least 2 years and is characterized by relatively typical depressive symptoms such as anorexia, insomnia, decreased energy, low self-esteem, difficulty concentrating, and feelings of hopelessness. Because dysthymic disorder is a mild chronic disorder, only two of these symptoms are necessary, but they must have persisted more or less continuously for at least a 2-year period.

Patients with dysthymia are chronically unhappy and miserable. Some of them also develop the relatively more severe major depressive syndrome; when the major depressive episode clears, these patients subsequently return to their chronic state of dysthymia. The coexistence of these mild and severe forms of depression is sometimes referred to as *double depression.*

A second mild mood syndrome is *cyclothymic disorder,* a condition in which the patient has mild swings between the two poles of depression and hypomania. While in the hypomanic phase, the person appears to be high, but not so high as to be socially or professionally incapacitated. During the depressed phase, the individual has some symptoms of depression, but these are not severe enough to meet criteria for a full major depressive episode (i.e., five symptoms persisting for 2 weeks). Thus, the individual with cyclothymic disorder tends to swing from high to low with a chronic mild instability of mood.

TABLE 6–3. DSM-IV-TR classification of mood disorders

Bipolar disorders	Depressive disorders
Bipolar disorder, manic	Major depression, single episode
Bipolar disorder, depressed	Major depression, recurrent
Bipolar disorder, mixed	Dysthymic disorder
Cyclothymic disorder	Depressive disorder not otherwise specified
Bipolar disorder not otherwise specified	

■ Classification and Subtypes

The mood disorders may be subdivided into two main groups. Patients who have depression only are also referred to as *unipolar*, because their illness affects only one "pole" on the continuum of mood states. The other group consists of those who are *bipolar*, characterized by mania (i.e., have a manic or hypomanic episode) either alone or in combination with depression (see Table 6–3). Thus, this classification initially subdivides the types of mood disorders into unipolar and bipolar types. This subdivision is based on its predictive power. These two subtypes of mood disorder typically have different familial patterns, require different treatments, and perhaps have a different pathophysiology and etiology.

The depressive disorders include major depressive disorder and dysthymic disorder as well as a residual category (*depressive disorder not otherwise specified*). Major depressive disorder is defined by the presence of at least one episode of major depression. The disorder can be further characterized by a variety of specifiers, as described later in this chapter. Dysthymic disorder is defined on the basis of the criteria enumerated earlier in this section. The residual category is used for the occasional odd case that does not fit any of the criteria but does seem to fit the overall syndrome.

The bipolar disorders include bipolar I disorder, bipolar II disorder, cyclothymic disorder, and bipolar disorder not otherwise specified. Bipolar I disorder is defined by the occurrence of at least one manic or mixed episode. Typically, bipolar I disorder is characterized by recurrent episodes of both mania and depression, which may be separated by intervals of months to years. Although the episodes may lead to psychosocial morbidity because of the effect of a severe recurrent illness on interpersonal relationships or work functioning, interepisode functioning may be good or even excellent.

Bipolar II disorder is characterized by periods of hypomania that typically occur either before or after periods of depression but also may occur independently. These mild manic episodes are not sufficiently severe to require hospitalization, although they may lead to personal, social, or work difficulties. During the mild bipolar phase, the patient is upbeat, shows signs of poor judgment, and has other indices of mania such as increased energy or insomnia, but the symptoms do not meet full criteria for a manic episode. Bipolar II disorder appears to breed true within families, in that relatives of bipolar II patients themselves have higher rates of bipolar II disorder than either bipolar I (i.e., criteria are met for a full manic episode) or unipolar major depression. Bipolar II patients also tend to have a high rate of comorbidity with other disorders, such as substance abuse. Patients with bipolar II tend to experience a greater burden of depressive symptoms than their bipolar I counterparts.

As previously defined, cyclothymic disorder is the mildest form of bipolar disorder.

■ Melancholia

The term *melancholic features* is used in DSM-IV-TR to describe a relatively severe form of depression that is more likely to respond to somatic therapy. The concept is based on an older historic distinction between endogenous and reactive depression, a distinction that was based on both presumed etiology and a characteristic clustering of symptoms. In the original definition of *endogenous depression,* it had no precipitating factors (*endogenous* means "grows from within"), whereas a *reactive depression* occurred in reaction to some stressful life event such as a divorce or loss of a job. The term *endogenous* is no longer used because increasing evidence has suggested that severe depressions also may be triggered by various physiological or psychological stressors.

Melancholia requires the presence of two specific characteristic features: pervasive loss of interest or pleasure and inability to respond to pleasurable stimuli. Three from a list of six additional features also are required: distinct quality of depressed mood, diurnal variation, terminal insomnia, severe psychomotor retardation or agitation, anorexia or weight loss, and excessive guilt. Many of these symptoms are predominantly somatic or vegetative, and sometimes this form of depression is referred to as *vegetative*. A substantial body of research has suggested that this clustering of symptoms predicts a good response to antidepressant medication or to electroconvulsive therapy (ECT).

■ Atypical Features

Unlike patients with melancholia, those with *atypical features* do not present with the classic vegetative symptoms such as insomnia, weight loss, or anorexia but instead have weight gain and hypersomnia. In addition, instead of having a nonreactive mood, they are quite responsive to their life situation, and they are particularly sensitive to slights or rejections. This rejection sensitivity often leads to difficulties in interpersonal relationships, with a stormy personal life characterized by being easily hurt, having many partners, and experiencing frequent breakups. Subjectively, these patients often express their somatic state by complaining of "leaden paralysis," the feeling that their arms and legs weigh them down and make activities difficult for them. Monoamine oxidase inhibitors (MAOIs) have proved particularly useful with this group of patients, and selective serotonin reuptake inhibitors (SSRIs) also may be effective.

■ Chronic, Postpartum, Catatonic, Seasonal, and Rapid-Cycling Specifiers

DSM-IV-TR also recognizes other aspects of a recent episode that also may be clinically important. The *chronic* specifier indicates that the full criteria for a major depressive episode have been present for 2 years; patients in this group have an illness that is refractory to treatment and clinically challenging.

The *postpartum onset* specifier identifies those patients who experience a depressive, manic, or mixed episode within the first 4 weeks postpartum. Although feeling a bit depressed after delivery is common (referred to as the postpartum blues), some women develop a full mood syndrome that requires medical attention with either somatic therapy or psychotherapy or both. At its most severe, the mood episode may become psychotic and/or life threatening to the mother or child; such severe abnormalities have been estimated to occur in 1 of 500 to 1 of 1,000 deliveries, and the risk of recurrence in subsequent deliveries is great— between 30% and 50% of cases.

The *catatonic features* specifier identifies a subgroup of patients who have catatonic features similar to those that historically have been observed primarily in schizophrenia (e.g., posturing, waxy flexibility, catalepsy, negativism, and mutism). The presence of this specifier serves to remind the clinician that such symptoms also may occur in other disorders and that they are not pathognomonic of schizophrenia.

Another useful descriptor in DSM-IV-TR recognizes that some depressed patients have a *seasonal pattern*. Clinicians have recognized for many decades that some individuals have a characteristic onset of mood symptoms in relation to changes of season, with depression typically occurring more frequently during the winter months and remissions or changes from depression to mania occurring during the spring. Light therapy is reported to be an effective treatment for seasonal affective disorder (i.e., depressive illness that recurs in winter months and tends to remit in the spring). Exposure to bright light (minimum of 2,500 lux for 2 hours each morning) alleviates depressive symptoms. Most patients who respond to light therapy tend to use it daily during the winter months. Patients can also be treated with standard antidepressant therapy. The U.S. Food and Drug Administration (FDA) recently approved an extended-release form of bupropion as a preventive treatment for seasonal affective disorder.

A *rapid-cycling* specifier identifies those patients who have had at least four major depressive, manic, hypomanic, or mixed episodes during the past 12 months. Rapid-cycling bipolar disorder is a particularly severe form of the disorder and is associated with a younger age at onset, more frequent depressive episodes, and greater risk for suicide attempts than other forms of the disorder.

■ Differential Diagnosis

When evaluating a patient with a mood disorder, the physician should always consider that the illness might result from some specific extrinsic factor that can induce a manic or depressive syndrome, such as drugs of abuse, sedatives, tranquilizers, antihypertensives, oral contraceptives, or glucocorticoids. General medical conditions such as hypothyroidism and systemic lupus erythematosus also may present with prominent depressive symptoms. If the episode of mood disorder is judged to be the result of a specific drug or medical illness, the disorder is diagnosed as secondary to it. Treatment usually involves withdrawing or reducing the drug or treating the underlying general medical illness.

Dysphoric mood may also occur in schizophrenia. In schizophrenia the dysphoric mood is more typically apathetic or empty, whereas in depression the dysphoric mood usually is experienced as intensely painful. The onset of schizophrenia usually is more gradual, and patients with schizophrenia also typically have a more severe deterioration in function than do patients with depression. Patients with schizophrenia and patients with major depression may both have psychotic symptoms; thus severe psychotic depression is sometimes difficult to distinguish from schizophrenia with acute onset. In this relatively difficult case, it is often best to treat the depression and to observe the course of illness over time. When psychotic symptoms persist after mood symptoms remit, then the diagnosis of schizophrenia or schizoaffective disorder is more likely.

The differential diagnosis between mania and schizophrenia is also quite important. Several features are useful in making this distinction. Personality and general functioning are usually satisfactory before and after a manic episode, even though mild disturbances in mood may occur. Although manic episodes may present with disorganized speech that is indistinguishable from the speech sometimes observed in schizophrenia, speech abnormalities in mania are always accompanied by a disturbance in mood and usually by overactivity and physical agitation. Manic patients may experience delusions or hallucinations, but these typically reflect the underlying disturbance in mood. (Mood-incongruent psychotic symptoms occur occasionally, making the differential diagnosis more difficult.) Additional guidelines that make the diagnosis of manic episode more likely include a family history of a mood disorder, good premorbid adjustment, and a previous episode of a mood disorder from which the patient completely or substantially recovered. When psychotic symptoms persist in the absence of an abnormality in mood, the diagnosis of schizophrenia or schizoaffective disorder is more likely.

People with bereavement may have many depressive symptoms and experience them for a sufficient duration to meet criteria for a depressive episode. Nevertheless, such patients are not given the diagnosis of depressive disorder because the presence of the symptoms is considered a normal reaction. The symptoms are usually self-limiting, clear spontaneously over time, have a different course and prognosis than major depression, and usually do not respond to antidepressant medication. When bereavement is accompanied by psychomotor retardation, suicidal ideation, or psychotic symptoms, a diagnosis of major depression may be appropriate. It is not uncommon for bereaved individuals to wish they had died instead of their loved one or to see fleeting images of the deceased.

■ Epidemiology

The recent National Comorbidity Study reported a lifetime prevalence of nearly 17% for major depression and about 2% for bipolar I and II disorders combined. Dysthymia has a prevalence of around 3%. Combined, these disorders affect just over one in five persons. Depression is more common in women than in men. The current ratio in the United States is approximately 2:1. Bipolar disorder also is more common in women than in men, with a ratio of approximately 3:2. This study also showed the median age at onset for major depression to be 32 years, for bipolar disorder 25 years, and for dysthymia 31 years. Men tend to have an earlier onset of bipolar disorder than women.

Data from the Epidemiologic Catchment Area (ECA) study showed that dysthymia is more common in women younger than 65, unmarried persons, and persons with low income. Dysthymia also may be quite common in elderly persons.

■ Etiology and Pathophysiology

The etiology of mood disorders is not well understood; however, genetic, social and environmental, and neurobiological factors may all play a role.

Genetics

Mood disorders tend to run in families, an observation confirmed by many investigators. However, familiality does not necessarily indicate genetic transmission, because role modeling, learned behavior, social environmental factors such as economic deprivation, and physical environmental factors such as prenatal and perinatal birth complications all may provide nongenetic contributions to the development of a disorder, and these contributions could themselves be familial. (For example, before the advent of antibiotics, tuberculosis tended to run in families for environmental rather than genetic reasons.)

Nearly all family studies show significantly increased rates of mood disorder, especially bipolar disorder, in the first-degree relatives of bipolar patients compared with control subjects. Unipolar patients tend to have much less bipolar illness among their first-degree relatives but a high rate of unipolar illness. Thus these disorders not only are familial but also tend to breed true. However, the fact that they do not breed perfectly true (i.e., bipolar illness *only* in the relatives of bipolar patients and unipolar illness *only* in the relatives of unipolar patients) also suggests that these two forms of mood disorder may not be totally distinct from each other. Twin and adoption studies have complemented these family studies and have provided evidence that mood disorders are genetic in addition to being familial. If one averages together all the twin studies of mood disorder (slightly fewer than 500 twin pairs), the overall monozygotic-to-dizygotic ratio is approximately 4:1 (65% vs. 14%).

Efforts to identify genes implicated in mood disorders face several challenges. There has been debate about the definition of the phenotype. One view treats bipolar and unipolar mood disorders as distinct phenotypes. Within bipolar disorder, it is not clear whether a narrow definition limited to bipolar I is preferable or whether a broader model that includes bipolar II should be used. Alternatively, some argue that all mood disorders, ranging from bipolar to unipolar, should be grouped together. Because depression is so common, including it undoubtedly introduces phenocopies. Genome-wide studies have implicated several chromosomal regions, including 9p, 10q, 14q, 18p-q, and 8q. Candidate genes showing replicated associations with bipolar disorder include the D-amino-acid oxidase gene *(G72)*, brain-derived neurotrophic factor gene *(BDNF)*, neuregulin 1 gene *(NRG1)*, and dysbindin *(DTNBP1)*. Genes associated with the regulation of circadian rhythm *(CLOCK, TIMELESS, PERIOD3)* have also been implicated. Additionally, a polymorphism in the serotonin transporter gene has been associated with a vulnerability to developing depression when experiencing stresses such as job loss or divorce. Clearly, the task of identifying genes for the mood disorders is difficult, and the search will continue for many years to come.

Social and Environmental Factors

One of the fundamental questions about the nature of depression is how to draw the line between a normal response to a painful personal life experience and a clinically significant depression. Everyone experiences transient episodes of sadness after breaking up with a girlfriend or boyfriend, getting a divorce, performing badly on an examination, or losing a loved one. Diagnostic criteria were developed to assist in drawing this line by suggesting that the sadness must persist for more than 2 months after a bereavement (i.e., loss of a loved one). However, the criteria do not help with disentangling the effects of less serious life experiences.

People who experience a loss or disappointment often develop symptoms similar to those of major depression: feelings of sadness, difficulties with sleep or appetite, indecisiveness, poor concentration, or guilt or self-criticism. We all know people who continue to have these symptoms for more than a few weeks after a personal loss or other psychosocial stressor. When the symptoms persist long enough, then the person who experienced the stressor does in fact meet criteria for major depression, and this person may respond well to treatment with an antidepressant. Therefore, it is intuitively obvious that psychosocial stressors may play a role in the etiology of depression. The crucial question is not "Do psychosocial and environmental factors play a role in precipitating depression?" but rather "What is the nature of the role that psychosocial and environmental factors play? Do they tip a predisposed person over the edge, or are they sufficient in and of themselves?"

A plausible model for the role of stressful life events is that they do induce a biological reaction (e.g., an outpouring of cortisol). Once this biological reaction is initiated, it is difficult to stop and may trigger or exacerbate a depressive syndrome, particularly in individuals who have been previously primed because of either a genetic diathesis or experiences that made them particularly vulnerable to stress. In fact, a tendency to be neurobiologically oversensitive to the effects of psychosocial stress may be one of the genetic factors that are transmitted within families, as suggested by the polymorphism that has been identified in the serotonin transporter gene. These individuals may be unable to increase serotonergic tone in their brains to help them cope with stress and therefore develop a depressive response. Early life events, such as harsh or abusive parenting during childhood, could create a diathesis by making a person more psychologically sensitive to rejection and more biologically sensitive to stress.

Neurobiology

The *catecholamine hypothesis*, perhaps the earliest formulation concerning the role of neurotransmitters in depression, suggested that depression is caused by a deficit of norepinephrine at crucial nerve terminals throughout the brain. This hypothesis received support from studies of the mechanism of action of antidepressant medications used during the 1970s and 1980s. Classic work by Julius Axelrod, which led to his Nobel Prize, demonstrated that antidepressants such as imipramine increase the amount of norepinephrine functionally available at nerve terminals by inhibiting reuptake. The MAOIs also increase the amount of norepinephrine available by inhibiting breakdown of norepinephrine through monoamine oxidase. Reserpine, which depletes monoamines, worsens depression.

The development of other types of antidepressant medications has indicated, however, that other neurotransmitters also may play a role in depression. The selective serotonin reuptake inhibitors (SSRIs) also are very effective treatments for depression, yet they do not act on the norepinephrine system. Instead, they appear to exert their therapeutic effect by increasing the amount of serotonin functionally available at nerve terminals. Furthermore, patients with severe depression have been found to have a decrease in a major serotonin metabolite, 5-hydroxyindoleacetic acid (5-HIAA), in their cerebrospinal fluid. In addition, numbers of serotonin type 2 (5-HT$_2$) receptors are decreased in postmortem brains of persons who have committed suicide.

Either a catecholamine hypothesis or a serotonin hypothesis is an oversimplification, although these hypotheses have been helpful. They have turned attention to examining the biological mechanisms of emotional and cognitive states and the role that these mental systems play in disease processes.

Neuroimaging Studies

Both structural and functional brain imaging techniques have been applied to study the mechanisms of mood disorders. A convergence of findings indicates that the subgenual prefrontal cortex (SGPFC) has particular importance among the various brain structures thought to play a role in depression. Positron emission tomography studies have demonstrated increased blood flow in this area when sadness is induced in non-ill subjects, and such changes are particularly marked in depressed patients. Lesions of this area block the extinction of fear conditioning in animal studies, and in humans the area is thought to be important in the evaluation of the consequences of social behavior. It may thus play a role in the heightened self-criticism and pessimistic ruminations that characterize depressive episodes. Several anatomic magnetic resonance studies have also found volumetric reductions in the SGPFC.

Efforts to characterize the projections of the SGPFC in primates have shown direct connections to a number of areas important to the pathophysiology of depressive disorders. Particularly plentiful are projections to the hypothalamus, a structure central to the regulation of the hypothalamic-pituitary-adrenal axis. Another magnetic resonance abnormality observed in some patients is an increased number of focal signal hyperintensities in white matter; the functional significance of this abnormality is unclear, but it has been noted in both bipolar and unipolar mood disorders.

Abnormalities in Neurophysiological Function

Neurophysiological abnormalities also have been extensively studied in mood disorders. The largest and most consistent body of data involves the use of sleep electroencephalography (EEG). (Sleep EEG, or polysomnography, is further discussed in Chapter 17.) Studies have consistently found that patients with depression have a variety of abnormal electroencephalographic findings during sleep, including decreased slow-wave sleep (i.e., deep sleep), a shortened time before the onset of rapid eye movement (REM) sleep (the period when dreams and nightmares occur), and longer periods of REM sleep, compared with subjects without depression. These three types of abnormality are referred to as decreased delta sleep, decreased REM latency, and increased REM density, respectively. All of these abnormalities in sleep EEG correspond with the subjective sleep complaints of depressed patients. A recent positron emission tomography study suggests that depressed patients, in contrast with control subjects, have a relative hypermetabolism in frontoparietal regions and thalamus during the transition from wakefulness to non-REM sleep, which may help to explain their sleep anomalies.

Abnormalities in Neuroendocrine Function

Neuroendocrine abnormalities also have been extensively explored in patients with depression. Early research in this area suggested that depressed patients have abnormal diurnal variation in cortisol production. The dexamethasone suppression test (DST) has been used extensively to explore the possibility of neuroendocrine dysregulation in depression and to attempt to determine the place on the hypothalamic-pituitary-adrenal axis where this abnormality might occur. Up to 70% of patients with severe depression have abnormal suppression of cortisol secretion after the administration of dexamethasone. Rates of dexamethasone nonsuppression in other psychiatric conditions, such as anorexia nervosa, dementia, and substance abuse, are also relatively high.

In addition to the hypothalamic-pituitary-adrenal axis, other aspects of the neuroendocrine system have been explored. Depressed patients have been shown to have a blunting of growth hormone output in response to insulin challenge as well as a blunted production of thyroid-stimulating hormone in response to thyrotropin-releasing hormone. The abnormalities across a variety of neuroendocrine target organs (e.g., adrenals, pancreas, thyroid) indicate that the problem is not in these organs, and the patterns of abnormal response to challenge suggest that it is also not in the pituitary. More likely, the abnormality is at the level of the hypothalamus, a brain region regulated largely through monoamine neurotransmitters.

■ Clinical Management

Treatment of Depression

Various medications are available to treat depression: tricyclics and other related compounds, MAOIs, SSRIs, and other antidepressants that are not easily categorized, such as bupropion and mirtazapine. These drugs are all thought to work by altering levels of various neurotransmitters at crucial nerve terminals in the central nervous system. They are largely similar in their overall effectiveness, and from 65% to 70% of persons who receive antidepressants will markedly improve. Unfortunately, and despite adequate treatment, some patients develop a tendency to become treatment refractory, a phenomenon called *tachyphylaxis.*

We generally recommend that treatment begin with one of the SSRIs because they are well tolerated and safe in overdose. Low dosages are generally effective, and frequent dosage adjustments are unnecessary. In particular, patients with cardiac conduction defects should receive an SSRI (or one of the other new agents). Likewise, impulsive or suicidal patients should receive an SSRI or one of the newer medications that are unlikely to be fatal in overdose. Most patients will actually start to improve relatively quickly, even within the first 1 or 2 weeks after starting medication. Although the SSRIs are relatively safe in overdose as compared with the older tricyclic antidepressants, they have also been reported to increase the risk for impulsive behavior and even suicidality. Therefore, patients treated with SSRIs need to be carefully monitored, and these agents should be used cautiously in teenagers.

Drug trials should last from 4 to 8 weeks. If the patient fails to respond within 4 weeks of treatment, the dosage should be increased or the patient should be switched to another drug, preferably from another class (e.g., providing a different balance of norepinephrine, serotonin, and acetylcholine).

One useful strategy to boost the effectiveness of antidepressants is to augment treatment with another drug. Augmentation with lithium carbonate is the best-researched option. Other agents have been used for augmentation and include triiodothyronine, a thyroid preparation; psychostimulants such as methylphenidate; pindolol, a beta-blocker; benzodiazepines; and antipsychotics. Aripiprazole, a second-generation antipsychotic (SGA), is approved by the FDA for use as augmenting agent. The combination of the SGA olanzapine and the SSRI fluoxetine is FDA approved for use in cases of treatment-resistant depression.

When the depressed patient is psychotic, we generally recommend co-administering an antipsychotic, such as one of the SGAs. Benzodiazepines co-administered with the antidepressant may help calm the anxious or agitated depressed patient relatively quickly.

For patients who are experiencing their first episode of depression, the drug should be continued for another 16–36 weeks after the patient is considered well. Thereafter, the clinician may decide to discontinue the medication while monitoring the patient closely. Because some antidepressants produce undesirable side effects such as weight gain, and because conservative prescription of medications is always a good clinical guideline, discontinuation should almost always be attempted in patients who do not have a history of recurrent depression. The medication should be discontinued gradually because many patients experience some mild withdrawal effects when tricyclics or SSRIs (except fluoxetine) are discontinued abruptly. Patients sometimes subjectively experience these withdrawal symptoms as a recurrence or relapse. Other symptoms that occur on abrupt withdrawal of antidepressants include insomnia and nervousness, nightmares, and gastrointestinal symptoms such as nausea or vomiting. Patients with recurrent depressions often will need long-term maintenance, typically at the full treatment dosage. Research shows that long-term maintenance will significantly reduce the risk of relapse and increase the patient's quality of life.

MAOIs may be used to treat those patients whose symptoms do not respond to the first-line antidepressants or who are unable to tolerate their side effects. MAOIs should be used with caution because they have potentially more dangerous side effects and interactions than do the other antidepressants. MAOIs may be particularly useful in patients characterized by *atypical depression*, with symptoms such as hypersomnia, increased appetite, and personality difficulties such as rejection sensitivity.

ECT is the treatment of choice for some patients with severe depression. Methods for administering and monitoring ECT, as well as its side effects, are described in more detail in Chapter 20. In general, indications for ECT include very severe depression, high potential for suicide, cardiovascular disease (which may preclude use of some antidepressants), and pregnancy. ECT is highly effective in producing a rapid remission of depressive symptoms. Patients will need maintenance antidepressant treatment after the course of ECT is completed.

Both repetitive transcranial magnetic stimulation (rTMS) and vagal nerve stimulation (VNS) are FDA approved to treat depressed adults who are treatment refractory. Neither treatment is widely available, and their respective roles in treating depression are not yet clear. With rTMS, magnetic pulses are applied to the scalp using a handheld coil. The magnetic field passes through the scalp and induces a current in underlying tissue, depolarizing neurons. Patients can experience headache, nausea, and dizziness. With VNS, a device is implanted under the skin of the chest wall and an electrode is connected to the vagus nerve. The device sends small electrical pulses to the vagus nerve on the left side of the neck, which in turn delivers these pulses to the brain. Problems include the discomfort of surgical implantation and adverse effects related to vagus nerve function, including hoarseness, cough, and dysphagia. Both treatments are thought to alter levels of neurotransmitters and functional activity of the central nervous system dysregulated in depression.

Key points to remember about depression

1. A hopeful, optimistic tone should be established at the initial interview.

   - The severity of the depressive syndrome should be assessed, remembering that there may be individual and cultural differences in the way depression is experienced and expressed.

   - Extensive psychological probing should not be attempted when the patient is deeply depressed.

   - Suicidal risk should be determined initially and reassessed frequently.

Key points to remember about depression *(continued)*

2. Moderate to severe depression should be treated aggressively with somatic therapy.

   • Severely depressed or suicidal patients may require hospitalization.

   • Severely depressed outpatients may need frequent (e.g., twice-weekly) brief (e.g., 10- to 15-minute) contacts for support and medication management until their depression lifts.

   • Most patients will require at least 16–20 weeks of maintenance medication following an initial episode and thereafter should be given a trial of decreasing or discontinuing the medication. If symptoms reemerge, medication should be reinstituted, and consideration should be given to long-term drug administration.

3. The clinician should determine whether psychosocial stressors are present that are contributing to the depressed mood and should counsel the patient on ways to cope with them.

4. Depressed patients tend to "get down" on themselves because they have been depressed; the clinician should help the patient learn to abandon negative or self-deprecating attitudes through cognitive-behavioral therapy or other psychotherapeutic techniques.

Treatment of Mania

Lithium, valproate, and carbamazepine are all approved by the FDA for the acute treatment of mania. Lamotrigine is approved for maintenance treatment of bipolar disorder. Several additional anticonvulsant drugs (including gabapentin and topiramate) have been used to treat bipolar patients but have had mixed results. In addition, all SGAs are approved to treat acute mania except clozapine, and several have received indications for maintenance treatment of bipolar disorder or as adjuncts to lithium or valproate. The rational use of these drugs, and their dosing, is found in Chapter 20.

Electroconvulsive therapy is highly effective in treatment of manic patients when medication is ineffective.

Key points to remember about mania

1. Somatic therapies should be used aggressively to treat manic symptoms as rapidly as possible.

2. The patient should be followed up closely as the mania "breaks" to determine whether a subsequent depression is emerging.

3. After an episode of mania, patients should receive maintenance medication; typically they will continue to take mood stabilizers for several years, and perhaps for the remainder of their lives, to prevent subsequent relapses.

4. Patients should be advised about the importance of getting sufficient sleep and of following sensible sleep hygiene measures (described in Chapter 17).

5. Even when they are stable, patients should be followed up regularly to ensure continued compliance with medication and to monitor blood levels (if applicable).

6. Manic episodes can have devastating personal, social, and economic consequences; patients will usually require (at a minimum) supportive psychotherapy to help them cope with these consequences and maintain their self-esteem.

7. Family members should be provided with both psychological support, as needed, and educational materials to help them understand the disorder, its symptoms, and the need for continued treatment.

8. Patients with bipolar illness are often appreciative of being told about the "good side" of their illness: its association with creativity and high achievement.

Other Treatments

Experiencing an episode of mood disorder is often a major blow to the patient's confidence and self-esteem. Consequently, most patients will require some supportive psychotherapy in addition to whatever medications are prescribed. During the acute episode, the clinician will typically let the depressive wound begin to heal. As the patient recovers, the clinician may begin to review with him or her the various social and psychological factors that may be causing distress or that may have worsened as a consequence of depression. Work, school performance, and interpersonal relationships all may be impaired because of a mood disorder. It is important to help patients assess these problems and recognize that the illness is responsible—rather than feeling that they themselves are responsible—and to instill confidence that they can now begin to restore and repair whatever injuries have occurred as a consequence of their episode of mood disorder.

Some depressed patients will respond well to brief psychotherapy alone. Both cognitive-behavioral therapy and interpersonal therapy are as effective as medication in the treatment of mild to moderately severe depression, and their combination with psychotherapy is even more powerful. Psychotherapy is described in greater detail in Chapter 19.

■ Self-Assessment Questions

1. What are the nine symptoms used to define a major depressive episode in DSM-IV-TR?

2. What is the difference between delusions that are mood congruent and those that are mood incongruent?

3. What is the lifetime prevalence for bipolar disorder and for major depressive disorder?

4. Review the evidence that suggests that mood disorders are familial and may be genetic.

5. Which neurotransmitter systems have been proposed to be dysfunctional in mood disorders?

6. Identify at least four genes that have been implicated as playing a role in mood disorders.

7. What is the difference between bereavement and a depressive episode?

8. Describe the first-line treatments for depression as well as the various alternative treatments and their indications.

9. Describe the first-line treatment for a manic episode. What alternative treatments are available?

CHAPTER 7

Anxiety Disorders

I stood stunned, my hair rose, the voice stuck in my throat.

Virgil

ANXIETY DISORDERS are a leading cause of distress and impairment. About one in four Americans has one of these conditions, which are characterized by excessive or irrational fear and worry. In 1871, Jacob DaCosta identified an anxiety syndrome among soldiers of the Union Army that he called *irritable heart*. Because chest pain, palpitations, and dizziness were the main symptoms, DaCosta thought the disorder represented a functional cardiac disturbance caused by an overexertion. DaCosta first described this syndrome in a soldier who developed the disorder during the Civil War. Shortly thereafter, the condition was identified in other settings and was variously referred to as *soldier's heart, effort syndrome,* or *neurocirculatory asthenia*.

While internists were emphasizing cardiovascular aspects of the anxiety syndrome, psychiatrists and neurologists focused their attention on its psychological aspects. Freud was one of the first to recognize that feelings related to earlier trauma could express themselves in symptoms and behaviors. He introduced the term *anxiety neurosis* to describe a disorder characterized by feelings of fearfulness, panic, and impending doom.

In DSM-III, in 1980, anxiety neurosis was divided into panic disorder and generalized anxiety disorder (GAD), based on new re-

TABLE 7–1. DSM-IV-TR anxiety disorders

Panic disorder
  With agoraphobia
  Without agoraphobia

Agoraphobia

Generalized anxiety disorder

Social phobia (social anxiety disorder)

Specific phobia

Obsessive-compulsive disorder

Posttraumatic stress disorder

Acute stress disorder

search findings and clinical observations suggesting that the two disorders were separable. At the same time, a new diagnosis, posttraumatic stress disorder (PTSD), was introduced. Acute stress disorder was added in 1994. In this chapter, we review panic disorder, agoraphobia, specific and social phobias, GAD, obsessive-compulsive disorder (OCD), and both PTSD and acute stress disorder. The anxiety disorders are listed in Table 7–1.

■ Panic Disorder and Agoraphobia

Panic disorder consists of recurrent, unexpected panic (or anxiety) attacks accompanied by at least 1 month of persistent concern about having another attack, worry about the implications of having an attack (e.g., dying, going crazy), or significant behavioral change related to the attacks (e.g., avoiding places where attacks had occurred). For an episode of anxiety to be defined as a panic attack, at least 4 of 13 characteristic symptoms, such as shortness of breath, dizziness, palpitations, and trembling or shaking, must occur (see Table 7–2). The clinician should determine that the attacks are not induced by a substance (e.g., caffeine) or a medical illness (e.g., hyperthyroidism) and that the anxiety is not better accounted for by another mental disorder. Panic disorder is further classified as occurring with or without agoraphobia. The DSM-IV-TR criteria for panic disorder without agoraphobia are shown in Table 7–3, and a description of agoraphobia follows.

TABLE 7–2.   DSM-IV-TR criteria for panic attack

Note: A Panic Attack is not a codable disorder. Code the specific diagnosis in which the Panic Attack occurs (e.g., 300.21 Panic Disorder With Agoraphobia).

A discrete period of intense fear or discomfort, in which four (or more) of the following symptoms developed abruptly and reached a peak within 10 minutes:

(1)   palpitations, pounding heart, or accelerated heart rate
(2)   sweating
(3)   trembling or shaking
(4)   sensations of shortness of breath or smothering
(5)   feeling of choking
(6)   chest pain or discomfort
(7)   nausea or abdominal distress
(8)   feeling dizzy, unsteady, lightheaded, or faint
(9)   derealization (feelings of unreality) or depersonalization (being detached from oneself)
(10) fear of losing control or going crazy
(11) fear of dying
(12) paresthesias (numbness or tingling sensations)
(13) chills or hot flushes

Agoraphobia is a disabling complication of panic disorder in which an individual fears being unable to get out of a place or situation quickly in the event of a panic attack. As a consequence of his or her fear, he or she avoids places or situations where this might occur (see Table 7–4). The term *agoraphobia* translates literally from Greek as "fear of the marketplace," and although many patients with agoraphobia are uncomfortable in shops and markets, their true fear is being separated from a source of security. Agoraphobic patients often fear having a panic attack in a public place, thereby embarrassing themselves, or having an attack and not being near a physician or medical clinic. They tend to avoid crowded places, such as malls, restaurants, theaters, and churches, because they feel trapped. Many have difficulty driving (i.e., because they fear being away from help should an attack occur), crossing bridges, and driving through tunnels. Many agoraphobic patients are able to go places they might otherwise avoid if accompanied by a trusted person. At its most severe, agoraphobia renders the person housebound. Common situations that either provoke or relieve anxiety in people with agoraphobia are shown in Table 7–5.

TABLE 7–3.   DSM-IV-TR diagnostic criteria for panic disorder without agoraphobia

A. Both (1) and (2):
  (1) recurrent unexpected Panic Attacks
  (2) at least one of the attacks has been followed by 1 month (or more) of one (or more) of the following:
    (a) persistent concern about having additional attacks
    (b) worry about the implications of the attack or its consequences (e.g., losing control, having a heart attack, "going crazy")
    (c) a significant change in behavior related to the attacks
B. Absence of Agoraphobia.
C. The Panic Attacks are not due to the direct physiological effects of a substance (e.g., a drug of abuse, a medication) or a general medical condition (e.g., hyperthyroidism).
D. The Panic Attacks are not better accounted for by another mental disorder, such as Social Phobia (e.g., occurring on exposure to feared social situations), Specific Phobia (e.g., on exposure to a specific phobic situation), Obsessive-Compulsive Disorder (e.g., on exposure to dirt in someone with an obsession about contamination), Posttraumatic Stress Disorder (e.g., in response to stimuli associated with a severe stressor), or Separation Anxiety Disorder (e.g., in response to being away from home or close relatives).

The following case illustrates how these common disorders affected one of our patients:

> Susan, a 32-year-old homemaker, came to the outpatient clinic for eval-uation of anxiety. She reported the onset of panic attacks at age 13, which she remembered as terrifying. She vividly recalled her first at-tack, which occurred during history class. "I was just sitting in class when my heart began to beat wildly, my skin began to tingle, and I be-gan to feel like I was dying. There was no need for me to feel nervous," she observed. Over the following 19 years, attacks became frequent and unrelenting, occurring up to 10 times daily. To Susan, the panic was dev-astating: "I grew up all those years feeling that I wasn't quite normal." The attacks made her feel different from others and kept her from hav-ing a normal social life.
>   Along with her fear of attacks, Susan began to avoid crowded places, particularly shopping centers, grocery stores, movie theaters, and restaurants. She was a regular churchgoer but would sit in a pew

TABLE 7–4. DSM-IV-TR criteria for agoraphobia

Note: Agoraphobia is not a codable disorder. Code the specific disorder in which the Agoraphobia occurs (e.g., 300.21 Panic Disorder With Agoraphobia or 300.22 Agoraphobia Without History of Panic Disorder).

A. Anxiety about being in places or situations from which escape might be difficult (or embarrassing) or in which help may not be available in the event of having an unexpected or situationally predisposed Panic Attack or panic-like symptoms. Agoraphobic fears typically involve characteristic clusters of situations that include being outside the home alone; being in a crowd or standing in a line; being on a bridge; and traveling in a bus, train, or automobile.

    Note: Consider the diagnosis of Specific Phobia if the avoidance is limited to one or only a few specific situations, or Social Phobia if the avoidance is limited to social situations.

B. The situations are avoided (e.g., travel is restricted) or else are endured with marked distress or with anxiety about having a Panic Attack or panic-like symptoms, or require the presence of a companion.

C. The anxiety or phobic avoidance is not better accounted for by another mental disorder, such as Social Phobia (e.g., avoidance limited to social situations because of fear of embarrassment), Specific Phobia (e.g., avoidance limited to a single situation like elevators), Obsessive-Compulsive Disorder (e.g., avoidance of dirt in someone with an obsession about contamination), Posttraumatic Stress Disorder (e.g., avoidance of stimuli associated with a severe stressor), or Separation Anxiety Disorder (e.g., avoidance of leaving home or relatives).

near an exit. Her phobic avoidance tended to wax and wane, and although she never became housebound, Susan would insist on having her husband or a friend accompany her when she went shopping.

Susan had not previously sought treatment and thought that no one could help her. On occasion, she had gone to the emergency department for evaluation, but she had never received a diagnosis of panic disorder. Because she believed that admitting her symptoms was a sign of weakness, she had not even told her husband of 15 years about her panic attacks.

Susan was given fluvoxamine and within 1 month was free of attacks; within 3 months, she was no longer avoiding crowded places. At a 6-month follow-up, she remained free of all anxiety-related symptoms. Susan reported feeling like a new person.

TABLE 7–5. Common situations that either provoked or relieved anxiety in 100 agoraphobic patients

Situations that provoke anxiety	%	Situations that relieve anxiety	%
Standing in line at a store	96	Being accompanied by spouse	85
Having an appointment	91	Sitting near the door in church	76
Feeling trapped at hairdresser, etc.	89	Focusing thoughts on something else	63
Increasing distance from home	87	Taking the dog, baby carriage, etc., along	62
Being at particular places in neighborhood	66	Being accompanied by friend	60
Having cloudy, depressing weather	56	Reassuring self	52
		Wearing sunglasses	36

Source. Adapted from Burns and Thorpe 1977.

Nine years later, Susan continued to be well, although she was now taking fluoxetine (20 mg/day). In the interim, she had divorced her husband, who had been unable to cope with a more confident and independent spouse. She eventually remarried, enrolled at a community college, and moved away from her small town.

Epidemiology, Clinical Findings, and Course

According to the National Comorbidity Survey, 5% of women and 2% of men have met criteria for panic disorder at some point in their life. The prevalence of agoraphobia is somewhat higher. Rates for panic disorder are elevated threefold in primary care patients and are even higher in specialty clinics. Among patients seeking cardiology evaluations for chest pain, the rate may exceed 50% in those found to have normal coronary arteries.

Panic disorder and agoraphobia each typically have an onset in the mid-20s, although age at onset may vary; nearly 8 in 10 panic patients develop the disorder before age 30 years. Women are more likely than men to develop agoraphobia. There are usually no precipitating stressors before the onset of either panic disorder or agoraphobia. Some patients, however, report that the attacks began after an illness, an accident, or the breakup of a relationship; developed postpartum; or occurred after using mind-altering drugs such as lysergic acid diethylamide (LSD) or marijuana.

The initial panic attack is alarming and may prompt a visit to an emergency department, where routine laboratory tests and electrocar-

TABLE 7–6. Specialists consulted depending on target symptoms of panic disorder

Specialist	Target symptoms
Pulmonologist	Shortness of breath, hyperventilation, smothering sensations
Cardiologist	Palpitations, chest pain or discomfort
Neurologist	Tingling and numbness, trembling, imbalance
Otolaryngologist	Dizziness, choking sensation, dry mouth
Gynecologist	Hot flashes, sweating
Gastroenterologist	Nausea, diarrhea, abdominal pain or discomfort
Urologist	Frequent urination

diograms generally produce normal results. Many patients undergo extensive, often unnecessary medical workups that focus on the target symptoms (see Table 7–6). Psychiatrists may be consulted when no obvious physical cause for the patient's symptoms is found.

Panic attacks tend to develop suddenly, peak within 10 minutes, and last 5–20 minutes. During attacks, patients hyperventilate; they appear fearful, pale, diaphoretic, and restless. Many patients report that their attacks last hours to days, but it is likely that their continuing symptoms represent anxiety that persists after an attack. Common symptoms of panic disorder and agoraphobia are presented in Table 7–7.

Panic disorder, with or without agoraphobia, is chronic, although symptoms fluctuate in frequency and severity. Total remission is uncommon, yet up to 70% of patients with panic disorder will experience some degree of improvement. Panic disorder patients are at increased risk for peptic ulcer disease and cardiovascular disease, including hypertension, and have higher death rates than expected. An increased risk of suicide is largely due to coexisting depression and substance misuse.

A number of other physical conditions have been found in patients with panic disorder including joint hypermobility syndrome, mitral valve prolapse, migraine, fibromyalgia, chronic fatigue syndrome, irritable bowel syndrome, asthma, allergic rhinitis, and sinusitis. It appears to share connective tissue, pain perception, and autoimmune abnormalities with these conditions. Mitral valve prolapse in patients with panic disorder may result from an interaction between lax connective tissue and noradrenergic activation of the circulation.

TABLE 7–8. Differential diagnosis of anxiety

Medical illnesses	Drugs
Angina	Caffeine
Cardiac arrhythmias	Aminophylline and related
Congestive heart failure	compounds
Hypoglycemia	Sympathomimetic agents (e.g.,
Hypoxia	decongestants and diet pills)
Pulmonary embolism	Monosodium glutamate
Severe pain	Psychostimulants and
Thyrotoxicosis	hallucinogens
Carcinoid	Alcohol withdrawal
Pheochromocytoma	Withdrawal from
Menière's disease	benzodiazepines and other
Psychiatric illnesses	sedative-hypnotics
Schizophrenia	Thyroid hormones
Mood disorders	Antipsychotic medication
Avoidant personality disorder	
Adjustment disorder with	
anxious mood	

occur in response to a recognizable stressor but are out of proportion to the stressor and cause impairment, the diagnosis of adjustment disorder with anxiety may be appropriate (see Chapter 13).

Clinical Management

Panic disorder generally is treated with a combination of medication and individual psychotherapy. Selective serotonin reuptake inhibitors (SSRIs) are the medications of choice and are effective in blocking panic attacks in 70%–80% of patients. The U.S. Food and Drug Administration (FDA) has approved fluoxetine, paroxetine, and sertraline for the treatment of panic disorder. The serotonin–norepinephrine reuptake inhibitor (SNRI) venlafaxine is also effective, and a long-acting formulation is also FDA approved. Although these medications are called antidepressants, they work for anxiety.

In the past, tricyclic antidepressants (TCAs) and monoamine oxidase inhibitors (MAOIs) were used, but SSRIs are safer and better tolerated. Benzodiazepines can be effective in blocking panic attacks, but they are potentially habit-forming. β-Adrenergic-blocking drugs, such as propranolol, are sometimes prescribed to patients with anxiety disorders but are much less effective than antidepressants or benzodiazepines. Drug treatment of panic disorder is discussed in more detail in Chapter 20.

In general, patients who respond well to pharmacotherapy tend to have milder anxiety symptoms, later age at onset, fewer panic attacks, and a relatively normal personality.

The antidepressant dosage depends on the specific medication but is usually similar to that used to treat major depression. Typical dosages for the SSRIs are fluoxetine, 20 mg/day; sertraline, 50 mg/day; paroxetine, 20 mg/day; and citalopram, 20 mg/day. Once panic attacks have remitted, the patient should continue taking medication for at least 1 year to prevent relapse. After this period, the medication may be gradually tapered and discontinued. Panic symptoms may recur, but some patients do not relapse after cessation of medication. When a patient relapses or panic attacks recur, the drug can be restarted. Some patients will need to take medication chronically.

Patients should avoid caffeine because it may contribute to anxiety in patients with anxiety disorders. Patients often fail to realize how much caffeine they are ingesting with coffee (50–150 mg), tea (20–50 mg), cola drinks (30–60 mg), and even milk chocolate (1–15 mg).

Cognitive-behavioral therapy also is effective in the treatment of panic disorder and is frequently combined with medication. Cognitive-behavioral therapy usually involves distraction and breathing exercises, along with education to help the patient make more appropriate attributions for distressing somatic symptoms. For example, patients learn that panic-induced chest pain will not cause a heart attack. Psychodynamic psychotherapy has also proven beneficial for the treatment of panic disorder.

A therapist can help to boost the patient's low morale and poor self-esteem and can help the patient to solve everyday problems. Books and other reading materials about panic disorder and agoraphobia can be recommended, and the patient can be referred to the Web site of the Anxiety Disorders Association of America.

Agoraphobia presents an additional challenge and is best treated with exposure therapy. This is the most effective intervention and in its most basic form consists of encouraging patients to gradually enter feared situations, such as a grocery store. Some patients may require direct supervision by a therapist during the process of exposure to the various feared situations.

■ Generalized Anxiety Disorder

Patients with GAD worry excessively about life circumstances, such as their health, finances, social acceptance, job performance, and marital adjustment. This worry is central to the diagnosis of GAD (see Table 7–9).

The diagnostic criteria require that GAD not be diagnosed when the symptoms occur exclusively during the course of another illness such as major depression or schizophrenia or when the generalized anxiety occurs in the context of panic disorder, social phobia, or OCD. The anxiety or worry in GAD should not relate solely to anxiety about having a panic attack, being embarrassed in social situations, being contaminated, or gaining weight (as in anorexia nervosa). The criteria also require that the individual have at least three of six symptoms, which include feeling restless or keyed up, being easily fatigued, having poor concentration, being irritable, having muscle tension, or experiencing poor sleep. The symptoms must be present more days than not and cause significant distress or impairment in social, occupational, or other important areas of functioning. Finally, the effects of a substance or a general medical condition should be ruled out as a cause of the symptoms. The condition must persist for 6 months or longer.

Epidemiology, Clinical Findings, and Course

GAD is relatively common, with a lifetime prevalence between 4% and 7% in the general population. Rates are higher in women, African-Americans, and persons younger than 30 years. The disorder often has an onset in the early 20s, yet persons at any age can develop the disorder. Few persons with GAD seek psychiatric treatment, although many seek evaluations from medical specialists for specific symptoms, such as muscle tension or sleep disturbance. The disorder is usually chronic, with symptoms that fluctuate in severity. Some patients who initially have generalized anxiety later develop panic disorder.

Patients with GAD appear worried. They are often restless, tremulous, and distractible, and they may appear tired from lack of sleep.

The most frequent complications of GAD are major depression and substance abuse. Many patients experience one or more episodes of major depression over the course of their illness, and some meet criteria for social phobia or specific phobia. Some patients use alcohol or drugs to control their symptoms, which can lead to substance abuse.

TABLE 7–9. **DSM-IV-TR diagnostic criteria for generalized anxiety disorder**

A. Excessive anxiety and worry (apprehensive expectation), occurring more days than not for at least 6 months, about a number of events or activities (such as work or school performance).
B. The person finds it difficult to control the worry.
C. The anxiety and worry are associated with three (or more) of the following six symptoms (with at least some symptoms present for more days than not for the past 6 months).   **Note:** Only one item is required in children.
   (1) restlessness or feeling keyed up or on edge
   (2) being easily fatigued
   (3) difficulty concentrating or mind going blank
   (4) irritability
   (5) muscle tension
   (6) sleep disturbance (difficulty falling or staying asleep, or restless unsatisfying sleep)
D. The focus of the anxiety and worry is not confined to features of an Axis I disorder, e.g., the anxiety or worry is not about having a Panic Attack (as in Panic Disorder), being embarrassed in public (as in Social Phobia), being contaminated (as in Obsessive-Compulsive Disorder), being away from home or close relatives (as in Separation Anxiety Disorder), gaining weight (as in Anorexia Nervosa), having multiple physical complaints (as in Somatization Disorder), or having a serious illness (as in Hypochondriasis), and the anxiety and worry do not occur exclusively during Posttraumatic Stress Disorder.
E. The anxiety, worry, or physical symptoms cause clinically significant distress or impairment in social, occupational, or other important areas of functioning.
F. The disturbance is not due to the direct physiological effects of a substance (e.g., a drug of abuse, a medication) or a general medical condition (e.g., hyperthyroidism) and does not occur exclusively during a Mood Disorder, a Psychotic Disorder, or a Pervasive Developmental Disorder.

TABLE 7–12. DSM-IV-TR diagnostic criteria for obsessive-compulsive disorder

A. Either obsessions or compulsions:

Obsessions as defined by (1), (2), (3), and (4):

  (1) recurrent and persistent thoughts, impulses, or images that are experienced, at some time during the disturbance, as intrusive and inappropriate and that cause marked anxiety or distress

  (2) the thoughts, impulses, or images are not simply excessive worries about real-life problems

  (3) the person attempts to ignore or suppress such thoughts, impulses, or images, or to neutralize them with some other thought or action

  (4) the person recognizes that the obsessional thoughts, impulses, or images are a product of his or her own mind (not imposed from without as in thought insertion)

Compulsions as defined by (1) and (2):

  (1) repetitive behaviors (e.g., hand washing, ordering, checking) or mental acts (e.g., praying, counting, repeating words silently) that the person feels driven to perform in response to an obsession, or according to rules that must be applied rigidly

  (2) the behaviors or mental acts are aimed at preventing or reducing distress or preventing some dreaded event or situation; however, these behaviors or mental acts either are not connected in a realistic way with what they are designed to neutralize or prevent or are clearly excessive

B. At some point during the course of the disorder, the person has recognized that the obsessions or compulsions are excessive or unreasonable. **Note:** This does not apply to children.

C. The obsessions or compulsions cause marked distress, are time consuming (take more than 1 hour a day), or significantly interfere with the person's normal routine, occupational (or academic) functioning, or usual social activities or relationships.

D. If another Axis I disorder is present, the content of the obsessions or compulsions is not restricted to it (e.g., preoccupation with food in the presence of an Eating Disorder; hair pulling in the presence of Trichotillomania; concern with appearance in the presence of Body Dysmorphic Disorder; preoccupation with drugs in the presence of a Substance Use Disorder; preoccupation with having a serious illness in the presence of Hypochondriasis; preoccupation with sexual urges or fantasies in the presence of a Paraphilia; or guilty ruminations in the presence of Major Depressive Disorder).

TABLE 7–12. DSM-IV-TR diagnostic criteria for obsessive-compulsive disorder *(continued)*

E. The disturbance is not due to the direct physiological effects of a substance (e.g., a drug of abuse, a medication) or a general medical condition.

Specify if:

With Poor Insight: if, for most of the time during the current episode, the person does not recognize that the obsessions and compulsions are excessive or unreasonable

TABLE 7–13. Varied content in obsessions

Obsession	Foci of preoccupation
Aggression	Physical or verbal assault on self or others (includes suicidal and homicidal thoughts); accidents; mishaps; wars and natural disasters; death
Contamination	Excreta, human or otherwise; dirt, dust; semen; menstrual blood; other bodily excretions; germs; illness, especially venereal diseases; AIDS
Symmetry	Orderliness in arrangements of any kind (e.g., books on the shelf, shirts in the dresser)
Sexual	Sexual advances toward self or others; incestuous impulses; genitalia of either gender; homosexuality; masturbation; competence in sexual performance
Hoarding	Collecting items of any kind, typically items with little or no intrinsic value (e.g., string, shopping bags); inability to throw things out
Religious	Existence of God; validity of religious stories, practices, or holidays; committing sinful acts
Somatic	Preoccupation with body parts (e.g., nose); concern with appearance; belief in having disease or illness (e.g., cancer)

Source. Adapted from Akhtar et al. 1975.

TABLE 7–14. Frequency of common obsessions and compulsions in 560 patients with obsessive-compulsive disorder

Obsessions	%	Compulsions	%
Contamination	50	Checking	61
Pathological doubt	42	Washing	50
Somatic	33	Counting	36
Need for symmetry	32	Need to ask or confess	34
Aggressive impulse	31	Symmetry and precision	28
Sexual impulse	24	Hoarding	18
Multiple obsessions	72	Multiple compulsions	58

Source. Adapted from Rasmussen and Eisen 1998.

tionships. In addition, the person must recognize that the obsessions and compulsions are unreasonable, and the clinician will have determined that the symptoms are not due to another Axis I disorder, such as major depression, nor are they caused by the effects of a substance or general medical condition.

Many psychiatrically normal individuals—especially children—will have occasional obsessional thoughts or repetitive behaviors, but these tend not to cause distress or interfere with living. In fact, in many ways rituals add needed structure to our lives (e.g., daily routines that have probably changed little in years). These rituals are viewed as desirable and are easily adapted to changing circumstances. To the obsessive-compulsive person, rituals are a distressing and unavoidable way of life.

The following case describes a patient treated in our clinic who endured the crippling effects of OCD:

Todd, a 24-year-old man, was accompanied to the clinic by his mother for evaluation of obsessions and compulsive rituals. The rituals had begun in childhood and included touching objects a certain number of times and rereading prayers in church, but these symptoms were not disabling. After graduating from college, he moved to a large Midwestern city to work as an accountant for a major firm. Soon after, he began to check the locks on his doors frequently and to check his automobile for signs of intruders. Eventually, he began to check the appliances, water faucets, and electrical switches in his apartment, fearing that they might be unsafe. Fearing contamination, he also developed extensive grooming and bathing rituals. Because of his time-consuming rituals, he was often late for work, and in fact his workload became too much for him. He would find himself adding columns of numbers over and over to make sure that he had "done it right." He eventually quit his accounting job.

Todd moved back into his parents' home. His rituals became even more extensive and eventually took up nearly his entire day. The rituals mostly involved bathing (he showered for a half hour and had to wash his body in a specific order), dressing in a certain way, and repeating activities, such as walking in and out of doorways a certain number of times.

Todd was a slender, unkempt young man with a scraggly beard, long hair, and unclipped fingernails. His shoelaces were untied, and he wore several layers of clothing. His rituals had become so time-consuming that he had found it easier not to shave or wash at all. He wore the same clothes every day for the same reason.

Todd began treatment with fluoxetine (20 mg/day), and his daily dosage was gradually increased to 80 mg. Within 2 months, his rituals were reduced to less than 1 hour per day and his grooming improved. After 6 months, Todd still had minor rituals but reported that he felt like his old self. He had obtained a job and was coaching track at a nearby high school.

Ten years later, Todd remained well. Attempts to stop the medication had always led to an increase in symptoms. In the interim, Todd had received a law degree, had married, and had developed a growing law practice.

Epidemiology, Clinical Findings, and Course

OCD typically begins in the late teens or early 20s, and most persons with the disorder will have developed it by age 30 years. Onset is generally gradual but may occur relatively suddenly and in the absence of any obvious stressor.

The Epidemiologic Catchment Area study showed that 2%–3% of the general population meet criteria for OCD at some point during their lives. Men and women are equally likely to develop OCD, although men tend to have an earlier onset.

In a study of 250 patients, 85% were reported to have a chronic course, 10% a progressive or deteriorating course, and 2% an episodic course with periods of remission. Because these and other data were collected before effective treatments were available, future outcome studies may show a more favorable course. A study of youth with OCD seems to bear this out. At a 5-year follow-up, most of the subjects still had obsessive-compulsive symptoms, but they were much less severe, and 6% of the youth had achieved full remission.

Mild or typical symptoms and good premorbid adjustment have been associated with good outcome; early onset and the presence of a personality disorder have been associated with poor outcome. Obsessive-compulsive symptoms are usually worsened by depressed mood and stressful events. Recurrent episodes of major depression occur in 70%–80% of OCD patients.

Etiology and Pathophysiology

The cause of OCD is unknown, but many experts favor a neurobiological model. Evidence supporting this model includes the fact that OCD occurs more often in persons who have various neurological disorders, such as epilepsy, Sydenham's chorea, and Huntington's chorea, as well as in cases of brain trauma. OCD has been linked to birth injury, abnormal electroencephalographic findings, abnormal auditory evoked potentials, growth delays, and abnormal neuropsychological test results. Recently, a type of OCD has been identified in children after a group A β-streptococcal infection. These children not only develop obsessions and compulsions but also have emotional lability, separation anxiety, and tics.

The neurotransmitter serotonin has been the focus of much interest, perhaps because antidepressant drugs that block its reuptake are effective in treating OCD, whereas other antidepressants are ineffective. Other evidence supporting the "serotonin hypothesis" is indirect but is consistent with the view that either levels of the neurotransmitter or variations in the number or function of serotonin receptors are disturbed in patients with OCD.

Brain imaging studies have provided evidence of basal ganglia involvement in some persons with OCD. Studies using positron emission tomography (PET) or single photon emission computed tomography (SPECT) scanning in OCD patients have found increased glucose metabolism in the caudate nuclei and the orbital cortex of the frontal lobes, abnormalities that partially reverse with treatment. One hypothesis is that basal ganglia dysfunction leads to the complex motor programs involved in OCD, whereas the prefrontal hyperactivity may be related to the tendency to worry and plan excessively. As discussed in Chapter 3, the prefrontal cortex has important connections with the basal ganglia.

Finally, OCD appears to have a considerable genetic component; family studies show it runs in families, while twin studies show high concordance rates in identical versus nonidentical twins. It appears linked to Tourette's disorder.

Behaviorists have explained the development of OCD in terms of learning theory. They believe that anxiety, at least initially, becomes paired with specific environmental events (i.e., classical conditioning), for example, becoming dirty or contaminated. The person then engages in compulsive rituals, such as compulsive hand washing, to decrease the anxiety. When the rituals successfully reduce the anxiety, the compulsive behavior is reinforced and is more likely to be repeated in the future (i.e., operant conditioning).

Differential Diagnosis

OCD overlaps with many other psychiatric syndromes that must be ruled out, including schizophrenia, major depression, PTSD, hypochondriasis, anorexia nervosa, Tourette's disorder, and obsessive-compulsive personality disorder. Schizophrenia is the most important disorder to exclude, because obsessional thoughts can resemble delusional thinking. In most patients the distinction between obsessions and delusions is clear-cut. Obsessions are unwanted, resisted, and recognized by the patient as having an internal origin, whereas delusions are typically not resisted and are looked on as having an external origin.

The obsessions reported by patients with OCD must be distinguished from the morbid preoccupations and guilty ruminations of some patients with major depression (e.g., "I have sinned!"). In such patients, the ruminations are viewed as reasonable, although perhaps exaggerated, and are seldom resisted. Whereas the depressed patient tends to focus on past events, the obsessional patient focuses on the prevention of future events.

Other disorders need to be ruled out as well. Tourette's disorder, characterized by vocal and motor tics, may coexist with OCD. PTSD is characterized by recurrent, intrusive thoughts that may suggest obsessional thinking. Anorexia nervosa also resembles OCD in that both disorders involve ritualistic behavior; however, the patient with anorexia views the behavior as desirable and rarely resists it. Some patients with anorexia nervosa also meet criteria for OCD and, in addition to their food-related rituals, will have symptoms typical of OCD, such as frequent hand washing and checking.

Obsessive-compulsive personality disorder and OCD should not be confused. Obsessive-compulsive personality is characterized by perfectionism, orderliness, and obstinacy, which in fact most persons with OCD do not have; they are more likely to have dependent, avoidant, or passive-aggressive character traits. Admittedly, distinguishing between the two disorders can sometimes be difficult. For example, we saw a 45-year-old man whose wife was "sick and tired" of his book collecting, which had "taken over" their house. He saw nothing wrong with his hobby, which he enjoyed. He pointed out that many of the books were quite valuable. In this case, the patient viewed his obsessive-compulsive traits as desirable and had not resisted them. Based on his history of a rigid and aloof demeanor, miserliness, and perfectionism, in addition to the collecting, he received a diagnosis of obsessive-compulsive personality disorder. (A further discussion of this personality disorder is found in Chapter 10.)

Clinical Management

The treatment for OCD generally involves the combined use of behavior therapy and medication. Behavior therapy involves exposure paired with response prevention. For example, a patient might be exposed to a dreaded situation, event, or stimulus by various techniques (e.g., imaginal exposure, systematic desensitization, flooding) and then prevented from carrying out the compulsive behavior that usually results. A compulsive washer may be asked to handle "contaminated" objects (e.g., a dirty tissue) and then be prevented from washing his or her hands.

The SSRIs are particularly effective in OCD, and several are approved by the FDA for that indication, including fluoxetine, fluvoxamine, paroxetine, and sertraline. Clomipramine, a TCA that is a relatively specific serotonin reuptake blocker, is also approved to treat OCD but because of its side effects is used less frequently. Venlafaxine may also be effective, as one randomized clinical trial suggests. The addition of an antipsychotic may boost the likelihood of response of patients whose illness appears refractory to SSRIs. Typically, higher dosages of the SSRIs are required to treat OCD than to treat major depression, and response is often delayed. For that reason, patients should have relatively lengthy trials (i.e., 12–16 weeks).

Research shows that nearly half of patients with treatment-refractory illness benefit from cingulotomy, the most commonly used psychosurgical procedure. Patients should not be referred for psychosurgery unless they fail to respond to proven therapies. Promising alternatives are deep brain stimulation and gamma knife surgery. None of these options is widely available.

Apart from behavior therapy, individual psychotherapy is beneficial in helping to restore a patient's low morale and self-esteem, in helping the patient solve day-to-day problems, and in encouraging treatment compliance.

Family therapy also has a role in managing OCD. Family members are often ignorant about OCD and get drawn into their relative's rituals in a misguided effort to be helpful. A mother, for example, may be asked to assist in her daughter's cleaning and checking rituals ("Is the stove turned off? Can you check it for me, please?"). In family therapy, the relatives can learn to accept the illness, learn to cope with its manifestations, and learn how not to encourage obsessive-compulsive behavior.

■ Posttraumatic Stress Disorder

PTSD occurs in persons who have experienced, witnessed, or been confronted with an event involving actual or threatened death, serious physical injury, or a threat to physical integrity. Examples of such events include combat, physical assault, rape, and disasters (e.g., home fires). The three major elements of PTSD are 1) reexperiencing of the trauma through dreams or recurrent and intrusive thoughts, 2) emotional numbing such as feeling detached from others, and 3) symptoms of autonomic hyperarousal such as irritability and exaggerated startle response. Two subtypes are specified: *acute* if the duration of symptoms is less than 3 months, and *chronic* if symptoms last 3 months or longer. If onset is delayed more than 6 months after the stressor, that delay is specified. The DSM-IV-TR criteria for PTSD are included in Table 7–15.

Epidemiology, Clinical Findings, and Course

PTSD has a prevalence of nearly 7% in the general population. Most men with the disorder have experienced combat. Fifteen percent of veterans of the Vietnam War suffered from PTSD. For women, the most frequent precipitating event is a physical assault or rape. The disorder can occur at any age, and even young children may develop the disorder, as occurred after the terrorist attacks of September 11, 2001, or several of the more recent school shooting incidents. The frequency of PTSD among survivors of catastrophes varies, but in one well-studied tragedy, the Cocoanut Grove nightclub fire that occurred in Boston in 1942, 57% of the patients still had a posttraumatic syndrome 1 year later.

We recently saw a woman in our psychiatric clinic who had developed PTSD after a sexual assault:

> Megan, a 21-year-old college student, presented for evaluation of depression and flashbacks. At a fraternity party 3 months earlier, she had become interested in one of the men. The man suggested they go elsewhere to have sexual relations. Although intoxicated, Megan objected,

TABLE 7–15. DSM-IV-TR diagnostic criteria for posttraumatic stress disorder

A. The person has been exposed to a traumatic event in which both of the following were present:
  (1) the person experienced, witnessed, or was confronted with an event or events that involved actual or threatened death or serious injury, or a threat to the physical integrity of self or others
  (2) the person's response involved intense fear, helplessness, or horror. **Note:** In children, this may be expressed instead by disorganized or agitated behavior
B. The traumatic event is persistently reexperienced in one (or more) of the following ways:
  (1) recurrent and intrusive distressing recollections of the event, including images, thoughts, or perceptions. **Note:** In young children, repetitive play may occur in which themes or aspects of the trauma are expressed.
  (2) recurrent distressing dreams of the event. **Note:** In children, there may be frightening dreams without recognizable content.
  (3) acting or feeling as if the traumatic event were recurring (includes a sense of reliving the experience, illusions, hallucinations, and dissociative flashback episodes, including those that occur on awakening or when intoxicated). **Note:** In young children, trauma-specific reenactment may occur.
  (4) intense psychological distress at exposure to internal or external cues that symbolize or resemble an aspect of the traumatic event
  (5) physiological reactivity on exposure to internal or external cues that symbolize or resemble an aspect of the traumatic event
C. Persistent avoidance of stimuli associated with the trauma and numbing of general responsiveness (not present before the trauma), as indicated by three (or more) of the following:
  (1) efforts to avoid thoughts, feelings, or conversations associated with the trauma
  (2) efforts to avoid activities, places, or people that arouse recollections of the trauma
  (3) inability to recall an important aspect of the trauma
  (4) markedly diminished interest or participation in significant activities

TABLE 7–15. **DSM-IV-TR diagnostic criteria for posttraumatic stress disorder** *(continued)*

    (5) feeling of detachment or estrangement from others

    (6) restricted range of affect (e.g., unable to have loving feelings)

    (7) sense of a foreshortened future (e.g., does not expect to have a career, marriage, children, or a normal life span)

D. Persistent symptoms of increased arousal (not present before the trauma), as indicated by two (or more) of the following:

    (1) difficulty falling or staying asleep

    (2) irritability or outbursts of anger

    (3) difficulty concentrating

    (4) hypervigilance

    (5) exaggerated startle response

E. Duration of the disturbance (symptoms in Criteria B, C, and D) is more than 1 month.

F. The disturbance causes clinically significant distress or impairment in social, occupational, or other important areas of functioning.

Specify if:

    Acute: if duration of symptoms is less than 3 months

    Chronic: if duration of symptoms is 3 months or more

Specify if:

    With Delayed Onset: if onset of symptoms is at least 6 months after the stressor

but the man persisted. He forced her into another room, tore off her clothing, and raped her. Later, feeling embarrassed and humiliated, Megan chose not to tell her friends, nor did she seek a medical evaluation. She thought that the police would ignore what they might consider consensual sex.

Although she never missed a class or her part-time clerical job, Megan became depressed and anxious and began to experience episodes of anger and irritability. She ruminated about the rape, would recall its unpleasant details, and withdrew from her friends. Several concerned friends convinced her to seek help.

Based on the history and symptoms, PTSD was diagnosed and explained to Megan. She was referred for group therapy at a local rape crisis advocacy center. Fluoxetine (20 mg/day) was prescribed to treat symptoms of depression and anxiety. With treatment, Megan gradually improved and was able to overcome her symptoms of PTSD.

PTSD generally begins soon after experiencing the stressor, but its onset may be delayed for months or years. The disorder is chronic for many, but symptoms fluctuate and typically worsen during stressful periods. Rapid onset of symptoms, good premorbid functioning, strong social support, and the absence of psychiatric or medical comorbidity are factors associated with a good outcome. Many patients with PTSD develop comorbid psychiatric disorders such as major depression, other anxiety disorders, or alcohol and drug abuse.

Etiology and Pathophysiology

The major etiological factor leading to PTSD is a traumatic event, which by definition must be severe enough to be outside the range of normal human experience. Business losses, marital conflicts, and the death of a loved one are not considered stressors that cause PTSD. In general, the more severe the trauma, the greater the risk of developing PTSD. In wartime situations, for example, certain experiences are linked to the development of the disorder: witnessing a friend being killed, witnessing atrocities, or participating in atrocities.

A person's age, history of emotional disturbance, level of social support, and proximity to the stressor are all factors that affect the likelihood of developing PTSD. Eighty percent of young children who sustain burn injuries, for example, show symptoms of posttraumatic stress 1–2 years after the injury, but only 30% of adults who sustain similar injuries do so. Persons who have received prior psychiatric treatment are more likely to develop PTSD, presumably because the previous illness reflects the person's greater vulnerability to stress. Persons with adequate social support are less likely to develop PTSD than are persons with poor support.

Certain biological abnormalities, such as decreased rapid eye movement latency in Stage IV sleep, have been found in persons with PTSD, and these abnormalities may play a role in its development. Recent research suggests that the sustained levels of high emotional arousal can lead to dysregulation of the hypothalamic-pituitary-adrenal axis. The noradrenergic and serotonergic pathways in the central nervous system also have been implicated in the genesis of PTSD.

Brain imaging is also helping researchers to understand the underlying neurobiology of PTSD. Reduced hippocampal volume and increased metabolic activity in limbic regions, particularly the amygdala, are the most replicated findings. These findings may help to explain the role of disturbed emotional memory in PTSD.

Differential Diagnosis

The differential diagnosis for PTSD includes major depression, adjustment disorder, panic disorder, GAD, acute stress disorder, OCD, depersonalization disorder, factitious disorder, or malingering. In some cases, a physical injury may have occurred during the traumatic event, necessitating a physical and neurological examination.

Clinical Management

Both paroxetine (20–50 mg/day) and sertraline (50–200 mg/day) have been approved by the FDA for the treatment of PTSD, but the other SSRIs are probably effective as well. These drugs help to decrease depressive symptoms, to reduce intrusive symptoms such as nightmares and flashbacks, and to normalize sleep. A long-acting form of the SNRI venlafaxine also appears effective based on large clinical trials. Benzodiazepines (e.g., diazepam, 5–10 mg twice daily; clonazepam, 1–2 mg twice daily) may help reduce anxiety but should be used for short-term treatment (e.g., days to weeks) because of their potential for abuse. The α_1-adrenergic antagonist prazosin (10 mg/day) has shown promise in alleviating the intractable nightmares that some PTSD patients report.

Establishing a sense of safety and separation from the trauma is an important first step in the treatment of PTSD. Cultivating a therapeutic working relationship requires time for the patient to develop trust. Research has shown that cognitive-behavioral therapy is effective in reducing PTSD symptoms. With cognitive-behavioral therapy, patients are provided the skills to control anxiety and to counter dysfunctional thoughts (e.g., "I deserved to be raped"). Controlled exposure to cues associated with the trauma may be helpful in decreasing avoidance. Group therapy and family therapy are also useful and have been widely recommended for veterans of war. The Department of Veterans Affairs has organized groups for distressed veterans across the country.

■ Acute Stress Disorder

Acute stress disorder occurs in some individuals after a traumatic experience and is considered a precursor to PTSD. By definition, the individual must have at least three dissociative symptoms (e.g., emotional numbing, derealization, amnesia) and one or more intrusion, avoidance, or hyperarousal symptom; the symptoms must cause clinically significant difficulties in functioning and last from 2 days to 4 weeks (see Table 7–16).

The diagnosis was introduced in DSM-IV because research suggested that dissociative symptoms occurring immediately after a traumatic event (see criterion B) predicted the development of PTSD. For example, about 80% of motor vehicle accident survivors with acute stress disorder have PTSD at 6 months posttrauma. The goal was to enable clinicians to more accurately identify persons less likely to recover from their traumatic experience and to develop PTSD. However, recent research suggests that other symptoms may be more useful in predicting the onset of PTSD.

Because acute stress disorder was recently defined, there is little information about its prevalence, gender distribution, or risk factors. The differential diagnosis is between PTSD, brief psychotic disorder, a dissociative disorder, or an adjustment disorder. PTSD lasts more than 1 month, and although dissociative symptoms may be present, they are usually not prominent. Brief psychotic disorder lasts less than 1 month but is characterized by hallucinations, delusions, or bizarre behavior. Dissociative disorders do not necessarily occur in response to traumatic situations or involve emotional numbing, reexperiencing of the trauma, or signs of autonomic hyperarousal. An adjustment disorder occurs in response to stressful situations (e.g., personal bankruptcy) but not necessarily a traumatic event involving serious personal threats; adjustment disorders may last up to 6 months, and the diagnosis is mainly used when criteria for other Axis I disorders are not met. A diagnosis of acute stress reaction would preempt a diagnosis of adjustment disorder.

Research shows that cognitive-behavioral therapy involving exposure and anxiety management (e.g., relaxation training, re-breathing) can help prevent the progression to full-blown PTSD. When anxiety is severe, a brief course of a benzodiazepine may be helpful (e.g., clonazepam, 1–2 mg twice daily). There is some evidence that the administration of β-blockers immediately after a trauma may reduce the later development of symptoms of PTSD.

TABLE 7–16. DSM-IV-TR diagnostic criteria for acute stress disorder

A. The person has been exposed to a traumatic event in which both of the following were present:
  (1) the person experienced, witnessed, or was confronted with an event or events that involved actual or threatened death or serious injury, or a threat to the physical integrity of self or others
  (2) the person's response involved intense fear, helplessness, or horror
B. Either while experiencing or after experiencing the distressing event, the individual has three (or more) of the following dissociative symptoms:
  (1) a subjective sense of numbing, detachment, or absence of emotional responsiveness
  (2) a reduction in awareness of his or her surroundings (e.g., "being in a daze")
  (3) derealization
  (4) depersonalization
  (5) dissociative amnesia (i.e., inability to recall an important aspect of the trauma)
C. The traumatic event is persistently reexperienced in at least one of the following ways: recurrent images, thoughts, dreams, illusions, flashback episodes, or a sense of reliving the experience; or distress on exposure to reminders of the traumatic event.
D. Marked avoidance of stimuli that arouse recollections of the trauma (e.g., thoughts, feelings, conversations, activities, places, people).
E. Marked symptoms of anxiety or increased arousal (e.g., difficulty sleeping, irritability, poor concentration, hypervigilance, exaggerated startle response, motor restlessness).
F. The disturbance causes clinically significant distress or impairment in social, occupational, or other important areas of functioning or impairs the individual's ability to pursue some necessary task, such as obtaining necessary assistance or mobilizing personal resources by telling family members about the traumatic experience.
G. The disturbance lasts for a minimum of 2 days and a maximum of 4 weeks and occurs within 4 weeks of the traumatic event.
H. The disturbance is not due to the direct physiological effects of a substance (e.g., a drug of abuse, a medication) or a general medical condition, is not better accounted for by Brief Psychotic Disorder, and is not merely an exacerbation of a preexisting Axis I or Axis II disorder.

Key points to remember about anxiety disorders

1. Mild cases of panic may respond to cognitive-behavioral therapy, but many patients will need medication.

    - SSRIs are the drugs of first choice because of their effectiveness and tolerability. TCAs and MAOIs work well but are second-line treatments due to their many adverse effects and dangerousness in overdose.

2. The agoraphobic patient should be gently encouraged to get out and explore the world.

    - Progress will not occur unless the phobic patient confronts the feared places or situations. Some patients will need formal behavior therapy.

3. Patients with anxiety disorders should minimize intake of caffeine, a known anxiogenic.

4. Behavioral techniques (e.g., exposure, flooding, desensitization) will help most persons with social and specific phobias.

    - Some people with a social phobia respond well to medication. SSRIs and venlafaxine are the drugs of choice because of their effectiveness and tolerability.

5. GAD may respond to simple behavioral techniques (e.g., relaxation training), but many patients will need medication.

    - Buspirone, venlafaxine, and the SSRIs paroxetine and escitalopram are effective FDA-approved treatments.

    - Benzodiazepines, when used, should be prescribed for a limited time (e.g., weeks or months). Hydroxyzine is a relatively benign alternative.

6. OCD generally responds best to the combination of medication and behavior therapy.

    - Clomipramine, or one of the SSRIs, is effective. With SSRIs, higher dosages will be needed than for the treatment of depression.

    - The lag time to improvement on medication is months, not weeks as in the treatment of depression.

Key points to remember about anxiety disorders *(continued)*

- Some patients will benefit from referral to an experienced behavior therapist, particularly motivated patients with prominent rituals.

7. PTSD tends to be chronic, but many patients will benefit from a combination of medication and cognitive-behavioral therapy.

- Paroxetine and sertraline are approved for the treatment of PTSD. The other SSRIs are probably effective as well.

- Prazosin may be effective in treating disturbing dreams and nightmares.

- Many patients will benefit from the mutual support found in group therapy.

- Group therapy has become especially popular with veterans. Most veterans organizations can offer help in finding a group.

■ Self-Assessment Questions

1. When is anxiety normal, and when is it abnormal?
2. What is the relation between panic disorder and agoraphobia?
3. What is the irritable heart syndrome?
4. What are the findings in genetic studies of panic disorder?
5. What is the differential diagnosis of panic disorder?
6. What is the pharmacological treatment of panic disorder? GAD? Social phobia?
7. What are social and specific phobias? How do they differ?
8. What is the natural history of the different anxiety disorders?
9. How are obsessions distinguished from delusions?
10. What are some of the behavioral techniques used to treat OCD?
11. When does PTSD develop? What factors predispose to its development? How is it treated?
12. What behavioral treatments are useful in the various anxiety disorders?

CHAPTER 8

Somatoform, Dissociative, and Related Disorders

So it is that a patient can confront his doctor with his symptoms, and put on him the whole onus of their cure.

Mayer-Gross, Slater, and Roth, Clinical Psychiatry

SOMATOFORM DISORDERS are an important group of conditions characterized by physical symptoms that defy medical investigation. They also are surprisingly common. For example, up to 30% of primary care patients present with unexplained symptoms, and a substantial proportion of them have a somatoform disorder. Patients with these disorders behave as though they are ill, yet have no verifiable organic disease. They report symptoms, visit doctors, and take medication; some will claim disability. Consequently, they baffle and frustrate physicians, who must balance their concern to investigate the patient's complaints against the real concern of inadvertently encouraging the patient's help-seeking behavior. Somatoform disorder patients tend not to respond to medical reassurance, and for that reason many continue to seek care, request unnecessary tests and procedures, and take unneeded medication. Many visit primary care physicians rather than psychiatrists, motivated by the belief that their symptoms are medically based.

TABLE 8–4. Complaints reported by a patient with somatization disorder

Organ system	Complaint
Neuropsychiatric	"The two hemispheres of my brain aren't working properly." "I couldn't name familiar objects around the house when asked." "I was hospitalized with tingling and numbness all over, and the doctors didn't know why."
Cardiopulmonary	"I had extreme dizziness after climbing stairs." "It hurts to breathe." "My heart was racing and pounding and thumping....I thought I was going to die."
Gastrointestinal	"For 10 years I was treated for nervous stomach, spastic colon, and gallbladder, and nothing the doctor did seemed to help." "I got a violent cramp after eating an apple and felt terrible the next day." "The gas was awful—I thought I was going to explode."
Genitourinary	"I'm not interested in sex, but I pretend to be to satisfy my husband's needs." "I've had red patches on my labia, and I was told to use boric acid." "I had difficulty with bladder control and was examined for a tipped bladder, but nothing was found." "I had nerves cut going into my uterus because of severe cramps."
Musculoskeletal	"I have learned to live with weakness and tiredness all the time." "I thought I pulled a back muscle, but my chiropractor says it's a disc problem."
Sensory	"My vision is blurry. It's like seeing through a fog, but the doctor said that glasses wouldn't help." "I suddenly lost my hearing. It came back, but now I have whistling noises, like an echo."
Metabolic/ endocrine	"I began teaching half days because I couldn't tolerate the cold." "I was losing hair faster than my husband."

was concerned that her skin was becoming darker and that her scalp hair was falling out. An extended medical workup was negative.

Six years later, she was admitted to the psychiatric service. During the intervening years, she had received a total hysterectomy and oophorectomy, but apart from menstruation-related symptoms, she continued to have the same unrelenting physical complaints. Again, a protracted medical workup was negative.

Carol's remarkable history of illness spanning 27 years leaves little doubt that she had an unrecognized somatization disorder. Her complaints were consistent over the years and had led to many unnecessary evaluations and procedures. Despite the multiplicity of her complaints, many quite alarming, Carol remained fit and physically healthy.

The lifetime prevalence of somatization disorder is about 1% in the general population but higher in primary care. Many more have unexplained symptoms but not the number required for the diagnosis. The disorder is more common in rural areas and among less educated persons. The disorder is much more common in women, many of whom report histories of childhood sexual abuse. The disorder typically has an onset in the 20s and is established by age 30.

Somatization disorder is associated with repeated surgeries, alcohol or drug abuse, marital instability, and suicide attempts. Co-occurring mood and anxiety disorders are common. Between one-half and two-thirds of patients with somatization disorder meet criteria for a personality disorder (e.g., borderline personality disorder). The disorder is chronic, with fluctuations in the frequency and diversity of symptoms. Few persons with somatization disorder will experience significant improvement or have a full remission of symptoms.

Research shows that somatization disorder runs in families and that within these families there is an excess of both antisocial personality disorder and substance abuse. These findings have led to the hypothesis that, depending on the individual's gender, genetic and/or environmental factors may lead to one or another overlapping clinical syndrome.

The differential diagnosis of somatization disorder includes panic disorder, major depression, and schizophrenia. Patients with panic disorder typically report multiple autonomic symptoms (e.g., palpitations, shortness of breath), but they occur almost exclusively during panic attacks. Patients with major depression often report multiple physical complaints, but these are overshadowed by the dysphoria and vegetative symptoms of depression (e.g., appetite loss, lack of energy, insomnia). Schizophrenic patients sometimes have physical complaints, but they are often bizarre or delusional (e.g., "My spine is a set of twirling plates").

Conversion Disorder

Conversion disorder involves symptoms that suggest a neurological or general medical condition; pain is purposely excluded from the definition. (Patients whose major complaint is limited to pain receive a diagnosis of *pain disorder.*) In addition, the physician will have determined that the symptom is not under voluntary control and cannot, after appropriate investigation, be explained by a known neurological or medical illness. Psychological factors are associated with the symptoms, as suggested by their initiation after stressful events. Furthermore, the symptoms must not be intentionally produced or culturally sanctioned behaviors (see Table 8–5).

Conversion symptoms are surprisingly common. For example, an estimated 20%–25% of the patients admitted to neurology wards have conversion symptoms. In a survey of consecutive psychiatric consultations in a general hospital, 5% of the patients had conversion symptoms. Conversion symptoms are more frequent in women, in patients from rural areas, and in persons with less education or low socioeconomic status. Onset tends to be in late childhood or early adulthood. Onset in middle or late age suggests a medical condition.

Typical conversion symptoms include paralysis, abnormal movements, inability to speak (aphonia), blindness, and deafness. *Pseudoseizures* are also common and may occur in patients with genuine epileptic seizures. (Pseudoseizures are spells that resemble true seizures but are unaccompanied by abnormal brain waves.) Conversion symptoms usually conform to the patient's concept of disease rather than to recognized physiological patterns. For example, anesthesia may follow a stocking-and-glove pattern, not a dermatomal distribution. Conversion symptoms sometimes occur in patients with mood disorders, somatization disorder, or schizophrenia and in these situations are likely attributable to the primary disorder.

The diagnosis of conversion disorder is established by ruling out medical or neurological illness and by identifying psychological factors involved in the initiation of symptoms. This is usually not difficult when a patient's somatic complaints are inconsistent with physical examination findings and there is clear evidence of a psychological stressor. Research shows that some patients who receive a diagnosis of conversion disorder are later found to have medical or neurological illnesses that, in retrospect, accounted for their symptoms. For that reason, clinicians need to remain tentative in their diagnosis of conversion disorder.

There are many useful clues to help clinicians diagnose conversion disorder. Patients with conversion symptoms typically have a history of

TABLE 8–5.   DSM-IV-TR diagnostic criteria for conversion disorder

A. One or more symptoms or deficits affecting voluntary motor or sensory function that suggest a neurological or other general medical condition.

B. Psychological factors are judged to be associated with the symptom or deficit because the initiation or exacerbation of the symptom or deficit is preceded by conflicts or other stressors.

C. The symptom or deficit is not intentionally produced or feigned (as in Factitious Disorder or Malingering).

D. The symptom or deficit cannot, after appropriate investigation, be fully explained by a general medical condition, or by the direct effects of a substance, or as a culturally sanctioned behavior or experience.

E. The symptom or deficit causes clinically significant distress or impairment in social, occupational, or other important areas of functioning or warrants medical evaluation.

F. The symptom or deficit is not limited to pain or sexual dysfunction, does not occur exclusively during the course of Somatization Disorder, and is not better accounted for by another mental disorder.

Specify type of symptom or deficit:
   With Motor Symptom or Deficit
   With Sensory Symptom or Deficit
   With Seizures or Convulsions
   With Mixed Presentation

mental illness. For that reason, an unexplained pseudoneurological symptom in a patient with a significant psychiatric disorder is likely to represent a conversion symptom. Patients sometimes mimic symptoms based on prior experience with an illness or base them on illness symptoms modeled by an important person in their life (e.g., parent, grandparent). Many people with conversion disorder display an indifference toward their symptoms (*la belle indifférence*), but such indifference is not invariably present.

The etiology of conversion disorder is not well understood, but psychodynamic, biological, cultural, and behavioral factors have been suggested to play a role. According to psychodynamic views, patients with certain developmental predispositions respond to particular types of stress with conversion symptoms. The stress awakens unconscious conflicts, usually involving sexuality, aggression, or dependency. The high frequency of conversion symptoms in patients with brain injuries, however, suggests a biological etiology. A study of conversion disorder patients in Australia and Great Britain found that 64% had coexisting or antecedent brain disorders, such as epilepsy, tumor, or stroke, compared with only 6% of control subjects. Sociologists point out that some ethnic and social (generally non-European) groups are more likely to respond to emotional stress with conversion symptoms than are other groups.

A favorable outcome is generally associated with acute onset, a precipitating stressful event, good premorbid adjustment, and the absence of medical or neurological comorbidity. One follow-up study found that 83% of the inpatients and outpatients were well or improved at a 4- to 6-year follow-up. Another study found that 100% of the outpatients with conversion symptoms had an immediate favorable response to treatment, with only 20% having relapsed by 1-year follow-up. When conversion symptoms occur in the context of another psychiatric disorder, their outcome reflects the natural history of the primary disorder, such as major depression or somatization disorder.

Hypochondriasis

Hypochondriasis is a preoccupation with fears of having, or the belief that one has, a serious disease based on misinterpretation of bodily symptoms (Table 8–6). This preoccupation persists after appropriate medical evaluation has ruled out a medical disorder that could account for the symptoms; furthermore, other mental disorders such as schizophrenia, major depression, or somatization disorder have been ruled out as a cause of the disturbance. Hypochondriasis has a duration of 6 months or more.

Hypochondriacal patients show an abnormal concern with their health and tend to amplify normal physiological sensations and misinterpret them as signs of disease. These patients often fear having a particular disease (e.g., cancer, AIDS) and cannot be reassured despite careful and repeated examinations. Their preoccupation with the idea of having a serious illness directs attention away from other activities and undermines relationships. The following vignette illustrates a case of hypochondriasis seen in our hospital:

> Mabel, an 80-year-old retired schoolteacher, was admitted for evaluation of an 8-month preoccupation with having colon cancer. The patient had a history of single vessel coronary artery disease and diabetes mellitus (controlled by oral hypoglycemic agents) but was otherwise well. She had no history of mental illness. On admission, Mabel reported her concern about having colon cancer, which her two brothers had devel-

---

TABLE 8–6. **DSM-IV-TR diagnostic criteria for hypochondriasis**

A. Preoccupation with fears of having, or the idea that one has, a serious disease based on the person's misinterpretation of bodily symptoms.

B. The preoccupation persists despite appropriate medical evaluation and reassurance.

C. The belief in Criterion A is not of delusional intensity (as in Delusional Disorder, Somatic Type) and is not restricted to a circumscribed concern about appearance (as in Body Dysmorphic Disorder).

D. The preoccupation causes clinically significant distress or impairment in social, occupational, or other important areas of functioning.

E. The duration of the disturbance is at least 6 months.

F. The preoccupation is not better accounted for by Generalized Anxiety Disorder, Obsessive-Compulsive Disorder, Panic Disorder, a Major Depressive Episode, Separation Anxiety, or another Somatoform Disorder.

Specify if:

With Poor Insight: if, for most of the time during the current episode, the person does not recognize that the concern about having a serious illness is excessive or unreasonable

---

oped. As evidence of a possible tumor, she reported having diffuse abdominal pain and cited an abnormal barium enema examination 1 year earlier. (The examination had revealed diverticulosis.) Because of her concern about having cancer, Mabel had seen 11 physicians, but each in turn had been unable to reassure her that she did not have cancer.

Mabel was pleasant and cooperated well with the ward team. Her physical examination and routine admission laboratory tests were unremarkable. Despite her complaint, Mabel denied depressed mood and displayed a full affect. She reported sleeping less than usual but attributed this to her abdominal discomfort. She chose not to socialize with other patients, whom she characterized as "crazy." She remained preoccupied with the possibility that she had cancer, despite our reassurance. A benzodiazepine was prescribed for her sleep disturbance, but she refused any other type of psychiatric treatment.

Many people develop hypochondriacal concerns transiently in response to new or unexplained symptoms. Symptoms of this kind occur in 60%–80% of healthy persons in any given week; intermittent worry about illness occurs in 10%–20%. However, unlike patients with hypochondriasis, most people can be readily reassured that their symptoms are benign.

Arthur was a good student in high school but participated in relatively few activities. Although he had occasionally dated, he had not had a close relationship with a girl. He experienced a brief rebellious period during high school in which he stopped studying and smoked marijuana. After several months of this behavior, he began to feel depressed, apathetic, guilt-ridden, and paranoid. He did not meet criteria for major depression and did not have delusions or hallucinations. The episode passed when he stopped rebelling and using marijuana. He later completed 1 year of college but then dropped out to work and thus obtain money for cosmetic surgery. After the surgery, he planned to return to college. One day he hoped to attend medical school.

Arthur was a handsome young man with heavy, dark eyebrows but a perfectly normal jawline. He related his motivation for seeking surgery to his general pattern of pursuing perfection in all aspects of life. He considered himself well adjusted and normal and, in fact, superior to most people. He saw no need for psychiatric treatment and refused a medication trial.

Clinical Management of the Somatoform Disorders

There are several important principles that guide the treatment of somatoform disorders. First, the physician should follow the Hippocratic oath and "do no harm." Because symptoms are often embellished or misidentified (e.g., minor spotting during the menses may be reported as "gushing"), physicians frequently overreact and pursue the diagnostic equivalent of a "wild goose chase." It is no surprise that the symptoms of the various somatoform disorders prompt unnecessary diagnostic evaluations, surgical procedures, or medication prescriptions that have little relevance to the underlying condition. For that reason, it is essential that physicians who evaluate patients with multiple unexplained symptoms learn to identify and diagnose somatoform disorders. Physicians should understand that the patient's suffering is real and should be legitimized.

Second, physicians should see their somatizing patients regularly, preferably at scheduled visits. Implicit in this approach is the message that new symptoms are not required in order to see a physician. The physician should listen attentively and convey genuine concern without making detailed inquiries about the patient's symptoms. In refraining from focusing on the symptoms, the physician communicates the message that somatic complaints are not the most important or interesting feature about the patient. The physician's goal becomes one of helping the patient cope with the symptoms, and in doing so, to enable him or her to function at as high a level as possible. To this end, patients will benefit from receiving an explanation for their symptoms, appropriate advice regarding diet and exercise, and encouragement to return to meaningful activity and work.

Third, the physician should prescribe psychotropic medications and analgesics cautiously. Somatoform disorder patients sometimes request medications, but there is often little benefit from them. Medications are rarely indicated unless another psychiatric syndrome develops that may respond. For example, antidepressants may help relieve major depression or block panic attacks, yet they have little effect on an underlying somatization disorder. As a general rule, benzodiazepines should be avoided because of their abuse potential.

Finally, the most important therapeutic element is an empathic doctor–patient relationship. Ideally, the doctor should become the patient's primary and only physician. This will reduce the tendency for the patient to doctor-shop or to seek out costly and unnecessary tests and procedures.

These simple measures have been shown to lower health care costs in patients with somatization disorder. A group of patients receiving a psychiatric consultation with recommendations for conservative care (i.e., essentially these measures) had a 53% decline in health care costs, mostly as a result of fewer hospitalizations, and improved physical functioning. The patients' general health status and satisfaction with their health care were unchanged. Health care costs of control subjects did not change.

The patient with hypochondriasis may further benefit from individual psychotherapy that involves education about illness attitudes and selective perception of symptoms. Controlled trials have shown that cognitive-behavioral therapy (CBT) can help to correct faulty beliefs about illness and counter the patient's tendency to seek inappropriate care. Another option is medication; selective serotonin reuptake inhibitors (SSRIs) are reported to be effective in treating hypochondriasis. One particular form of hypochondriasis, *illness phobia,* has been reported to respond to the tricyclic antidepressant imipramine.

The treatment of conversion disorder is not well established, but symptom removal is the goal. Reassurance and gentle suggestion (for example, that gradual improvement may be expected) are appropriate measures, along with efforts to resolve stressful situations that may have prompted the symptoms. The spontaneous remission rate for acute conversion symptoms is high, so that even without any specific intervention, most patients will improve and probably not suffer any serious complications.

A treatment approach for persistent conversion symptoms using behavioral modification for psychiatric inpatients has been described. The

---

TABLE 8–8.   DSM-IV-TR dissociative disorders

Amnestic states
    Dissociative amnesia
    Dissociative fugue

Dissociative identity disorder (formerly multiple personality disorder)

Depersonalization disorder

Dissociative disorder not otherwise specified

---

way hypnosis"). An even more common example is the daydreaming that nearly all of us engage in at one time or another. These are both examples of normative dissociation, while hypnosis and meditation are examples of induced forms of dissociation. In these situations, it has been suggested that dissociation serves an adaptive function by allowing the mind to process the events of daily life. In some people, however, the dissociative process becomes distorted, and actively interferes with one's functioning and quality of life.

Amnestic States

Psychologically induced memory loss is called *dissociative amnesia* (see Table 8–9). The disorder is defined as one or more episodes of inability to recall important personal information, usually of a traumatic or stressful nature, that is considered too extensive to be explained by ordinary forgetfulness. With dissociative amnesia, the person is typically confused and perplexed. He or she may not recall significant personal information or even his or her own name. The amnesia typically develops suddenly and can last from minutes to days, or even longer. In one case series, 79% of the amnestic episodes lasted less than a week.

The prevalence of dissociative amnesia is unknown, but it has been reported to occur following severe physical or psychosocial stressors (e.g., natural disasters, war). In a study of combat veterans, between 5% and 20% were amnesic for their combat experiences. It has been estimated that from 5% to 14% of all military psychiatric casualties experience some degree of amnesia.

Dissociative fugue is characterized by amnesia with inability to recall one's past and the assumption of a new identity, which may be partial or complete (see Table 8–10). The fugue usually involves sudden, unexpected travel away from home or one's workplace, is not due to a dissociative identity disorder, and is not induced by a substance or a

---

TABLE 8–9. DSM-IV-TR diagnostic criteria for dissociative amnesia

A. The predominant disturbance is one or more episodes of inability to recall important personal information, usually of a traumatic or stressful nature, that is too extensive to be explained by ordinary forgetfulness.

B. The disturbance does not occur exclusively during the course of Dissociative Identity Disorder, Dissociative Fugue, Posttraumatic Stress Disorder, Acute Stress Disorder, or Somatization Disorder and is not due to the direct physiological effects of a substance (e.g., a drug of abuse, a medication) or a neurological or other general medical condition (e.g., Amnestic Disorder Due to Head Trauma).

C. The symptoms cause clinically significant distress or impairment in social, occupational, or other important areas of functioning.

TABLE 8–10. DSM-IV-TR diagnostic criteria for dissociative fugue

A. The predominant disturbance is sudden, unexpected travel away from home or one's customary place of work, with inability to recall one's past.

B. Confusion about personal identity or assumption of a new identity (partial or complete).

C. The disturbance does not occur exclusively during the course of Dissociative Identity Disorder and is not due to the direct physiological effects of a substance (e.g., a drug of abuse, a medication) or a general medical condition (e.g., temporal lobe epilepsy).

D. The symptoms cause clinically significant distress or impairment in social, occupational, or other important areas of functioning.

---

general medical condition (e.g., temporal lobe epilepsy). Like dissociative amnesia, fugue states are reported to occur in psychologically stressful situations, such as natural disasters or war. Personal rejections, losses, or financial pressures are reported to have preceded the fugue in some cases. Fugues can last for months and lead to a complicated pattern of travel and identity formation.

The case of a woman who had a fugue follows:

Carrie, a 31-year-old attorney from a small Midwestern town, was reported as missing for 4 days under mysterious circumstances. Carrie was known to have finished her day at work and to have exercised at a health spa but had failed to return home. Her car was found abandoned.

A search was mounted, and it was assumed that she had been abducted or murdered, especially after a headless corpse was found. Candlelight vigils were held, psychics were consulted, and friends blanketed the community with posters offering rewards for help in locating her.

One month after her disappearance, Carrie called her father from Las Vegas, where she had been the entire time. She was at a local hospital and claimed to have had amnesia. Carrie reported that she had been physically assaulted while jogging on the night of her disappearance. During the struggle, she had been knocked unconscious: "When I came to, I was dazed, confused, and disoriented." She felt that the assault prompted the amnesia, leading her to forget her past. She later hitchhiked to Las Vegas, where she was found wandering aimlessly. The police took her to a nearby hospital, where she claimed a new identity.

With the help of a psychologist who used hypnosis, Carrie quickly recovered her memory and her identity. She returned home and resumed her legal practice. Her family and friends had described her as a "creature of habit" and were as baffled as was Carrie about her amnesia. She had no history of mental illness.

The differential diagnosis of dissociative amnesia or fugue includes many medical and neurological conditions that can cause memory impairment (e.g., a brain tumor, closed head trauma, dementia) as well as the effects of a substance (e.g., alcohol-induced blackouts). Before assuming that the amnesia or fugue is psychologically motivated, medical and neurological conditions and substance abuse must be ruled out. A workup should include a thorough physical examination, mental status examination, toxicological studies, an electroencephalogram, and other tests when indicated (e.g., magnetic resonance imaging brain scan).

As a general rule, the onset and termination of amnestic and fugue states due to medical illness or a substance are unlikely to be associated with psychological stress. Memory impairment due to brain injury is likely to be more severe for recent than for remote events and to resolve slowly if at all; in these cases, memory only rarely recovers fully. Disturbances in attention, orientation, and affect are characteristic of many brain disorders (e.g., brain tumors, strokes, Alzheimer's disease) but are unlikely in dissociative amnesia. Memory loss from alcohol intoxication (blackouts) is characterized by impaired short-term recall and evidence of heavy substance abuse. *Malingering* involves claiming amnesia for behaviors that are alleged to be out of character when obvious reasons exist for secondary gain (e.g., claiming amnesia for a crime). Careful observation in a hospital setting can help to clarify the diagnosis.

There is no established treatment for dissociative amnesia or fugue, and recovery tends to occur spontaneously. For some persons, a safe environment such as that found in a psychiatric hospital may foster recovery. As the name *fugue* implies, the condition involves psychological flight from overwhelming circumstances, and once these circumstances are resolved, the dissociative fugue resolves as well. In fugue states, recovery of past memories and the resumption of the individual's former identity may occur abruptly (i.e., over several hours) but can take much longer. Both conditions can recur, particularly when the precipitating stressors remain or return. Hypnosis and interviews conducted under the influence of intravenous sodium amobarbital (narcoanalysis) have been reported to help patients recover missing memories. When memories return, patients should be helped to understand the reason for their memory loss and to reinforce healthy coping mechanisms.

Dissociative Identity Disorder (Multiple Personality Disorder)

Dissociative identity disorder (DID) is characterized by the presence of two or more distinct identities or personality states, each with its own relatively enduring pattern of perceiving, relating to, and thinking about the environment and self (see Table 8–11). A personality state is not as well developed or integrated in either thinking or behavior as an identity. In some cases, there may be at least two fully developed identities, whereas in others there may be only one distinct identity and one or more personality states. According to DSM-IV-TR, at least two identities or personality states recurrently take full control of the person's behavior. Although DID has been described for centuries, most lay conceptions are based on media portrayals, the most famous of which are found in *The Three Faces of Eve* and *Sybil*. Both provide detailed accounts of women with many strikingly different personalities.

The prevalence of DID is unknown, but it is likely uncommon. The number of reported cases has grown in the past few decades, and some experts believe that the disorder is common in both inpatient and outpatient settings. This reported increase in frequency has led some to question whether well-meaning therapists might unwittingly induce the phenomenon through attention, suggestion, and the process of hypnosis. These methods are thought by some to lead to the creation of additional personalities in suggestible patients. These same experts observe that many personalities disappear when ignored by the therapist.

From 75% to 90% of patients with DID are women. The disorder is thought to have a childhood onset, usually before age 9 years, and is of-

TABLE 8–11.   DSM-IV-TR diagnostic criteria for dissociative identity disorder

A. The presence of two or more distinct identities or personality states (each with its own relatively enduring pattern of perceiving, relating to, and thinking about the environment and self).
B. At least two of these identities or personality states recurrently take control of the person's behavior.
C. Inability to recall important personal information that is too extensive to be explained by ordinary forgetfulness.
D. The disturbance is not due to the direct physiological effects of a substance (e.g., blackouts or chaotic behavior during Alcohol Intoxication) or a general medical condition (e.g., complex partial seizures).   **Note:** In children, the symptoms are not attributable to imaginary playmates or other fantasy play.

ten chronic. DID may be familial; it has been described as occurring in multiple generations and among siblings.

The cause of DID is unknown. Some researchers believe that the disorder results from severe physical and sexual abuse during early childhood. They hypothesize that DID results from self-induced hypnosis, used by the individual to cope with abuse, emotional maltreatment, or neglect. Some compare DID to posttraumatic stress disorder (PTSD), a condition that develops in response to life-threatening situations. Like persons with PTSD, DID patients are reported to have smaller hippocampal and amygdalar volumes, suggesting that early traumatic experiences may affect neural circuitry alterations in brain areas associated with memory.

In one large case series, the mean number of personalities (or "alters") in DID patients was 7, and approximately one-half had more than 10. Different alters are reported to control an individual's behavior for varying lengths of time. The transition from one alter to another may be sudden or gradual. Switches have been observed with stressful situations, disputes among the alters, and psychological conflicts. Some alters seem to know about the other personalities, while others are unaware of them.

Some of the more common symptoms reported by patients with DID, as well as characteristics of their alters, are presented in Table 8–12.

The case of a patient with DID follows:

Cindy, a 24-year-old woman, was transferred to the psychiatry service to facilitate community placement. Over the years, she had received many different diagnoses, including chronic schizophrenia, borderline

TABLE 8–12. Common symptoms in 50 patients with dissociative identity disorder and characteristics of alternate personalities ("alters")

Symptoms	%	Alternate-personality characteristics	%
Markedly different moods	94	Amnestic personalities	100
Exhibiting an alter	84	Personalities with proper	98
Different accents	68	names (e.g., Nick, Sally)	
Inability to remember angry	58	Angry alternate personality	80
outbursts		Depressed alternate	74
Inner conversations	58	personality	
Different handwriting	34	Personalities of different ages	66
Different dress or makeup	32	Suicidal alternate personality	62
Unfamiliar people know	18	Protector alternate	30
them well		personality	
Amnesia for a previously	14	Self-abusive alternate	30
learned subject		personality	
Discovery of unfamiliar	14	Opposite-sexed alternate	26
possessions		personality	
Different handedness	14	Personality with nonproper	24
		names (e.g., "observer," "teacher")	
		Unnamed alternate	18
		personality	

Source. Adapted from Coons et al. 1988.

personality disorder, schizoaffective disorder, and bipolar disorder. DID was her current diagnosis.

Cindy had been well until 3 years before admission, when she developed depression, "voices," multiple somatic complaints, periods of amnesia, and wrist cutting. Her family and friends considered her a pathological liar because she would do or say things that she would later deny. Chronic depression and recurrent suicidal behavior led to frequent hospitalizations. Cindy had trials of antipsychotics, antidepressants, mood stabilizers, and anxiolytics, all without benefit. Her condition continued to worsen.

Cindy was a petite, neatly groomed woman who cooperated well with the treatment team. She reported having nine distinct alters that ranged in age from 2 to 48 years; two were masculine. Cindy's main concern was her inability to control the switches among the alters, which made her feel out of control. She reported having been sexually abused by her father as a child and described visual hallucinations of him threatening her with a knife. We were unable to confirm the history of sexual abuse but thought it likely, based on what we knew of her chaotic early home life.

Nursing staff observed several episodes in which Cindy switched to one of her troublesome alters. Her voice would change in inflection and tone, becoming childlike when Joy, an 8-year-old alter, took control. Arrangements were made for individual psychotherapy, and Cindy was discharged.

At a follow-up 3 years later, Cindy still had many alters but was functioning better, had fewer switches, and lived independently. She continued to see a therapist weekly and hoped to one day integrate her many alters.

Patients with DID often meet criteria for other psychiatric disorders. Like Cindy, many have unexplained physical complaints and fulfill criteria for somatization disorder. Headaches and amnesia ("losing time") are particularly common symptoms. Borderline personality disorder, found in up to 70% of DID patients, is diagnosed on the basis of mood instability, identity disturbance, deliberate self-harm, and other symptoms characteristic of the disorder. Many DID patients report psychotic symptoms such as auditory hallucinations ("voices"), and many will have a past diagnosis of schizophrenia, schizoaffective disorder, or psychotic mood disorder. These diagnoses need to be ruled out.

Patients with DID tend to report that the voices originate within their heads, are not experienced with the ears, and are not associated with mood changes; insight generally is preserved. By contrast, patients with psychotic disorders usually report that auditory hallucinations "come from the outside," have the quality of a percept (as opposed to one's own thoughts), and are accompanied by changes in mood; insight is minimal. Hallucinations that accompany DID are probably best considered *pseudohallucinations*—that is, hallucinations that are a product of one's own mind and are accompanied by the realization that the experience is due to illness and is not real.

There is no standard treatment for DID, but many clinicians recommend long-term individual psychotherapy to help patients integrate their many alters. When in a crisis, DID patients may benefit from inpatient hospitalization. Once stable, they may benefit from the structure found in a partial hospital or residential treatment program. At least one study has shown that motivated patients treated by experienced therapists can achieve integration and remission of symptoms. Other aspects of treatment remain controversial. Hypnosis or narcoanalysis have been recommended to help access the different alters in the con-

---

TABLE 8–13. DSM-IV-TR diagnostic criteria for depersonalization disorder

---

A. Persistent or recurrent experiences of feeling detached from, and as if one is an outside observer of, one's mental processes or body (e.g., feeling like one is in a dream).
B. During the depersonalization experience, reality testing remains intact.
C. The depersonalization causes clinically significant distress or impairment in social, occupational, or other important areas of functioning.
D. The depersonalization experience does not occur exclusively during the course of another mental disorder, such as Schizophrenia, Panic Disorder, Acute Stress Disorder, or another Dissociative Disorder, and is not due to the direct physiological effects of a substance (e.g., a drug of abuse, a medication) or a general medical condition (e.g., temporal lobe epilepsy).

---

text of psychotherapy. CBT has also been used to help patients achieve reintegration. All experts agree that therapy is lengthy and challenging.

Although the core features of DID do not respond to medication, typical patients have mood and anxiety symptoms that may respond to drug therapy. For example, antidepressants may relieve coexisting major depression and block panic attacks.

Depersonalization Disorder

Depersonalization disorder is characterized by feeling detached from oneself or one's surroundings, as though one were an outside observer; some patients experience a dreamlike state (see Table 8–13). A patient with depersonalization may feel as though he or she were cut off from his or her thoughts, emotions, or identity. Another may feel like a robot or automaton. Depersonalization may be accompanied by *derealization*, a sense of detachment, unreality, and altered relation to the outside world.

The prevalence of depersonalization disorder is unknown, but it is more common in women. Many people who are otherwise normal transiently experience mild depersonalization. For example, depersonalization may occur when a person is sleep deprived, travels to unfamiliar places, or is intoxicated with hallucinogens, marijuana, or alcohol. In a study of college students, one-third to one-half reported having experienced transient depersonalization. Persons exposed to life-threatening situations, such as traumatic accidents, may also experience depersonalization. For these reasons, depersonalization disorder is diagnosed only when it is persistent and causes distress.

The disorder starts in adolescence or early adulthood but rarely after age 40 years. Many persons vividly recall their first episode of depersonalization, which may begin abruptly. Some report a precipitating event, such as smoking marijuana. The duration of depersonalization episodes is highly variable, but they can last hours, days, or even weeks. Although depersonalization disorder is typically experienced as chronic and continuous, some persons experience periods of remission. Exacerbations may follow psychologically stressful situations, such as the loss of an important relationship.

The cause of depersonalization disorder is unknown. Freud postulated that depersonalization allows a person to deny painful or unacceptable feelings. It also could represent an adaptive response to life-threatening danger, perhaps serving as a buffer against extreme emotions such as fear. The fact that depersonalization frequently accompanies several central nervous system disturbances (e.g., partial complex seizures, tumors, stroke, encephalitis, migraine) suggests a biological basis. One recent theory holds that the state of increased alertness seen in depersonalization disorder results from activation of the prefrontal attentional systems combined with reciprocal inhibition of the anterior cingulate, causing "mind emptiness."

Psychiatric disorders in which depersonalization symptoms sometimes occur must be ruled out, such as schizophrenia, major depression, phobias, panic disorder, obsessive-compulsive disorder, and drug abuse. Medical illness (e.g., partial complex seizures, migraine), sleep deprivation, and drug-induced states need to be ruled out as well.

There are no standard treatments for depersonalization, but benzodiazepines may be helpful in reducing the accompanying anxiety (e.g., diazepam, 5 mg three times daily). SSRIs and clomipramine have been reported to relieve symptoms of depersonalization, although in a controlled trial fluoxetine proved ineffective. Patients also have been reported to benefit from hypnotherapy or CBT to help control their episodes of depersonalization. With CBT, patients learn to confront their distorted thoughts and challenge their feelings of unreality.

Key points to remember about dissociative disorders

1. Medical causes (e.g., tumors, temporal lobe epilepsy) must be ruled out as a cause of the amnesia, dissociation, or depersonalization.

Key points to remember about dissociative disorders *(continued)*

2. The therapist should be patient and supportive. In most cases of amnesia, return of memory is rapid and complete.

3. Patients with DID are especially challenging, and therapy may be long-term. The clinician may want to refer the patient to a therapist experienced in treating DID.

   • It may be best to help the patient gradually learn about the number and nature of his or her alters.

   • A goal with these patients should be to help them function better and to bring about better communication among the alters.

4. Medications have no proven benefit in treating dissociative disorders, although antidepressants may help some patients with depersonalization disorder.

   • Benzodiazepines may help to reduce the anxiety that often accompanies depersonalization.

■ Factitious Disorders and Malingering

Factitious disorders and malingering are conditions in which physical or emotional illness or amnesia is mimicked. Factitious disorders have their own category in DSM-IV-TR, whereas malingering is grouped with the V-code conditions. These are conditions not attributed to mental illness but are a focus of attention or treatment.

Factitious Disorders

Factitious disorders involve the intentional production (or feigning) of physical or psychological symptoms. Patients with factitious disorders have no obvious external incentive for the behavior, such as economic gain. Rather, they are thought to be motivated by an unconscious desire to occupy the sick role.

Some persons with the disorder appear to make hospitalization a way of life and have been called "hospital hobos" or "peregrinating problem patients." The term *Munchausen syndrome* also has been used to describe patients who move from hospital to hospital simulating various illnesses. The name *Munchausen* comes from the fictitious wander-

TABLE 8–14.   Methods used to produce symptoms in patients with a factitious disorder

Method	%
Injection or insertion of contaminated substance	29
Surreptitious use of medications	24
Exacerbation of wounds	17
Thermometer manipulation	10
Urinary tract manipulation	7
Falsification of medical history	7
Self-induced bruises or deformities	2
Phlebotomy	2

Source.   Adapted from Reich and Gottfried 1983.

ings of the nineteenth-century Baron von Münchhausen, known for his tall tales and fanciful exaggeration. Cases of Munchausen syndrome by proxy have also been observed. In this instance, a parent induces (or simulates) illness in his or her child so that the child is repeatedly hospitalized.

The frequency of factitious disorder is unknown because many cases go undetected. In one study involving persons with a fever of unknown origin, up to 10% of the fevers were diagnosed as factitious. Most cases of factitious disorder involve the simulation of physical illness. Patients typically use one of three strategies to feign illness: 1) they report symptoms suggesting an illness, without having them; 2) they produce false evidence of an illness (e.g., a factitious fever produced by applying friction to a thermometer to raise the temperature); or 3) they intentionally produce symptoms of illness (e.g., by injecting feces to produce infection or taking warfarin orally to induce a bleeding disorder). Some of the more common methods for producing symptoms are presented in Table 8–14.

A factitious mental illness is probably much less common. The diagnosis can be extremely difficult to make because of the lack of objective physical or laboratory abnormalities associated with psychiatric disorders. In a follow-up of nine patients with factitious psychosis, the patients remained emotionally disturbed and had poor social functioning.

Factitious disorders are chronic and begin in early adulthood. They often develop in people who have had experience with hospitalization

TABLE 8–15.   Differentiating among the somatoform disorders, factitious disorders, and malingering

Disorder	Mechanism of illness production	Motivation for illness production
Somatoform disorders[a]	Unconscious	Unconscious
Factitious disorder	Conscious	Unconscious
Malingering	Conscious	Conscious

[a]Includes somatization disorder, conversion disorder, hypochondriasis, and pain disorder.
Source. Adapted from Eisendrath 1984.

or severe illness involving either themselves or someone close to them (e.g., a parent). The disorder can severely impair social and occupational functioning and is usually associated with the presence of a personality disorder (e.g., borderline personality disorder). In one study, most of the factitious disorder patients had worked in health care occupations. Most had maladaptive personality traits, but none had a diagnosis of a major mental disorder, such as depression or schizophrenia. Nearly all were women.

Some experts believe that the patient with factitious disorder consciously produces the signs or symptoms of physical illness to obtain medical care. Patients are aware of their role in producing signs and symptoms of illness yet are unaware of their motivation for doing so. According to one interpretation, factitious disorder patients have experienced emotional deprivation at the hands of absent or inattentive parents but received love and attention from health care givers. By producing illness, these patients re-create the nurturing atmosphere that they experienced earlier in their lives from caregivers.

The differentiation of factitious disorder from somatoform disorders and malingering, based on presumed psychological mechanisms, is shown in Table 8–15.

The diagnosis of a factitious disorder requires almost as much inventiveness as is shown by the patient in producing symptoms. Clues to the diagnosis include a lengthy and involved medical history that does not correspond to the patient's apparent health and vigor, a clinical presentation that too closely resembles textbook descriptions, a sophisticated medical vocabulary, demands for specific medications or treatments, and a history of excessive surgeries. Previous hospital charts should be gathered and prior clinicians contacted when a factitious disorder is suspected.

In one intriguing case reported in the literature, the authors were able to document at least 15 different hospitalizations in a 2-year period and found that medical evaluations had included repeated cardiac catheterizations and angiograms. Complications from the procedures had eventually resulted in the loss of a limb. In this particular patient, clues to the diagnosis included the manner in which the patient presented his story, the absence of family or friends at the hospital, the presence of multiple surgical scars, and an absence of distress despite complaints of crushing retrosternal pain.

The treatment of factitious disorder is difficult and frustrating. The first task is to make the diagnosis so that additional and potentially harmful procedures can be avoided. Because many of these patients are hospitalized on medical and surgical wards, a psychiatric consultation should be obtained. The psychiatrist can help make the diagnosis and educate the treatment team about the nature of factitious disorders. Once sufficient evidence has been assembled to support the diagnosis, the patient should be confronted in a nonthreatening manner by the attending physician and the consulting psychiatrist. In a follow-up of 42 patients with factitious disorder, 33 were confronted. None signed out of the hospital or became suicidal, but only 13 acknowledged causing their disorders. Nevertheless, most improved after the confrontation, and 4 became asymptomatic. The authors reported that their lawyers had advised that room searches could be justified legally and ethically in the pursuit of a diagnosis. Like the suicidal patient whose belongings may be searched for dangerous objects, the factitious disorder patient also has a potentially life-threatening condition that justifies such measures.

Malingering

Malingering is the intentional production of false or grossly exaggerated physical or psychological symptoms motivated by external incentives, such as avoiding military conscription or duty, avoiding work, obtaining financial compensation, evading criminal prosecution, obtaining drugs, or securing better living conditions.

Unlike factitious disorder, in which symptoms are produced for presumably unconscious reasons, malingering is intentional for reasons that are apparent to the malingerer. Most malingerers are male, and most have obvious reasons to feign illness. Many are prisoners, factory workers, or persons living in unpleasant situations (e.g., homeless persons). An illness may provide an escape from a harsh reality, while the hospital may offer a temporary sanctuary.

Malingering should be suspected when any of the following clues are present: medicolegal context of presentation (e.g., the person is being referred by his or her attorney for examination); marked discrepancy between the person's claimed disability and objective findings; lack of cooperation during the diagnostic evaluation and noncompliance with the treatment regimen; and the presence of an antisocial personality disorder. Symptoms reported by malingering patients are often vague, subjective, and unverifiable.

There is some debate about the correct approach to take with the malingerer. Some experts believe that malingering patients should be confronted after sufficient evidence has been collected to confirm the diagnosis. Others feel that confrontations will simply disrupt the doctor–patient relationship and make the patient even more alert to possible future detection. Clinicians who take the second position feel that the best approach is to treat the patient as though the symptoms were real. The symptoms can then be given up in response to treatment without the patient losing face.

■ Self-Assessment Questions

1. How is somatization disorder diagnosed? Hypochondriasis? Pain disorder?

2. What do family studies of somatization disorder show?

3. What are the risk factors for conversion disorder?

4. What is the natural history of the different somatoform disorders?

5. How does somatization disorder differ from hypochondriasis?

6. What are the common features of body dysmorphic disorder?

7. How are the somatoform disorders managed?

8. How does dissociative amnesia differ from dissociative fugue?

9. What is the differential diagnosis of the dissociative disorders?

10. What is a current etiological theory of DID?

11. What is depersonalization, and how common is it?

12. How are the somatoform disorders, factitious disorders, and malingering similar? How are they different?

CHAPTER 9

Alcohol- and Drug-Related Disorders

I persevered in my abstinence for ninety hours. . . . Then I took—ask me not
how much; say, ye severest, what would ye have done?

Thomas De Quincey, Confessions
of an English Opium Eater

A LITERAL CORNUCOPIA of psychoactive drugs is readily
available in the United States, many of them used inappropriately,
leading to abuse and addiction. Alcohol is perhaps the oldest and
most important of these, but many other substances also have been
around since antiquity. Many of the newer drugs are a product of
modern organic chemistry techniques, and additional drugs continue to be synthesized at a dizzying pace.

The problems resulting from the misuse of alcohol or other drugs
appear more extensive today than in the past, probably because of the
increased availability of a growing number of substances that are subject to experimentation and use. Drug-related problems cut across
social and economic boundaries. All age groups are affected, but particularly prone are adolescents and young adults. Because of the near-
epidemic abuse of alcohol and other drugs and the understandable
public concern, the federal government has responded by increasing
research funding. Tough federal and state laws mandating heavy

TABLE 9–1. Categories of substance use disorders

Alcohol	Hallucinogens
Sedatives, hypnotics, and anxiolytics	Phencyclidine
Barbiturates	Cannabis
Nonbarbiturates (e.g., meprobamate)	
Benzodiazepines	Inhalants
Opioids	Other substances
Heroin	Nicotine
Oxycodone	Caffeine
Codeine	Anabolic steroids
Hydrocodone	Nitrate inhalants
Morphine	Nitrous oxide
Stimulants	
Amphetamines	
Methylphenidate	
Cocaine	

penalties for both drug possession and drug distribution have been enacted. One unintended consequence has been the rapid growth in arrests and incarceration for drug-related offenses. Presidential commissions have been appointed, and since 1989 a drug "czar" has been in place to coordinate drug containment efforts. At the same time, the disease concept of substance abuse has taken hold, encouraging problem drinkers and drug abusers alike to seek help in a humane and nonjudgmental way. Nonetheless, receiving appropriate treatment in an overburdened and poorly funded system is an ongoing challenge.

In this chapter, we review the major categories of substance use disorders: alcohol; sedatives, hypnotics, and anxiolytics; opioids; central nervous system (CNS) stimulants; hallucinogens; phencyclidine (PCP); cannabis; and inhalants. Nicotine, caffeine, anabolic steroids, nitrate inhalants, and nitrous oxide also are discussed in this chapter. (See Table 9–1 for a list of the categories and substances of abuse.)

■ Definition

The concept of a general drug-dependent syndrome is embedded in DSM-IV-TR and has been endorsed by the World Health Organization. For this reason, all substance use disorders, including alcohol abuse and

TABLE 9–2. DSM-IV-TR diagnostic criteria for substance abuse

A. A maladaptive pattern of substance use leading to clinically significant impairment or distress, as manifested by one (or more) of the following, occurring within a 12-month period:

   (1) recurrent substance use resulting in a failure to fulfill major role obligations at work, school, or home (e.g., repeated absences or poor work performance related to substance use; substance-related absences, suspensions, or expulsions from school; neglect of children or household)

   (2) recurrent substance use in situations in which it is physically hazardous (e.g., driving an automobile or operating a machine when impaired by substance use)

   (3) recurrent substance-related legal problems (e.g., arrests for substance-related disorderly conduct)

   (4) continued substance use despite having persistent or recurrent social or interpersonal problems caused or exacerbated by the effects of the substance (e.g., arguments with spouse about consequences of intoxication, physical fights)

B. The symptoms have never met the criteria for Substance Dependence for this class of substance.

dependence, follow the same set of criteria (Tables 9–2 and 9–3). The definition of *substance abuse* requires a maladaptive pattern of substance use leading to significant impairment or distress, as manifested in at least one of four problem areas (e.g., job, physical hazard, legal, interpersonal), occurring during a 12-month period. Furthermore, the person has never met criteria for substance dependence.

The definition of *substance dependence* requires that the person have at least three of seven problem behaviors at any time during a 12-month period. The criteria focus on substance use behavior, impairment caused by substance use, and the development of tolerance or withdrawal. Substance dependence is subtyped as occurring with or without physiological dependence (i.e., evidence of either withdrawal or tolerance). These criteria are geared toward separating individuals whose use of a substance is hazardous (dependence) from those whose use is merely harmful (abuse). The distinction is not always clear, and considerable overlap exists between abuse and dependence. These disorders are probably better thought of as lying along a continuum, with dependence at the severe end of the spectrum. In this chapter, the terms *alcoholic* and *alcoholism* will be used interchangeably with alcohol dependence.

TABLE 9–3.   DSM-IV-TR diagnostic criteria for substance dependence

A maladaptive pattern of substance use, leading to clinically significant impairment or distress, as manifested by three (or more) of the following, occurring at any time in the same 12-month period:
(1) tolerance, as defined by either of the following:
    (a) a need for markedly increased amounts of the substance to achieve intoxication or desired effect
    (b) markedly diminished effect with continued use of the same amount of the substance
(2) withdrawal, as manifested by either of the following:
    (a) the characteristic withdrawal syndrome for the substance (refer to Criteria A and B of the criteria sets for Withdrawal from the specific substances)
    (b) the same (or a closely related) substance is taken to relieve or avoid withdrawal symptoms
(3) the substance is often taken in larger amounts or over a longer period than was intended
(4) there is a persistent desire or unsuccessful efforts to cut down or control substance use
(5) a great deal of time is spent in activities necessary to obtain the substance (e.g., visiting multiple doctors or driving long distances), use the substance (e.g., chain-smoking), or recover from its effects
(6) important social, occupational, or recreational activities are given up or reduced because of substance use
(7) the substance use is continued despite knowledge of having a persistent or recurrent physical or psychological problem that is likely to have been caused or exacerbated by the substance (e.g., current cocaine use despite recognition of cocaine-induced depression, or continued drinking despite recognition that an ulcer was made worse by alcohol consumption)
Specify if:
    With Physiological Dependence: evidence of tolerance or withdrawal (i.e., either Item 1 or 2 is present)
    Without Physiological Dependence: no evidence of tolerance or withdrawal (i.e., neither Item 1 nor 2 is present)
Course specifiers:
    Early Full Remission
    Early Partial Remission
    Sustained Full Remission
    Sustained Partial Remission
    On Agonist Therapy
    In a Controlled Environment

■ Alcohol-Related Disorders

Nearly two-thirds of American adults occasionally drink alcoholic beverages, whereas 12% are heavy drinkers—that is, they drink almost every day and become intoxicated several times a month. Drinkers tend to be young, relatively prosperous, well educated, and urban. The lifetime prevalence for alcohol dependence is almost 14%; in any given 6-month period, 5% of persons will meet criteria for lifetime alcohol dependence. In hospitals, the prevalence is far greater. From 25% to 50% of medical-surgical patients in general hospitals are alcohol dependent, and an estimated 50%–60% of psychiatric inpatients in some settings have coexisting alcoholism or some other drug use disorder.

There are about two to three alcoholic men for each alcoholic woman, and the usual age at onset is between 16 and 30 years. Onset in men occurs earlier than in women, although the medical complications of alcoholism progress more rapidly in women. People in certain occupations are prone to alcoholism, including waitstaff, bartenders, longshoremen, and writers. Other groups prone to alcoholism include people with antisocial personality disorder and people with anxiety or mood disorders.

A simple classification for alcoholism has been developed based on demographic and clinical distinctions. *Type I* alcoholic persons are characterized by an adult onset; gradually increasing consumption; personality characteristics of guilt, worry, dependency, and introversion; little or no family history of alcoholism; equal prevalence in men and women; and a better response to treatment than Type II alcoholism.

Type II alcoholic persons are characterized by early onset; personality characteristics of impulsivity, distractibility, and recklessness; presence of antisocial personality disorder; a strong family history of alcoholism; male gender; and poor treatment response.

Diagnosis

Alcohol use disorders can usually be diagnosed on the basis of a careful history and mental status examination. Because many alcoholic persons deny their illness or underestimate the extent of their drinking, it is helpful to gather information from family members or other informants when alcoholism is suspected. The four-question CAGE test is a simple screen for the presence of alcohol abuse or dependence (see Table 9–4). Any positive or overly defensive answer suggests that a problem exists.

Blood alcohol concentration can be useful in detecting alcohol abuse or dependence. In fact, blood alcohol levels can be roughly correlated to

TABLE 9-4.   CAGE: Screening test for alcohol abuse or dependence

C	Have you felt the need to CUT DOWN on your drinking?
A	Have you felt ANNOYED BY CRITICISM of your drinking?
G	Have you felt GUILTY (or had regrets) about your drinking?
E	Have you felt the need for an EYE-OPENER in the morning?

Source.   Adapted from Ewing 1984.

level of intoxication. The following levels apply to persons without tolerance to alcohol:

0–100 mg/dL: A sense of well-being, sedation, tranquility
100–150 mg/dL: Incoordination, irritability
150–250 mg/dL: Slurred speech, ataxia
>250 mg/dL: Passing out, unconsciousness

With even higher concentrations—greater than 350 mg/dL—an individual can become comatose and die. The presence of few clinical symptoms of intoxication in a person with a level of 150 mg/dL or higher is strong evidence of alcoholism.

Alcohol is the only drug for which intoxication has been legally defined on the basis of a laboratory test. In many jurisdictions, a motor vehicle operator is considered legally under the influence at a blood alcohol concentration of 0.08 g per 100 mL, equivalent to 80 mg/dL. In hospitals and clinics, blood samples are used to test for blood alcohol levels, but breath testing for alcohol has become a standard part of the roadside assessment for driving impairment.

Other laboratory measures are useful but not diagnostic. Alcoholic persons may develop increased high-density lipoprotein cholesterol, increased lactate dehydroxygenase, decreased low-density lipoprotein cholesterol, decreased blood urea nitrogen, decreased red blood cell volume, and increased uric acid level. Mean corpuscular volume is increased in up to 95% of alcoholic persons. Thirty percent of alcoholic persons have evidence of an old rib or vertebral fracture on chest X-ray (compared with 1% of control subjects). Liver enzymes are frequently abnormal. γ-Glutamyltransferase (GGT) is increased in about 75% of alcoholic persons and may be the earliest laboratory sign of alcoholism. Transaminase (aspartate aminotransferase and alanine aminotransferase) levels also are increased. One study showed that a combination of elevated serum GGT and elevated erythrocyte mean corpuscular volume identified 90% of alcoholic patients.

Clinical Findings

Because both drinking patterns and symptoms vary widely, there is no standard or general clinical picture of the alcoholic person. In its earliest stages, alcoholism is difficult to identify because symptoms are few, and the alcoholic person may deny excessive drinking. Family members and coworkers are often in the best position to identify early symptoms, which may include a subtle change in work habits or productivity, lateness or unexplained absences, or minor personality changes such as irritability or moodiness.

As alcoholism progresses, minor physical changes can occur, including the development of acne rosacea (an enlarged, reddened nose); the development of palmar erythema (reddened palms associated with higher estrogen levels circulating in the blood of alcoholic persons); or the development of painless enlargement of the liver consistent with fatty infiltration, the earliest form of alcoholic liver disease. Other early manifestations of early alcoholism include unexplained respiratory or other infections, unexplained bruises, periods of amnesia (blackouts), minor traumatic accidents (e.g., unexplained falls at home), complaints by others about the drinker's driving skills, or an arrest (or accident) related to driving while intoxicated. Advancing signs of liver disease can develop, such as jaundice or ascites. Testicular atrophy, gynecomastia, and Dupuytren's contractures can occur. At this point, alcoholism is likely to disrupt the person's life and to lead to job loss, marital discord, and family problems.

The following patient illustrates many of the clinical symptoms and findings of alcoholism and is an example of a person with Type I alcoholism:

> Ed, a 66-year-old attorney, was brought to an alcohol rehabilitation unit by his wife and son. On arrival, he smelled of alcohol and was mildly disheveled. In a belligerent manner, and slurring his words, Ed said that he would not stay. His wife intervened and told him firmly that she would file for divorce if he refused to stay and get help. He stayed.
>
> Ed had a 20-year history of excessive drinking. He had started drinking socially while in the Army. After his military service he had married, obtained his law degree, and established a successful career as a trial attorney. Although he sometimes enjoyed a single beer or cocktail after work, the drinking never progressed. Then, in his mid-40s, his alcohol consumption began to escalate. Ed would drink several beers or

cocktails in the evening and then fall asleep. He and his wife began to fight, mainly about his drinking, which he denied was a problem. A series of personal crises followed. Ed had an affair with a divorcée, separated from his wife, and eventually sought a divorce. He had a falling-out with his law partners and withdrew from his longtime friends. His drinking took a more serious turn. His caseload decreased as lawyers in his town became increasingly aware of his impairment. He began to drink in the morning, had several cocktails at lunch, and continued his drinking in the evening, finally passing out on the sofa. He continued to deny his alcoholism, even when confronted by his new wife and all his children. He pointed out that he was still able to work and was not a skid row bum.

His doctor became concerned. Ed was overweight and hypertensive and had developed the stigmata of alcoholism: spider angiomata, acne rosacea, and palmar erythema. The progression of his alcoholism was so gradual that by the time of hospital admission, no one could remember what Ed's personality had once been like.

The inpatient program consisted of individual, group, and family therapy sessions following an uneventful withdrawal. By the end of his 30-day stay, he was noticeably happier, was more optimistic, and looked forward to the future. Three years later, he was still abstinent, had developed a more satisfying relationship with his wife and children, and had reestablished his law practice.

Complications

Alcoholism can affect a person's medical and emotional health and lead to a broad range of social problems; these are summarized in Table 9–5. Medical problems range from benign fatty infiltration of the liver to fulminant liver failure. Almost all organ systems are affected by the heavy use of alcohol. The gastrointestinal tract is especially affected; early problems include gastritis and diarrhea. Peptic ulcers can develop or if present can be aggravated by the direct toxic effect that alcohol has on the mucosa. Fatty infiltration of the liver occurs in almost all alcoholic persons; cirrhosis will develop in about 10% of heavy drinkers. Pancreatitis can occur, leading to impaired digestion or diabetes mellitus. Cardiomyopathy, thrombocytopenia, anemia, and myopathy all have been reported.

The CNS and peripheral nervous system may be damaged by the direct and indirect effects of alcohol. Peripheral neuropathy commonly occurs in a stocking-and-glove distribution, probably the result of an alcohol-induced vitamin B deficiency. Cerebellar damage can cause dysarthria and ataxia. Wernicke's encephalopathy can result from thiamine deficiency and consists of nystagmus, ataxia, and mental confusion (which usually reverses with an injection of thiamine). The Wernicke-

TABLE 9–5. Medical and psychosocial hazards associated with alcoholism

Drug interactions	**Alcohol withdrawal syndromes**
Gastrointestinal	Uncomplicated alcohol
Esophageal bleeding	withdrawal (the "shakes")
Mallory-Weiss tear	Withdrawal seizures
Gastritis	Alcoholic hallucinosis
Intestinal malabsorption	Alcohol withdrawal delirium
Pancreatitis	(delirium tremens)
Liver disease	**Infectious disease**
Fatty infiltration	Pneumonia
Alcoholic hepatitis	Tuberculosis
Cirrhosis	**Cardiovascular**
Nutritional deficiency	Cardiomyopathy
Malnutrition	Hypertension
Vitamin B deficiency	**Cancer**
Neuropsychiatric	Oral cavity
Wernicke-Korsakoff syndrome	Esophagus
Cortical atrophy/ventricular	Large intestine/rectum
dilation	Liver
Alcohol-induced dementia	Pancreas
Peripheral neuropathy	**Birth defects**
Myopathy	Fetal alcohol syndrome
Depression	**Psychosocial**
Suicide	Accidents
Endocrine system	Crime
Testicular atrophy	Spouse and child abuse
Increased estrogen levels	Job loss
	Divorce, separation
	Legal entanglements

Korsakoff syndrome occurs when cognitive and memory impairment endures, although it may be reversible in one-third of patients. This syndrome involves an anterograde amnesia characterized by the presence of *confabulation,* in which a patient invents stories to fill in memory gaps. The syndrome is associated with necrotic lesions of the mamillary bodies, thalamus, and other brain stem regions.

Severely alcoholic persons can develop a frank dementia as a result of either vitamin deficiency or the direct effects of alcohol, although the exact cause is unknown. Chronic alcoholism also has been associated with enlarged cerebral ventricles and widened cortical sulci, effects that may be partially reversible when the individual stops drinking. Careful neuropsychological testing of alcoholic persons generally reveals mild to moderate cognitive deficits that like the structural abnormalities, partially reverse with sobriety.

A *fetal alcohol syndrome* (FAS) has been described in children whose mothers are alcoholic. This syndrome is related to excessive maternal consumption of alcohol during pregnancy, especially when binge drinking produces a surge in blood alcohol levels. Abnormalities associated with this disorder include facial anomalies (i.e., small head circumference, epicanthic folds, indistinct philtrum, small midface), low IQ, and behavior problems. FAS affects about one to two infants per 100,000 live births. Women should be warned that FAS can result from alcohol consumption during pregnancy.

Alcohol consumption is a frequent cause of traumatic injuries and contributes to more than one-half of all motor vehicle deaths each year. Household injuries also are common. This comes as no surprise, because alcoholic persons are often unsteady on their feet and accident prone, leading to falls, with resulting bruises, fractures, and lacerations. The highly publicized deaths of actors William Holden and Natalie Wood in the 1980s testify to the lethal nature of these accidents. Both sustained a fall while intoxicated, directly leading to their deaths. Subdural hematomas occur in many elderly alcoholic persons who fall and sustain head injuries; the impact tears the bridging veins within the skull.

Cancer rates of the mouth, tongue, larynx, esophagus, stomach, liver, and pancreas are increased. The precise role that alcohol plays in these cancers is uncertain because its effects are confounded by those of smoking and tobacco use. Alcohol interferes with male sexual function and can cause impotence and affect fertility by lowering serum testosterone levels. Increased circulating levels of female hormones (e.g., estrogen) can cause breast enlargement (gynecomastia) and a female escutcheon (pubic hair pattern) in men.

The psychiatric complications of alcoholism include acute intoxication, alcohol withdrawal disorders, amnestic syndromes such as Wernicke-Korsakoff syndrome, and/or alcohol-related dementia. Depression occurs in up to 60% of alcoholic patients; alcohol itself can induce depression through its direct effects on the brain. Depression can contribute to an increased risk of suicide, which occurs in 2%–3% of alcoholic persons. Alcoholic persons at greatest risk for suicide include those with a history of interpersonal loss within the past year, best defined as the loss of an intimate relationship.

Other problems associated with alcoholism are largely social and occupational: marital and family problems that can lead to domestic abuse, separation, and divorce; work-related problems such as absenteeism and job loss; and legal entanglements stemming from arrests for public intoxication, drunk driving, or bar fights. Alcoholism also increases the risk that individuals have for abuse of or dependence on other substances.

Course and Outcome

In a review of 10 large studies, the researchers concluded that 2%–3% of alcoholic persons become abstinent each year and about 1% return to asymptomatic or controlled drinking. These findings were true for both treated and untreated samples, supporting the hypothesis that alcoholism is self-limiting for some persons. In the 10 studies, 46%–87% of the subjects remained alcoholic at follow-up; 0%–33% were asymptomatic drinkers; and 8%–39% had achieved abstinence.

Etiology and Pathophysiology

Strong evidence has supported a role for genetics in the etiology of alcoholism. Family studies have consistently shown high rates of the disorder among first-degree relatives of alcoholic persons. Nearly 25% of the fathers and brothers of alcoholic persons are themselves alcoholic. The relatives of alcoholic persons also have high rates of drug dependence, antisocial personality disorder, and mood and anxiety disorders. Typically, depression occurs in the female relatives of alcoholic persons, and alcohol dependence, drug dependence, or antisocial personality disorder occurs in the male relatives.

Twin and adoption studies also support the role of genetic factors in the development of alcohol use disorder. Identical twins have a higher concordance rate for alcoholism than do nonidentical twins. Adoption studies have shown that the biological relatives of alcoholic adoptees are more likely to have alcoholism than are the relatives of control adoptees. Genetic transmission may be gender specific: in men, alcoholism tends to run in families; in women, alcoholism tends to occur sporadically.

Molecular genetic techniques are now being used to search for an alcoholism gene (or genes). The best-replicated findings are genes encoding for the alcohol-metabolizing enzymes that are protective against the development of alcoholism. An example is the *ADH2*2* allele, which is common among Asian populations and may help to explain their lower prevalence of alcohol disorders. It is likely that multiple genes conferring vulnerability interact with multiple environmental risk factors.

One key genetically influenced risk factor may be a person's level of response (or sensitivity) to alcohol. In studies of offspring of alcoholic persons, those with a low level of response are likely to drink more to produce the desired effect and are at greater risk for alcoholism. A low level of response to alcohol (in response to challenge doses of alcohol) also is associated with less impairment of motor performance, less body sway, and increased alpha-wave activity and low P3 wave amplitude on the electroencephalogram.

Behaviorists have suggested that learning plays an important role in the genesis of alcoholism and point to the fact that children tend to imitate their parents' drinking patterns. Boys are encouraged to drink more than girls, reinforcing the gender difference in alcoholism. Learning processes also may contribute to the development of the disorder through the repeated experience with alcohol withdrawal; relieving the symptoms with alcohol only encourages further drinking.

Clinical Management

Alcohol-induced disorders often require medical intervention. Intoxication is the most common disorder and rarely requires more than simple supportive measures, such as decreasing external stimuli and removing the source of alcohol. When respiration is compromised by excessive alcohol intake, intensive care may be required.

Treatment of alcohol withdrawal depends on the syndrome an alcoholic person develops. Students should understand that alcohol withdrawal, while typically following abrupt cessation of alcohol consumption, can also develop in alcoholic persons who simply reduce their usual high intake.

Uncomplicated alcohol withdrawal (the "shakes") begins 12–18 hours after the cessation of drinking and peaks at 24–48 hours, then subsides within 5–7 days, even without treatment. Minor symptoms include anxiety, tremors, and nausea and vomiting; heart rate and blood pressure may be increased.

Alcoholic withdrawal seizures ("rum fits") occur 7–38 hours after the cessation of drinking and peak between 24 and 48 hours. The patient may have a single burst of one to six generalized seizures; status epilepticus is rare. Withdrawal seizures occur primarily in chronic, long-term alcoholic patients.

Alcoholic hallucinosis—vivid and unpleasant auditory, visual, or tactile hallucinations—begins within 48 hours of cessation of drinking and occurs in the presence of a clear sensorium. The hallucinations typically last about 1 week but have been reported to become chronic in some persons. Like withdrawal seizures, they are a sign of severe alcoholism. The most dramatic withdrawal syndrome is *alcohol withdrawal delirium* (delirium tremens, or "DTs"). Delirium tremens occurs in about 5% of hospitalized alcoholic patients but in about one-third of those who have had withdrawal seizures. Manifestations include delirium (confusion and disorientation, perceptual disturbances, sleep cycle disturbance, agitation), mild fever, and autonomic hyperarousal. The delirium may begin 2–3 days after the drinking stops or after a significant reduction of intake. Symptoms peak 4 or 5 days later. The syndrome typically lasts about 3 days but can persist for weeks. With good supportive care, death is rare, although mortality rates of up to 15% were reported in the past.

In treating alcoholic persons, the clinician should ask patients to describe their past symptoms that developed when they either stopped drinking or cut back from their usual heavy drinking. The most common symptom patients typically describe is the "shakes," and far fewer will have had seizures, hallucinations, or delirium tremens. Some patients will misidentify their shakes as "DTs"; however, few people know what delirium tremens is (including some physicians!). If a patient had developed an alcohol withdrawal delirium, he or she most likely would not remember it. For that reason, students might ask patients whether a doctor had ever told them that during withdrawal they were agitated, confused, or required tranquilizers, seclusion, or restraint.

The following case illustrates the dramatic nature of alcohol withdrawal delirium and its management:

> Dave, a 34-year-old unemployed veteran, requested admission for alcohol withdrawal treatment. He had a 10-year history of alcoholism and had experienced delirium tremens, alcoholic blackouts, and withdrawal seizures. He had been admitted many times for alcohol withdrawal and rehabilitation services and was well known at the hospital for his unpleasant and critical attitude.
>
> Dave had been drinking heavily—about 1 quart of liquor daily— since his last inpatient stay 3 months earlier, particularly during the week before seeking help. He was tremulous, hypertensive, and diaphoretic. The "Librium protocol" (i.e., chlordiazepoxide taper, described later) was instituted. To the chagrin of the treatment team, Dave insisted on leaving the hospital against medical advice the next day. He claimed that he had "more important things" to do. The night before, nursing staff had noted that he was mildly intrusive and had wandered into other patients' rooms.
>
> Dave was brought back to the hospital the next day by the police. He had been found wandering aimlessly around town. He was noticeably

paranoid and thought that unnamed persons were plotting against him. He was also disoriented; he knew where he was but was unable to give the date or the year. By the next morning, Dave was globally confused. He also was febrile, had very high diastolic blood pressure, and was diaphoretic. Because of his belligerence and physical restlessness, he was placed in seclusion, and restraints were used for his protection. Over the next 2 days, he received nearly 1,200 mg of chlordiazepoxide, but he remained loud and agitated. Intravenous hydration was required because of his poor oral intake. The nurses observed him playing an imaginary game of chess with unseen partners.

On the third day of hospitalization, Dave awakened and was fully oriented. He remained suspicious but was no longer hallucinating. He gradually returned to his baseline over the next week and was discharged.

The management of alcohol withdrawal consists of general support (i.e., adequate food and hydration, careful medical monitoring), nutritional supplementation, and the use of benzodiazepines. Persons with a history of uncomplicated withdrawal and a physician who is familiar with the patient probably can be managed as outpatients. Treatment may include 25–50 mg of chlordiazepoxide four times daily, tapered slowly over the next 4–5 days.

Alcoholic patients with comorbid medical or psychiatric illness, impaired ability to follow instructions, inadequate or absent social support, or a history of severe withdrawal symptoms require careful monitoring and may need to be hospitalized. Patients should receive an adequate diet plus oral thiamine (100 mg), folic acid (1 mg), and multivitamins. Thiamine (100–200 mg intramuscularly) can be administered if oral intake is not possible and should be given before any situation in which glucose loading is required, because glucose can deplete thiamine stores. Chlordiazepoxide should be administered in dosages ranging from 25 to 100 mg orally four times daily on the first day, with a 20% per day decrease in dosage over 4–5 days. (A specific protocol is recommended in Table 9–6.) Additional doses can be given for breakthrough signs or symptoms (e.g., tremors or diaphoresis).

Chlordiazepoxide and the other benzodiazepines are the preferred drugs for withdrawal because of their safety and cross-tolerance with alcohol. Chlordiazepoxide is most often recommended because of its long half-life and low cost, but other benzodiazepines work just as well. Intermediate- or short-acting benzodiazepines (e.g., lorazepam, oxazepam) are generally preferred in patients with liver damage or in elderly patients because these benzodiazepines lack metabolites and are renally excreted. Diazepam can be given to interrupt seizures should status epilepticus occur. Other drugs, including carbamazepine, cloni-

---

TABLE 9–6. Management of alcohol withdrawal syndromes

---

1. Chlordiazepoxide protocol

   - 50 mg every 4 hours × 24 hours, then
   - 50 mg every 6 hours × 24 hours, then
   - 25 mg every 4 hours × 24 hours, then
   - 25 mg every 6 hours × 24 hours

   The protocol should be started when 3 of the following 7 parameters are met: systolic blood pressure >160 mm Hg, diastolic blood pressure >100 mm Hg, pulse >110 beats/min, temperature >38.3°C, nausea, vomiting, or tremors.
   The dose should be held if any of the following signs are present: nystagmus, sedation, ataxia, slurred speech, or the patient is asleep.

2. Thiamine: 50–100 mg orally or intramuscularly × 1; folic acid: 1 mg/day orally

3. Haloperidol: 2–5 mg/day; or risperidone: 2–6 mg/day for patients with alcoholic hallucinosis

4. For delirium tremens:

   - 10 mg of intravenous diazepam (or 2–4 mg of lorazepam), followed by 5-mg doses (or 1–2 mg of lorazepam) every 5–15 minutes until calm; once stabilized, the dosage may be tapered slowly over 4 or 5 days
   - Seclusion and restraints as necessary
   - Adequate hydration and nutrition

---

dine, propranolol, and valproate, have been used to treat alcohol withdrawal, but their role in treating the disorder is not yet clear.

Delirious patients require additional care; this may include seclusion and restraints. To facilitate patient care, 10 mg of intravenous diazepam (or 2–4 mg of lorazepam) may be given, followed by 5-mg doses every 5–15 minutes (or 1–2 mg of lorazepam) thereafter until the patient is calm. Once the patient has stabilized, the benzodiazepine dosage should be tapered slowly over the next 4 or 5 days. Intravenous hydration also may be necessary, although most alcoholic patients are overhydrated, not dehydrated, as is commonly believed. Any electrolyte disturbance should be corrected, and the patient should be examined for injuries or evidence of a physical illness (e.g., pneumonia).

A small dose of haloperidol (2–5 mg/day), or one of the second-generation antipsychotics (e.g., risperidone, 2–6 mg/day), may help relieve the frightening hallucinations of the patient with alcoholic hallucinosis. The medication usually is discontinued when the hallucinations stop.

Rehabilitation

Efforts at rehabilitation can begin once alcohol detoxification has been accomplished. Rehabilitation has two goals: 1) that patients remain sober, and 2) that coexisting disorders be identified and treated. Perhaps two-thirds of alcoholic patients have additional psychiatric diagnoses (including mood or anxiety disorders) and will benefit from their treatment. Because alcoholism itself can cause depression and most alcohol-induced depressions lift with sobriety, antidepressants are probably needed only for patients who remain depressed after 2–4 weeks of sobriety.

The first step toward rehabilitation occurs when the physician diagnoses alcohol abuse or dependence. Patients should be told that their disorder is significant and potentially life threatening and that treatment is recommended. Receiving a diagnosis may be the single most important step in leading the alcoholic person to change.

Patients should be encouraged to attend Alcoholics Anonymous (AA), a worldwide self-help group for recovering alcoholic persons founded in 1935. AA uses a program of 12 steps; new members are asked to admit their problems, to give up a sense of personal control over the disease, to make personal amends, and to help others to achieve sobriety. The meetings provide a blend of acceptance, belonging, forgiveness, and understanding.

A team approach is used for the hospitalized alcoholic patient. Group therapy enables patients to see their own problems mirrored in others and to learn better coping skills. With individual therapy, alcoholic persons can learn to identify triggers that prompt drinking and learn more effective coping strategies. Family therapy is often important because the family system that has been altered to accommodate the patient's drinking may end up reinforcing it. These issues can be addressed in family therapy. Inpatient programs also provide education about the harmful effects of alcohol.

Motivational interviewing techniques are being increasingly used with alcoholic persons to help persuade them to make their own case for change (i.e., to abandon alcohol). Avoiding confrontation, the therapist seeks to achieve clarity about the patient's motivation for change, impediments that stand in the way of making needed change, and possible actions that might bring about change.

The U.S. Food and Drug Administration (FDA) has approved the use of three drugs—disulfiram, naltrexone, and acamprosate—for the treatment of alcohol dependence. Disulfiram inhibits aldehyde dehydrogenase, an enzyme necessary for the metabolism of alcohol. Inhibiting this enzyme leads to the accumulation of acetaldehyde when alcohol is consumed. Acetaldehyde is toxic and induces noxious symptoms, such as nausea, vomiting, palpitations, and hypotension. Disulfiram should be prescribed only after careful consideration and with the full cooperation of the patient. The usual dosage is 250 mg once daily. Because patients taking disulfiram are aware of the potential adverse reaction, they are motivated to avoid alcohol.

Naltrexone, a μ-opioid antagonist, appears to reduce the pleasurable effects of and craving for alcohol. The recommended daily dosage is 50 mg. The drug is generally well tolerated but can produce nausea, headache, anxiety, or sedation. (The drug carries a black box warning that it not be given to people with severe liver disease and that its use requires periodic monitoring of liver enzymes.) Acamprosate, a glutamate receptor modulator, also reduces craving. Although it is generally well tolerated, some patients report headache, diarrhea, flatulence, and nausea. The recommended dosage is two 333-mg tablets three times a day, a dosing schedule that may limit its acceptance. Both naltrexone and acamprosate help patients to maintain abstinence, thereby reducing the risk of relapse. For those who are chronically noncompliant, naltrexone is also available in an extended-release injectable formulation that is administered monthly.

A large government-supported multicenter trial found that naltrexone, when given with a modest program of medical management, was as effective as specialized behavioral treatment in preventing relapse. The researchers concluded that naltrexone along with medical management could be easily delivered in most health care settings, thus serving alcohol-dependent persons who might otherwise not receive treatment.

Rehabilitation programs for alcoholic patients have shifted from traditional inpatient to residential and outpatient settings. Outcome studies have shown that these programs are effective for most patients. In general, patients likely to benefit have a stable marriage and home life, are employed, have fewer comorbid psychiatric disorders (especially antisocial personality disorder), and have no family history of alcoholism. Nearly 50% of treated alcoholic persons relapse, most commonly during the first 6 months following treatment. Even though relapse is common, treatment should be viewed as beneficial and cost-effective. Treatment has the potential to reduce the medical and social complications of alcoholism as well as the excessive mortality associated with the disorder.

Key points to remember about the management of alcoholism

1. The alcoholic person needs acceptance, not blame.

2. Although it is tempting to refuse treatment to the chronic alcoholic person based on his or her history of failure, it is always possible that the next rehabilitation effort may work. The clinician must not give up!

3. Treatment of alcohol withdrawal syndromes should take place in an inpatient setting if the patient has a history of severe "shakes," hallucinations, seizures, or delirium tremens. Other patients— perhaps the majority—can be treated on an outpatient basis.

   • Chlordiazepoxide is standard treatment, but other benzodiazepines (e.g., lorazepam, clonazepam) work just as well.

4. The clinician should manage the patient's other comorbid disorders (e.g., panic disorder, depression); when untreated, these disorders may contribute to relapse.

5. The patient should be referred to AA to provide ongoing social support and encouragement from persons similarly affected.

6. The family should be included in the treatment process.

   • Alcoholism affects every member of the family, and unresolved issues may lead to relapse.

   • Family members should be encouraged to attend Al-Anon, a support group for relatives of alcoholic persons.

■ Drug-Related Disorders

Substance misuse is widespread in the United States. It is probably impossible to know its true extent, because drug abusers may not cooperate with surveys and because much use is recreational and not necessarily accompanied by signs or symptoms of abuse or dependence. The Epidemiologic Catchment Area survey found that the lifetime prevalence of the combined category of drug abuse and dependence ranged from 5.5% to 5.8%. In the National Comorbidity Survey Replication study, lifetime prevalence of drug abuse was estimated at 8%, whereas lifetime drug dependence was estimated at 3%. In these surveys, drug abuse and dependence were more common in men, young persons, and those with low incomes.

These data do not show the true extent of illicit drug use. Surveys show, for example, that marijuana has been used by more than one-quarter of Americans and is regularly smoked by about 20 million persons. Up to 50% of high school students admit to having smoked marijuana. Cocaine achieved great popularity in the 1980s, particularly among young urban professionals, and nearly one-quarter of young Americans have used it, including nearly 7% of high school seniors. A 2007 household survey found that nearly 6 million Americans admitted to using cocaine in the year before the survey. Patterns of use change, however, reflecting the fluctuating popularity of drugs, their availability, and their cost. Opioids and barbiturates peaked in popularity long ago, but the estimated number of persons addicted to heroin in 2007 was about 200,000. Cocaine is more widely available and less expensive than in the past. Crack, a freebased derivative of cocaine, is even cheaper, and its use has become epidemic in inner cities and elsewhere. Another factor in drug use is the introduction of new substances to the black market. Many drugs are easily synthesized in basement laboratories and are widely available at low prices. Methamphetamine (meth) is a recent example. A stimulant that is inhaled or injected, methamphetamine can be synthesized from battery acid, drain cleaner, paint thinner, and pseudoephedrine, an over-the-counter cold remedy.

Among the more worrisome trends is the use of multiple drugs of abuse. As a general rule, the use of one substance greatly increases the chance that a person will use another. Some drugs are deliberately combined to produce a desired effect (e.g., a speedball, consisting of a combination of cocaine and heroin). The extent of combined drug use is only now becoming apparent. In DSM-IV-TR, this pattern of use is classified as *polysubstance dependence*—that is, three or more drugs have been repeatedly used, but no single agent has predominated.

Etiology

The confluence of genes and individual biology, the person's environment, and the drug itself leads to drug use disorders. No single factor determines whether a person will become addicted to drugs.

Some users appear to have an inherited vulnerability to drug abuse. Research shows that dependence on certain substances (e.g., tobacco, narcotics, alcohol) is familial; adoptees born to substance-abusing parents and placed in drug-free homes show an increased likelihood of drug use. Genetic factors are estimated to contribute to 40%–60% of the variability in the risk for addiction. The neurobiologic mechanisms by which environmental factors interact with genes to create vulnerability to addiction are just beginning to be studied.

Although no single personality pattern is associated with drug abuse, the frequency of personality disorders among drug abusers is very high. Antisocial and borderline personality disorders appear to predispose to drug use. Narcissistic traits have been identified as a possible risk factor in cocaine abusers. Other psychological characteristics seen in drug abusers include hostility, low frustration tolerance, inflexibility, and low self-esteem. Several longitudinal studies have shown that many of these traits (e.g., aggressiveness and rebelliousness manifested in childhood) precede and predict the use of psychoactive substances.

Other medical and psychiatric disorders have been linked with drug abuse, including chronic pain, anxiety disorders, and depression. Many patients experiencing physical or emotional pain often seek relief through drugs or alcohol and are at high risk for abuse or dependence.

Research has begun to identify the neurobiologic substrates of drug abuse and dependence. Dopamine pathways that form part of the CNS "reward system" have been identified in the ventral tegmental region of the forebrain and in the nucleus accumbens. All drugs of abuse appear to target the brain's reward system by flooding the circuit with dopamine. Dopamine facilitates conditioned learning, thereby involving memory circuits as well. The association of drug-induced pleasurable experiences with increases in CNS dopamine likely results in strong conditioning. This may account for the enhanced excitement reported by drug users that characterizes compulsive use.

The pharmacological properties of the drug itself may contribute to abuse. Some agents (e.g., opioids, sedatives, hypnotics, anxiolytics) can produce rapid relief of anxiety. Stimulants generally relieve boredom and fatigue and provide a sensation of energy and increased mental alertness. Hallucinogens provide a temporary escape from reality. These properties all contribute to their abuse. Substances that do not give pleasure to the user (e.g., chlorpromazine, haloperidol) are rarely abused. In general, drugs with rapid onset and briefer action (e.g., heroin, cocaine) are preferred. Methods of administration that enhance the rapidity of onset—for example, sniffing, smoking, or intravenous use—are often exploited to provide an added kick. Tolerance and withdrawal symptoms also contribute to abuse. Users quickly learn that higher doses of some substances are needed to get the same effect and that the drug itself can be used to prevent unpleasant withdrawal symptoms.

Societal and family values influence the use of illicit drugs. When parents smoke cigarettes, drink alcoholic beverages, or use drugs, their offspring are more prone to use these substances, perhaps through learning the implicit lesson that their use is socially acceptable. People whose friends use drugs are more likely to use them as well, which suggests that peers influence a person's choices. Susceptibility to peer influence has been associated with the lack of a close bond with one's parents, a large amount of time spent away from home, and increased reliance on peers as opposed to parents.

Laws also can affect illicit drug use. Antidrug laws have been tried with mixed success for centuries. The grand experiment called Prohibition in the United States during the 1920s is one of the best examples, perhaps because it was such a policy failure. Antidrug laws are generally more successful in authoritarian regimes where behavior can be monitored more effectively than in more open and pluralistic societies, such as the United States.

Diagnosis

The diagnosis of a substance use disorder requires a careful history, a thorough physical examination, and a detailed mental status examination. The assessment of addicted persons is rarely easy, because few will spontaneously report their drug use. More commonly, these persons will present for evaluation of a medical complaint or for emotional distress. A careful interview may help to uncover social, marital, occupational, or legal problems that may have contributed to the drug use. The clinician should remember that drug use can lead to the development of depression, mania, or psychosis. Likewise, many drug-addicted persons will have comorbid psychiatric disorders, such as major depression, bipolar disorder, or an anxiety disorder, that should be diagnosed and treated. Personality disorders—particularly antisocial and borderline personality disorders—are common in drug-addicted persons and may contribute to continued drug use.

Additional history obtained from relatives or friends, or from other physicians, will help fill in the gaps. Even patients who are straightforward about their abuse may minimize its extent. Once the physician's suspicion has been raised about drug use, he or she should inquire specifically about each class of commonly abused drugs and record the patient's pattern of use.

A physical examination will offer signs of intoxication and withdrawal, depending on when the individual presents at a hospital or clinic (see Table 9–7). The clinician should be forthright and nonjudgmental with these patients and help them to obtain needed services.

Laboratory testing for drugs has become a routine part of the workup in emergency departments for patients who are unresponsive or

TABLE 9–7.   Signs of drug intoxication

Signs	Sedatives, hypnotics, or anxiolytics	Stimulants	Opioids	Cannabis
Eyes	Nystagmus; miosis when severe	Mydriasis, which may require protective sunglasses	Miosis prominent	Injected conjunctivae
Vital signs	Stage dependent; chronic user has increased blood pressure	Increased—or sometimes decreased—heart rate and blood pressure, varied arrhythmias	Bradycardia, risk of respiratory depression and pulmonary edema	Tachycardia
Neurological	Incoordination to unsteady gait, slurred speech	Dyskinesia, dystonia, muscle weakness, seizures	Slurred speech	Impaired coordination
Psychomotor	Agitation, combativeness	Agitation (sometimes retardation) and stereotyped behaviors	Activity usually outside normal range; may be increased or decreased	Passive
Sensorium	Impaired concentration and memory; stupor to coma	Confusion to coma	Impaired attention and memory; drowsiness to coma	Impaired attention, memory, and sense of time
Autonomic	Diaphoresis, flushed face and skin	Diaphoresis, chills	None	Dry mouth

TABLE 9–7. Signs of drug intoxication *(continued)*

Signs	Sedatives, hypnotics, or anxiolytics	Stimulants	Opioids	Cannabis
Gastro-intestinal	Poor nutrition	Nausea, vomiting, marked weight loss, poor nutrition	Constipation, poor nutrition	Increased appetite
Skin and mucosa	Dental neglect	Needle marks and tracks, ulcerated nasal septum, dental neglect	Needle marks and tracks, dental neglect	None

Source. Adapted from Barber and O'Brien 1995.

confused; tests are also routinely used now during insurance examinations, in the workplace, in the military, and in the criminal justice system. Intoxication and overdosage are the most common indications to test for drugs, but drug testing should be considered when assessing a patient presenting with alterations in mood or behavior. Most testing involves sampling blood or urine. Urine drug screenings are easily performed and are generally reported as positive or negative for a particular substance. Most screenings cover the major drugs of abuse. Due to contamination, morning sampling should be avoided, and if sample dilution or substitution is suspected, direct observation of voiding may be indicated. Cannabis, which is fat soluble, can be detected in urine up to 3 weeks after the last use.

The following patient treated at our hospital illustrates many of the symptoms that beset substance abusers, as well as some of the factors that lead to the abuse. Laura's story also points out the dilemma that caregivers face with uncooperative patients and the lack of satisfactory solutions:

> Laura, a 21-year-old American Indian nursing assistant, was referred to the hospital for evaluation of polydrug abuse. She had been adopted at an early age into a middle-class family. Her adoptive parents took care to ensure that she was adequately clothed and fed but provided little emotional nurturing. Laura was sexually molested for several years by one of her adoptive brothers, and at age 12 she became pregnant by him. She carried the baby to term and gave it up for adoption.
>
> Laura had an extensive drug abuse history. She started using marijuana and drinking alcoholic beverages at age 12, was using amphetamines by age 14, and later used cocaine and crack. She also admitted to having tried an assortment of other drugs, including PCP, lysergic acid diethylamide (LSD), and heroin. To pay for her drug use, Laura sold drugs and later engaged in prostitution.
>
> In the 6 months before her hospitalization, she had begun to inject cocaine intravenously, sometimes in combination with heroin (a "speedball," she called it). She reported that she enjoyed the sexual feelings she received from the injections but had actually lost interest in sexual activity with her boyfriend. She admitted using unclean needles despite knowing that they could transmit HIV. Her boyfriend was a drug dealer with an extensive prison record and worked as her pimp.
>
> Laura had received prior psychiatric treatment for depression and had had several prior admissions for drug detoxification, one following a suicide attempt. She had never stayed in the hospital very long and usually left against medical advice.
>
> Laura was referred to our hospital under a court order and told us she had no plans to stop using drugs. She was eventually transferred to a drug rehabilitation center. The referral was based on our hope that at some point the treatment would "take." Our alternative was to do nothing.

Sedative, Hypnotic, and Anxiolytic Use Disorders

Sedatives, hypnotics, and anxiolytics have been used to provide sedation, induce sleep, relieve anxiety, prevent seizures, relax muscles, and induce general anesthesia. All sedatives, hypnotics, and anxiolytics are cross-tolerant with one another and with alcohol. They are also capable of producing physical and psychological dependence and symptoms of withdrawal. Classes of these compounds include the barbiturates, the nonbarbiturate sedative-hypnotics (e.g., meprobamate), and the benzodiazepines.

The history of sedative-hypnotics dates to 1903, when barbital, the first barbiturate, was introduced. Later, other sedative-hypnotics (e.g., meprobamate) were synthesized; benzodiazepines first became available in the 1960s. Because of their wide margin of safety, the benzodiazepines have largely displaced barbiturates and the earlier nonbarbiturate sedative-hypnotics from the market. An overdose of barbiturates is potentially fatal, but the benzodiazepines produce almost no respiratory depression, and the ratio of lethal to effective dosage is extraordinarily high. Although the barbiturate and nonbarbiturate sedative-hypnotics are effective in providing both sedation and hypnosis (e.g., sleep induction), they are rarely used today. The main indication for phenobarbital now is as an anticonvulsant. The benzodiazepines are among the most widely prescribed medications in the United States, and about 15% of the general population is prescribed a benzodiazepine in any given year. Research has shown that most prescriptions for benzodiazepines are appropriate, and only a small percentage of patients abuse the drugs. Nonetheless, prescribing practices contribute to the problem of sedative-hypnotic abuse, and physicians have an obligation to monitor and, if necessary, limit the use of these drugs (see Table 9–8). Further information about the rational use of sedative-hypnotics is found in Chapter 20.

Sedative-hypnotic abuse involves a maladaptive pattern of use leading to clinically significant impairment, as indicated by one or more independent indications of inappropriate use or problems directly attributable to the substance at any time during a 12-month period. Dependence requires the presence of three or more problem behaviors (out of seven) at any time in the same 12-month period, including manifestations of tolerance and withdrawal. (Please refer to Tables 9–2 and 9–3 for the criteria for abuse and dependence, respectively.)

TABLE 9–8. Rational prescribing of sedative-hypnotic agents

1. Avoid or limit prescriptions to patients if risk for substance abuse is suggested by

   • A history of alcohol abuse or dependence

   • A history of drug abuse or dependence

   • The presence of an antisocial or borderline personality disorder

   • A strong family history of substance abuse or dependence

2. Learn to recognize "red flag" presentations by patients seeking prescription drugs, as suggested by

   • Dramatic claims of need for a scheduled drug

   • Reports of lost prescriptions

   • Frequent requests for early refills

   • Requests for a specific scheduled drug, reports of allergies to other drugs, or use of nonscheduled drugs for pain relief or anxiety

   • Obtaining prescriptions from many physicians ("doctor-shopping")

Source. Courtesy of William R. Yates, M.D.

Sedative, hypnotic, and anxiolytic dependence can lead to medical and social complications, occupational problems (e.g., job loss), and impaired relationships. Drug-dependent persons sometimes turn to crime to obtain drugs. Not much is known about the natural history of sedative, hypnotic, and anxiolytic dependence, but like alcoholism, the course probably is chronic and relapsing.

Sedative, hypnotic, and anxiolytic intoxication, withdrawal, and withdrawal delirium vary little from drug to drug, although withdrawal symptoms may be more intense with the shorter-acting drugs (e.g., alprazolam) and more prolonged with the longer-acting ones (e.g., phenobarbital). The syndromes are similar to those seen with alcoholism, which is not surprising because these drugs are cross-tolerant. As in alcohol withdrawal, symptoms may occur when the substance is abruptly withdrawn or the dosage is reduced.

The symptoms of sedative, hypnotic, and anxiolytic intoxication are dose related. Lethargy, impaired mental functioning, poor memory, irritability, self-neglect, and emotional disinhibition all may occur in intoxicated persons. As intoxication progresses, slurred speech, ataxia, and impaired coordination can develop. With higher dosages, death can occur as a result of respiratory depression, a complication that rarely occurs with the benzodiazepines.

Withdrawal from sedatives, hypnotics, and anxiolytics should be carefully monitored. Conservative management may consist of very slow withdrawal of the drug over many days or weeks. Many patients will need formal detoxification in the hospital to forestall the development of significant withdrawal symptoms.

Abrupt drug discontinuation leads to anxiety, restlessness, and a feeling of apprehension in the first 24 hours. Coarse tremors soon develop, and deep tendon reflexes become hyperactive. Weakness, nausea and vomiting, orthostatic hypotension, sweating, and other signs of autonomic hyperarousal occur. On the second or third day after discontinuation, grand mal seizures can occur. The seizures generally consist of a single convulsion or burst of several convulsions; status epilepticus rarely develops. A withdrawal delirium, associated with confusion, disorientation, and visual and somatic hallucinations, sometimes develops at this stage. Barbiturate withdrawal can be especially serious and without medical intervention can result in death.

A gradually tapering schedule should be developed for those being withdrawn from sedatives, hypnotics, or anxiolytics. If the patient's usual maintenance dose is known, that will serve as the starting point. A pentobarbital (or diazepam) tolerance test can be performed in those who are unreliable or in whom the dose is difficult to determine (see Table 9–9). The test should be administered to a patient who is not currently intoxicated and should be medically monitored in the hospital.

Once the level of tolerance has been established, the patient is withdrawn using diazepam or another long-acting benzodiazepine. Long-acting barbiturates such as phenobarbital can also be used, but their use is relatively uncommon. With diazepam, the daily dosage is decreased by 10 mg from an initial level equal to the intoxicating dosage. If phenobarbital is used, the initial dose is determined by substituting 30 mg of phenobarbital for every 100 mg of pentobarbital administered during the tolerance test. For example, if the patient is tolerant to 400 mg of pentobarbital, the starting dose of phenobarbital is 120 mg. During withdrawal, the daily dosage of phenobarbital is decreased by 30 mg. On these schedules, the patient will be somewhat uncomfortable during the withdrawal period. If signs of withdrawal worsen or if the patient becomes somnolent or intoxicated, the schedule can be adjusted and the patient can be given more diazepam (or phenobarbital), or the schedule can be stretched out. Some patients will present at the hospital already experiencing withdrawal symptoms, in which case pentobar-

TABLE 9–9.   Pentobarbital-diazepam tolerance test

1. Pentobarbital 200 mg (or diazepam 20 mg) is administered orally.
    Evaluate in 2 hours:

    •   No tolerance—the patient is asleep but arousable

    •   Tolerance to 400–500 mg of pentobarbital (or 40–50 mg of
        diazepam)—the patient is grossly ataxic and has a coarse
        tremor or lateral nystagmus

    •   Tolerance to 600 mg of pentobarbital (or 60 mg of diazepam)—
        the patient is mildly ataxic

    •   Tolerance to 800 mg of pentobarbital (or 80 mg of diazepam)—
        the patient has slight nystagmus

    •   Tolerance to 1,000 mg of pentobarbital (or 100 mg of
        diazepam)—the patient is asymptomatic

2. If the patient remains asymptomatic, an additional oral dose of
    pentobarbital 200 mg (or diazepam 20 mg) is given.

    •   Failure to become symptomatic at this dose suggests a daily
        tolerance of >1,600 mg of pentobarbital (or 160 mg of
        diazepam)

bital or diazepam should be administered in sufficient dosages to make
them comfortable before withdrawal is initiated.

Certain general rules apply to patients given these drugs. The drugs
should be targeted at specific symptoms or syndromes (e.g., generalized anxiety disorder), and their use should be limited to weeks or
months when possible. The drugs should be prescribed at the minimum
dosage necessary to control the patient's symptoms. Because of the
proven safety and efficacy of benzodiazepines, there is no reason to prescribe the more dangerous barbiturates or the other nonbarbiturate sedative-hypnotics.

Opioid Use Disorders

The opioids include morphine, heroin, hydrocodone, oxycodone, co-
deine, tramadol, and meperidine. These drugs are commonly used for
pain control. Heroin is the only one not available by prescription in the
United States. There is a growing awareness of the widespread misuse
of prescription pain relievers, and it is important to note that there are
over five times as many persons dependent on prescription opioid pain
relievers than on heroin.

Opioid abuse is more common in urban settings, among men, and among African Americans. Among those who are dependent on prescription pain relievers, there is a slight female preponderance. Opioid abuse is more common among health care professionals than among other occupations, probably because of the availability of these drugs in medical settings. Many persons who are addicted to opioids have other mental illnesses, including other addictions or a mood or anxiety disorder. Antisocial personality disorder is common among opioid users. Many users turn to crime because of the relatively high cost of opioid drugs.

The natural history of opioid addiction is variable and depends on both availability and exposure to its use. In a 12-year follow-up of opioid-addicted patients treated in a federal treatment center, 98% returned to using opioids within 12 months of release. A follow-up study in London found a relapse rate of 53% within 6 months. A 24-year follow-up of persons addicted to narcotics in California confirmed that substance abuse and criminal involvement continued over the years and that cessation of drug use was uncommon. However, a study of military veterans who had used opioids in Vietnam found that fewer than 2% continued their use after returning home. These discrepant findings suggest that there may be more than one type of opioid user.

Opioid addiction is associated with high mortality rates because of inadvertent fatal overdoses, accidental deaths, and suicide. Although it is unlikely that addicted persons will outgrow their habit over the years, the death rate is so high that there are relatively few older abusers.

Opioid users need to be carefully evaluated because they are likely to have comorbid medical illness. Opioid-dependent persons also are at high risk for developing medical conditions resulting from malnutrition and use of dirty needles—for example, hepatitis B and C infection, HIV infection, pneumonia, skin ulcers at injection sites, and cellulitis.

Persons addicted to opioids inject, snort, or smoke these drugs, producing both euphoria and a sense of well-being. Drowsiness, inactivity, psychomotor retardation, and impaired concentration follow. Physical signs that occur after a heroin-addicted person "shoots up" (which may occur three or more times a day) include flushing, pupillary constriction, slurred speech, respiratory depression, hypotension, hypothermia, and bradycardia. Constipation, nausea, and vomiting are also frequent.

Tolerance eventually develops to most of these drug effects, including the initial euphoria. Sexual interest diminishes, and in women, menstruation may cease. In the chronic user, depending on dosage and drug potency, withdrawal symptoms begin approximately 10 hours after the last dose with short-acting opioids (e.g., morphine, heroin) or after a longer period with longer-acting substances (e.g., methadone). Minor withdrawal symptoms include lacrimation, rhinorrhea, sweating, yawning, piloerection, hypertension, and tachycardia. Symptoms that indicate more severe withdrawal include hot and cold flashes, muscle and joint pain, nausea, vomiting, and abdominal cramps. Seizures sometimes occur during meperidine withdrawal. Psychological symptoms of withdrawal include severe anxiety and restlessness, irritability, insomnia, and decreased appetite.

Patients addicted to opioids should be gradually withdrawn under medical supervision using methadone, a long-acting opioid. The initial methadone dosage is determined by the presenting signs and symptoms of withdrawal (see Table 9–10). The dose is then repeated in 12 hours, and supplemental doses of 5 mg or 10 mg are given as needed if withdrawal symptoms are not suppressed. Once the 24-hour dosage is determined, the dosage is tapered at the rate of 20% per day for short-acting opioids or 10% per day for long-acting opioids. Methadone should be given in two to three divided doses daily, and the patient's vital signs should be recorded before each dose. It is unusual for a starting dose to exceed 40 mg during the initial 24 hours of withdrawal. Withdrawal from short-acting substances (e.g., heroin, morphine) typically takes 7–10 days. Withdrawal from longer-acting substances (e.g., methadone) proceeds more slowly (e.g., 2–3 weeks).

Another drug used to withdraw patients from opioids is clonidine, which provides good suppression of the autonomic signs of withdrawal. Patients do better with an abrupt switch to clonidine when the methadone dosage is first stabilized at 20 mg or less daily. At the first sign of opioid withdrawal, the patient is given 0.3–0.5 mg (0.006 mg/kg) of clonidine, which is repeated at bedtime. For the next 4 days, the patient receives 0.9–1.5 mg/day in three to four divided doses. The dose should be withheld if the diastolic blood pressure falls below 60 mm Hg or marked sedation occurs. On days 6–8, the dosage can be decreased by 50%, and on day 9, clonidine can be discontinued altogether. For long-acting opioids, clonidine reduction should occur on days 11–14, with discontinuation on day 15.

Other adjunctive therapies are often helpful. Benzodiazepines can treat very mild cases of withdrawal and can help relieve anxiety and promote needed sleep. Mild analgesics, such as the nonsteroidal anti-inflammatory drugs, can relieve muscle aches and pain. Gastrointestinal distress can be treated with dicyclomine.

It is not uncommon to find patients tolerant to different substances (e.g., both a sedative-hypnotic and an opioid). When this situation oc-

TABLE 9–10. Methadone (MTD) withdrawal dosing schedule

Signs and symptoms	Initial MTD dose, mg
Lacrimation, rhinorrhea, diaphoresis, yawning, restlessness, insomnia	5
Dilated pupils, piloerection, muscle twitching, myalgias, arthralgias, abdominal pain	10
Tachycardia, hypertension, tachypnea, fever, anorexia, extreme restlessness, nausea	15
Diarrhea, vomiting, dehydration, hyperglycemia, hypotension	20

Source. Adapted from Perry et al. 2006.

curs, it is safest to stabilize the patient on a dosage of methadone and withdraw the sedative-hypnotic first because sedative-hypnotic withdrawal is potentially the more dangerous syndrome.

Participation in a federally licensed methadone maintenance program continues to be the major alternative to complete cessation of use. With this approach, methadone is administered orally (e.g., 60–100 mg/day). Because of its long half-life (22–56 hours) and its wide distribution in the body, the drug has few subjective effects and produces almost no withdrawal symptoms. The rationale for methadone maintenance is that by switching addicted persons to methadone, their drug hunger is alleviated so that they are less preoccupied with drug-seeking behavior. This approach has been successful, and most people enrolled in these programs have significant decreases in opioid and nonopioid drug use, criminal activity, and depressive symptoms. They also show increases in gainful employment and stability in social relationships. Many programs espouse the view that methadone is a transitional treatment that will eventually lead to total abstinence, and at least one well-designed study has shown that methadone maintenance programs produce better results than detoxification. Methadone programs also emphasize ongoing individual and group psychotherapy; this helps keep addicted persons in the program and provides new skills to help them cope with day-to-day problems without resorting to drugs.

There are now several alternatives to methadone maintenance. Naltrexone, a long-acting opioid antagonist, is FDA approved to treat opioid dependence. The drug is usually given after the acute withdrawal process is complete at dosages of 50–100 mg/day, or 100–150 mg three times weekly. Its use is intended to block the pleasurable effects of opioid drugs thereby making their use less attractive. Buprenorphine (Subutex), a mixed opioid agonist–antagonist, and a combination of buprenorphine and naloxone (Suboxone) are FDA approved to treat opioid dependence. The prescription use of these agents is limited to specially trained physicians who meet certain requirements.

Central Nervous System Stimulant Use Disorders

CNS stimulants include dextroamphetamine, methylphenidate, methamphetamine, phenmetrazine, and cocaine. The action of these drugs is to elevate mood, increase energy and alertness, decrease appetite, and improve task performance. These drugs also cause autonomic hyperarousal, which leads to tachycardia, elevated blood pressure, and pupillary dilation. Amphetamines were first used in the 1930s and have been prescribed to treat depression, obesity, sleep disorders, and attention-deficit/hyperactivity disorder.

The abuse potential of stimulants was recognized relatively early, and illicit use of these drugs is widespread. Because of their overuse in the 1970s as diet pills, changes in the regulation of their legitimate distribution were made to stem the tide of abuse. Even though their legal use has declined, many of these drugs are easy to synthesize, and their illegal use continues to grow. The use of methamphetamine has reached epidemic proportions. Many states have responded by restricting the sale and distribution of pseudoephedrine-containing products, the major ingredient for "meth."

Cocaine differs structurally from the amphetamines but has similar stimulant effects. Derived from the coca plant, which is indigenous to certain countries in South America, cocaine has legitimate medical use as a local anesthetic. Cocaine has always had a following in the United States, and it was used in the late nineteenth century in a variety of elixirs and tonics, including the original Coca-Cola formulation. Freud was one of its earliest advocates. However, cocaine became increasingly associated with sudden death, emotional and domestic problems, and addiction. It was finally declared illegal in the Harrison Act of 1914. Cocaine remains a popular recreational drug, although its use has generally been restricted to affluent groups because of its high cost. A low-cost derivative, crack, became available in the 1980s.

The clinical syndromes produced by the CNS stimulants include those of abuse and dependence, intoxication, delirium, psychosis,

TABLE 9–11. Common psychological and physical symptoms in 32 freebase cocaine abusers

Psychological symptoms	%	Physical symptoms	%
Paranoia	63	Blurred vision	34
Visual hallucinations	50	Coughing	34
Craving	47	Muscle aches	34
Asocial behavior	41	Dry skin	28
Impaired concentration	38	Tremors	28
Irritability	31	Weight loss	25
Bad dreams	31	Chest pains	22
Hyperexcitability	28	Episodic unconsciousness	16
Violence	28	Difficult urination	16
Auditory hallucinations	25	Respiratory problems	9
Lethargy	25	Edema	9
Depression	25	Seizures	3

Source. Adapted from Vereby and Gold 1988.

mood disorders, and withdrawal. Amphetamine intoxication and cocaine intoxication are quite similar and are diagnosed on the basis of their recent use, maladaptive behavior, and evidence of autonomic hyperarousal. Cocaine intoxication also has the potential to induce tactile hallucinations (e.g., "coke bugs").

Psychological symptoms of intoxication include a sense of euphoria, disinhibition, sexual arousal, enhanced feelings of mastery, and improved self-esteem. Depending on how the drug is administered (e.g., intranasally, intravenously), users may experience a rapid onset of euphoria, or "rush." By smoking a purified cocaine base that has been freed from its salts and cutting agents by a chemical process (i.e., freebasing), users report an even more rapid but short-lived high. Table 9–11 presents a list of common psychological and physical symptoms seen in freebase cocaine abusers.

Stimulant intoxication can induce aggression, agitation, and impaired judgment. Transient psychosis can occur, involving persecutory delusions similar to those seen in patients with schizophrenia. The psychosis usually subsides 1–2 weeks after the drug use stops. If a stimulant-induced psychosis persists, a diagnosis of schizophrenia should be considered as long as it is clear that there is no continuing source of the drug. Delirium is a rare complication that gradually resolves once the drug has been discontinued. Cocaine also has been associated with serious medical complications, such as acute myocardial infarction due to coronary artery constriction and anoxic brain damage due to cocaine-induced seizures.

Cessation or reduction of amphetamine (or cocaine) use may lead to a withdrawal syndrome often referred to as a "crash." Symptoms include fatigue and depression, nightmares, headache, profuse sweating, muscle cramps, and hunger. Withdrawal symptoms usually peak in 2–4 days. Intense dysphoria can occur, peaking between 48 and 72 hours after the last dose of the stimulant.

Because amphetamine intoxication and amphetamine-induced psychotic disorder are generally self-limiting, no specific treatment is necessary. Benzodiazepines (e.g., diazepam, lorazepam) can be used to treat agitation or anxiety. Antipsychotics have been used to treat the symptoms of stimulant-induced psychosis but may be unnecessary because the psychosis is generally short-lived once the offending drugs have been stopped. Elimination of the drug can be accelerated by acidifying the urine with ammonium chloride, but this step is rarely necessary. A withdrawal depression that persists longer than 2 weeks can be treated with antidepressants, although their use in these cases has not been systematically evaluated. Some of the effects of stimulant abuse persist long after usage has stopped, including subtle deficits in attention and motor skills.

No medications have been consistently effective in treating stimulant dependence. Desipramine and other antidepressants, the dopamine agonists bromocriptine and amantadine, and even disulfiram have been used to treat cocaine dependence, but their success has been mixed. Cognitive-behavioral therapy has also been studied and appears promising.

Hallucinogen Use Disorders

Hallucinogens are a diverse group of compounds; most are synthetic, but two (peyote, mescaline) are of botanical origin. These drugs can induce psychotic-like experiences, including hallucinations, perceptual disturbances, and feelings of unreality. Some persons believe that hallucinogens bring them closer to God or can expand their minds. The drugs achieved popularity in the late 1960s and early 1970s when psychedelic experiences were romanticized and self-styled drug gurus such as the late Timothy Leary advocated their use. Their use continues, although they are probably not as popular now.

Because they are sympathomimetics, hallucinogens can cause tachycardia, hypertension, sweating, blurry vision, pupillary dilation, and tremors. They affect several neurotransmitter systems, including the dopamine, serotonin, acetylcholine, and γ-aminobutyric acid (GABA) systems. Tolerance develops rapidly to the euphoric and psychedelic effects of hallucinogens. Hallucinogens are probably not physically addicting, but many persons become psychologically dependent on them.

The hallucinogens differ in quality and duration of their subjective effects. As the prototype, LSD is short acting and rapidly absorbed. Onset of action occurs within an hour of ingestion, and effects last between 8 and 12 hours. In addition to autonomic hyperarousal, the drug causes varied psychological effects, including profound alterations in perception (e.g., colors may be experienced as brighter and more intense), and senses appear heightened. Emotions seem to intensify, and many users report becoming more introspective. Many users claim that their use leads to spiritual and philosophical insight. In DSM-IV-TR this reaction is referred to as *hallucinogen intoxication.* In fact, these properties led psychiatrists to experiment with LSD and other hallucinogens in the early 1960s for therapeutic purposes, such as to facilitate communication, improve insight, and increase self-esteem.

"Bad trips" occasionally occur, in which patients become markedly anxious or paranoid. Another undesirable outcome is the *flashback,* a brief reexperiencing of the drug's effects that occurs in situations unrelated to taking the drug. Flashbacks consist of visual distortions, geometric hallucinations, and misperceptions. In DSM-IV-TR, flashbacks that cause marked distress are diagnosed as *hallucinogen persisting perception disorder.* The disorder is usually self-limiting, but it may become chronic in rare cases.

Chronic psychosis has been reported in some hallucinogen users, and it was once thought that these drugs could induce schizophrenia. Although these drugs can cause psychotic episodes in some people, it is likely that users who develop schizophrenia probably would have developed the illness regardless of their hallucinogen use.

Several new "designer" drugs have grown in popularity during the past decade, including methylenedioxymethamphetamine (MDMA), better known as Ecstasy. Mainly used by youth and young adults, it first appeared at "raves" around 1995. Its use has grown dramatically, perhaps because of its acute reinforcing effects. It induces an intense feeling of attachment and connection to others and high energy, which makes users feel that they can dance all night or for days on end. Other effects include altered time perception, peacefulness, euphoria, increased desire for sex, and heightened sensory perceptions—but the drug can also lead to anxiety, depression, and psychosis. Cognitive and memory deficits have been described in chronic users.

Although there is no known withdrawal syndrome for hallucinogens, benzodiazepines have been used to help calm users who experience an adverse reaction when "talking them down" (i.e., explaining that their reaction is due to the drug and providing reassurance) does not work. Overdose can result in a medical emergency due to hyperpyrexia, tachycardia, arrhythmias, stroke, dehydration, or even death.

Phencyclidine Use Disorder

PCP, the prototypical arylcyclohexylamine, has become a significant drug of abuse since the late 1960s. Common street terms for the drug include *angel dust* and *crystal*. PCP originally was developed as an anesthetic agent for animals, and although it affects several neurotransmitter systems, its mechanism of action is unknown. The drug may produce intoxication, delirium, psychosis, or mood disorders and has been known to cause flashbacks. Because PCP is easy to manufacture and is relatively cheap, it is often used to adulterate other illicit compounds.

PCP can be administered in several different ways (e.g., orally, intravenously, intranasally). Onset of action occurs in as little as 5 minutes and peaks in about 30 minutes. Users report euphoria, derealization, tingling sensations, and a feeling of warmth. With moderate dosages, bizarre behavior can occur, along with myoclonic jerks, confusion, and disorientation. Higher dosages can produce coma and seizures. Death can result from respiratory depression. Unlike hallucinogen users, who tend to have dilated pupils, PCP users have normal or small pupils. Chronic psychotic episodes can follow its use. PCP can also cause long-term cognitive deficits.

Treatment may be required for adverse reactions. Diazepam can be used to treat agitation, but severe behavioral disturbances may require use of a short-term antipsychotic, preferably one with a relative lack of anticholinergic side effects (e.g., haloperidol, risperidone). Phentolamine or other antihypertensive drugs can be used to reduce elevated blood pressure. Ammonium chloride can be used to acidify the urine to promote the drug's elimination, although its use is generally unnecessary.

Cannabis Use Disorders

The active ingredient in marijuana is thought to be delta-9-tetrahydrocannabinol (THC). Marijuana is a hemp plant (*Cannabis sativa*) that has been used for centuries for medicinal and recreational purposes. The plant contains varying amounts of THC; plants used today tend to have much higher THC concentrations than in the past. Marijuana achieved popularity among the drug subculture in the 1960s and 1970s and remains the most widely used illicit drug in the United States. Often thought of as relatively benign, marijuana use is common in people with other psychiatric disorders and can precipitate episodes of psychosis in vulnerable persons. Marijuana abuse or dependence also is associated with increased risk for misuse of other drugs.

Marijuana is generally smoked as a cigarette ("joint"), causing intoxication within 10–30 minutes. THC and its metabolites are highly lipid soluble and accumulate in fat cells; the half-life is approximately 50 hours. Intoxication can last 2–4 hours depending on the dosage, although behavioral changes may continue for many hours. Oral ingestion (e.g., from adding marijuana to baked goods) produces a slower onset of action but leads to more powerful intoxicant effects.

Marijuana intoxication can lead users to feel a sense of euphoria and serenity. Users also report feeling that time has slowed. Users develop increased appetite and thirst, feel that their senses are heightened, and report improved self-confidence. Unwanted effects include conjunctivitis (red eyes), tachycardia, dry mouth (cotton mouth), and coughing fits. Many psychological effects reported by marijuana users are similar to those reported by LSD users, such as the development of perceptual distortions, sensitivity to sound, and a feeling of oneness with the environment. But they also can develop feelings of anxiety and paranoia (e.g., hyperalertness, suspiciousness), impaired attention, and decreased motor coordination. Marijuana rarely causes dangerous psychological or physical reactions.

Marijuana has been shown to impair the transfer of material from immediate to long-term memory. Electroencephalographic studies show a suppression of rapid eye movement (REM) sleep and diffuse slowing of background activity. It is often difficult to isolate the effects of marijuana because many of its regular users also take other drugs.

Professional help usually is not needed to treat the adverse effects of marijuana. Benzodiazepines (e.g., diazepam) may help to calm highly anxious users. There is emerging consensus that a withdrawal syndrome occurs when chronic use of marijuana stops. Symptoms include hypersomnia, feeling weak/tired, psychomotor retardation, yawning, depression, and anxiety.

Inhalant Use Disorders

The inhalants are a group of compounds that produce psychoactive vapors. Inhalants include airplane glue, paint thinner, nail polish remover, gasoline, and many other substances found in aerosol cans (e.g., hair spray, room deodorizers). The active substances in the inhalants include toluene, acetone, benzene, and other organic hydrocarbons. Methods of inhalation may vary, but usually a substance is sprayed into a plastic bag and inhaled.

The use of volatile solvents is widespread, and it is estimated that 1 in 10 persons younger than 17 years has experimented with them. Because they are widely available and cheap, inhalants are mostly used by young persons who have trouble gaining access to other psychoactive substances.

Most users of inhalants are male. Latinos and American Indians are overrepresented among inhalant users. Although experimentation with inhalants is extremely common, regular use is found primarily among the low-income groups, children of alcoholic parents, and children from abusive or chaotic homes.

Inhalants act as CNS depressants and produce intoxication similar to that of alcohol but of shorter duration. Effects can last 5–45 minutes and include feelings of excitation, disinhibition, and euphoria. Adverse effects include dizziness, slurred speech, and ataxia. Inhalants also may induce an acute delirium characterized by impaired concentration and disorientation. Hallucinations and delusions have been reported with their use. Other effects include loss of appetite, lateral nystagmus, hypoactive reflexes, and double vision. At higher dosages, patients may become stuporous or comatose.

Inhalants do not cause a specific withdrawal syndrome. Because inhalants often contain high concentrations of heavy metals, permanent neuromuscular and brain damage can occur, along with serious risk of damage to the kidneys, liver, and other organs from benzene and other hydrocarbons.

Other Substance Use Disorders

Nicotine

Nicotine is a highly addictive drug found in cigarettes, chewing tobacco and snuff, and other tobacco products. About 25% of adult Americans smoke, although smoking is even more frequent in certain groups (e.g., minority groups, low-income persons, less-educated persons). Rates among psychiatric patients are also very high. For example, alcohol- or drug-dependent patients are highly likely to smoke, and nearly 90% of schizophrenic patients smoke.

Smoking has been implicated as a cause of lung cancer, emphysema, and cardiovascular disease. Snuff and chewing tobacco have been associated with oropharyngeal cancers. Secondary smoke has been associated with respiratory and cardiovascular diseases.

Dependence on nicotine develops quickly and is often reinforced by peer pressure. Society has clearly changed its views on smoking, and in recent years, smokers' rights have been increasingly limited.

Nicotine withdrawal usually begins within 1 hour after the last cigarette is smoked and peaks within 24 hours. Withdrawal may last weeks or months and consists of nicotine craving, irritability, anxiety, restlessness, and decreased heart rate. Weight gain and depression often follow smoking cessation.

There are several FDA-approved treatments for smoking cessation. These options include nicotine transdermal patches and nicotine-containing gum, lozenges, and inhalers; bupropion, an antidepressant marketed as Zyban; and varenicline (Chantix), a newer option that may be more effective than nicotine replacement or bupropion.

Because the consequences of tobacco use are so potentially harmful, all physicians have a responsibility to urge their patients, particularly young patients, not to smoke or to use tobacco products and to assist patients who do use them to quit.

Caffeine

Caffeine is found in coffee, tea, chocolate, cola drinks, and many over-the-counter pain and cold remedies. Use of caffeine is nearly universal.

The mild stimulant effects of caffeine occur at dosages of 50–150 mg (i.e., one cup of coffee). These effects include increased alertness and improved verbal and motor performance. At higher dosages, unless tolerance has been achieved, signs of intoxication occur, including restlessness, irritability, and insomnia. Massive doses can lead to seizures and coma. Withdrawal from caffeine can induce headaches, lethargy, irritability, and depression. Higher daily dosages are more likely to lead to withdrawal.

Because caffeine is well known to aggravate anxiety syndromes such as panic disorder or generalized anxiety disorder, students should always ask patients about their caffeine intake. Chronic use can itself cause excessive anxiety; in DSM-IV-TR, this condition is called *caffeine-induced anxiety disorder.* Caffeine intake can contribute to excess gastric acidity and thereby worsen esophageal and gastric disorders, and can exacerbate fibrocystic breast disease in women. Caffeine also is probably the most common and underrecognized cause of insomnia.

Once caffeinism is diagnosed, treatment consists of reducing or gradually eliminating caffeine from the diet. Decaffeinated cola drinks, tea, and coffee are now widely available.

Anabolic Steroids

Anabolic steroids are widely abused by athletes who believe that their performance and muscle mass will be enhanced by their use. Although these drugs may initially produce a sense of well-being, this feeling is later replaced by anergy, dysphoria, and irritability. Frank psychosis can develop, as can serious medical problems, including liver disease.

Nitrate Inhalants

Nitrate inhalants ("poppers") produce an intoxicated state character-ized by a feeling of fullness in the head, mild euphoria, a change in time perception, relaxation of the smooth muscles, and possibly an increase in sexual feelings. These drugs carry the possible risk of immune sys-tem impairment, respiratory system irritation, and a toxic reaction that may lead to vomiting, severe headaches, and hypotension.

Nitrous Oxide

Nitrous oxide ("laughing gas") can cause intoxication characterized by light-headedness and a floating sensation that quickly clear once the administration of gas stops. Temporary confusion or paranoia can occur when this substance is used regularly.

Clinical Management of Drug Use Disorders

As in the treatment of alcohol abuse and dependence, treatment of drug use disorders can be thought of as having two phases—an acute phase and a continuation phase. In the acute phase, detoxification is the major goal. This goal may be difficult to achieve in some patients, such as those with potentially serious withdrawal syndromes (e.g., barbiturate or opioid abusers). Detoxification may be easier in others (e.g., mari-juana abusers) who have no specific withdrawal syndrome. Hospital-ization is necessary for safe detoxification in some patients so that tolerance can be determined and a slow drug taper can be monitored under medical supervision. The circumstances of detoxification should be determined by the patient and physician working together.

Many persons addicted to drugs have serious medical conditions that the physician also must address during this phase of treatment. For example, a heroin-addicted person may have an antecubital cellulitis and be seropositive for HIV; a cocaine-addicted person may have an eroded nasal septum (from sniffing the drug) that has become second-arily infected.

Psychiatric comorbidity is also important to assess during the acute phase of treatment. Many, if not most, substance abusers have additional mental illnesses that can have a profound effect on their treatment outcome. Abuse of other substances is the most common comorbidity, followed by mood disorders, anxiety disorders, and personality disorders. Comorbidity complicates treatment efforts and reduces the likelihood of success. Examples include the amphetamine abuser who develops a suicidal depression during withdrawal and the heroin-addicted person with an antisocial personality disorder whose use seems, in part, motivated by his membership in a street gang that celebrates drug use.

The continuation phase of treatment consists of efforts to rehabilitate the patient and to prevent future misuse of drugs. The success of this phase is almost completely dependent on the motivation of the patient because there is no way to truly assess or enforce compliance—except, of course, by frequent and random drug screening tests and threats of punishment for noncompliance. Such strict enforcement is neither possible nor desirable, except in the military, in certain professions (e.g., pilots), and in authoritarian societies.

Multimodal approaches are necessary for rehabilitation. Individual psychotherapy is important to help patients learn about their motivation for using drugs and to learn alternative methods for handling stressful situations. Group therapy, especially in the hospital, is useful in confronting patients with the seriousness of their problem and how the drug significantly affects their lives. Peer groups are unequaled in their ability to achieve confrontation. At least among cocaine-dependent persons, the combination of individual and group psychotherapy works best at preventing relapse, as one recent study showed.

Among other approaches, cognitive-behavioral therapy may help the patient reverse habits that lead to or promote drug use or may correct cognitive distortions (e.g., "If I don't use drugs, I won't be popular"). Social skills training may help some patients break a cycle of getting in with the wrong crowd and learn to meet and be accepted by more appropriate peers. Family therapy and marital counseling are necessary adjuncts in other patients. Examples include the teenager whose inhalant use has disrupted his family life and the young man whose marriage is coming apart because of his cocaine addiction.

Contingency management, a form of behavior therapy, is used in some programs to encourage a drug-free lifestyle. With contingency management, people are "rewarded" (or positively reinforced) for appropriate behavior. For example, each time a person submits a clean urine sample, he or she receives a voucher that can be exchanged for retail goods or services. Research shows that low-cost rewards can be effective in reducing drug use.

Medical approaches for the continuation phase of treatment can be important. Methadone maintenance for those persons addicted to opioids has been popular for years and seems to have an established role in the treatment of at least some opioid addiction. The user is given a carefully monitored substitute addiction that allows him or her to function in society. Buprenorphine is another recent alternative for the maintenance phase of treatment. Patients with comorbid psychiatric disorders may, of course, benefit from ongoing treatment of anxiety, depression, or psychosis.

Self-help groups have become an integral part of a comprehensive treatment approach to substance use disorders. AA has led the way for the creation of sister groups, such as Cocaine Anonymous, Narcotics Anonymous, and Drugs Anonymous. These groups, now available in many parts of the United States, are organized along the same lines as AA and follow a 12-step model. They provide an atmosphere of mutual support in which recovering addicted persons can share their experiences.

Key points to remember about drug use disorders

1. The clinician should not allow his or her personal beliefs and attitudes about drug abuse to interfere with the care of the addicted patient.

   - Patients need a consistent yet firm approach.
   - The clinician should neither condemn addicted persons nor condone their behavior.

2. The clinician should assess the patient for medical and psychiatric comorbidity. Many addicted persons have potentially serious medical problems that require treatment, significant addictions to other substances, and co-occurring mood and anxiety disorders, or a personality disorder.

3. The clinician should be prepared for relapses during the continuation phase of treatment. Relapse is nearly inevitable, but it does not represent failure of the treatment program. The clinician must be there to help the patient get back on the wagon.

4. Support groups can be very helpful to the patient, and referral to community-based organizations is essential.

■ Self-Assessment Questions

1. What is the benefit to the disease concept of alcoholism?
2. How is alcohol dependence diagnosed?
3. How do Type I and Type II alcoholic persons differ?
4. What are the clinical findings in the earliest stage of alcoholism? Middle stage? Late stage?
5. List the medical complications of alcoholism. What laboratory abnormalities are associated with alcoholism?
6. What are the major alcohol withdrawal syndromes, and how are they treated?
7. Discuss the role of disulfiram, naltrexone, and acamprosate in the treatment of alcoholism.
8. What are the predictors of good outcome for alcohol rehabilitation efforts?
9. How widespread are drug abuse and dependence, and what are their risk factors?
10. What appear to be the two types of sedative-hypnotic abusers?
11. Describe the withdrawal syndrome from sedatives, hypnotics, and anxiolytics. Why are barbiturates especially dangerous? Describe the pentobarbital-diazepam tolerance test.
12. Describe the opioid withdrawal syndrome and how it differs from sedative-hypnotic withdrawal.
13. What are the psychological effects of cocaine use?
14. What drugs are used to treat opioid dependence?
15. What are the symptoms of PCP intoxication?
16. What are the long-term consequences of marijuana use?
17. Why are the inhalants potentially dangerous?
18. Why do athletes abuse anabolic steroids?
19. What are the approved treatments for smoking cessation?
20. What is contingency management?

CHAPTER 10

Personality Disorders

All is caprice, they love without measure those whom they will soon hate without reason.

Thomas Sydenham

MALADAPTIVE CHARACTER traits have been recognized since Cain killed his brother Abel. In ancient Greece, Hippocrates observed and classified many of the mental illnesses that are recognized today. Although he had no category for personality disorders, he described four temperaments believed to embody the elements of earth, air, fire, and water: the optimistic sanguine, the irritable choleric, the sad melancholic, and the apathetic phlegmatic. Variations of this simple classification of temperament were used right up to the twentieth century; the German psychiatrist Kraepelin, in fact, described the personalities he found in manic-depressive patients and their relatives as depressive, hypomanic, or irritable, terms that correspond to the melancholic, sanguine, and choleric temperaments.

Formal attempts to list the variety of personality types took root with the publication of DSM-I in 1952, in which seven different types of personality disturbances were described. With the arrival of DSM-III in 1980, personality disorders were accorded new status on a separate axis in the multiaxial evaluation system; criteria for 11 different personality disorders were enumerated, including several new disorders created in response to clinical and research observations. The list of personality disorders was pared to 10 in DSM-IV, which was published in 1994, and did not change with the text revision, DSM-IV-TR, published in 2000 (see Table 10–1).

Personality disorders are defined in DSM-IV-TR as an enduring pattern of inner experience and behavior that deviates markedly from the expectations of the individual's culture, is pervasive and inflexible, has an onset in adolescence or early adulthood, is stable over time, and leads to distress or impairment. As a general rule, personality disorders are representative of long-term functioning and are not limited to episodes of illness. A personality disorder is not diagnosed, for instance, in a person who develops transient personality changes during an episode of major depression.

These disorders are coded on Axis II in order to separate them from the major mental disorders, which are coded on Axis I. A person can— and often does—have both Axis I and Axis II disorders, with some exceptions. For example, personality disorders are not diagnosed in persons with chronic psychotic disorders (e.g., schizophrenia). These conditions are so devastating to the personality that the concept of personality disorder becomes meaningless.

The purpose of creating a separate axis for personality disorders was to separate them from major (Axis I) mental disorders. To some clinicians, coding personality disorders on Axis II devalues their importance and promotes the impression that they are lesser disorders that can be ignored in favor of the "major disorders." Yet for many patients, the preponderant problem is a personality disorder, not the dysthymia, panic disorder, or adjustment disorder coded on Axis I.

The 10 personality disorders are divided among three clusters. Each cluster is characterized by phenomenologically similar disorders, or personality disorders whose criteria overlap. Cluster A consists of the eccentric disorders—paranoid, schizoid, and schizotypal personality disorders. They are characterized by a pervasive pattern of abnormal cognition (e.g., suspiciousness), self-expression (e.g., odd speech), or relating to others (e.g., reclusiveness). Cluster B consists of the dramatic disorders—borderline, antisocial, histrionic, and narcissistic personality disorders. They are characterized by a pervasive pattern of violating social norms or the rights of others (e.g., criminal behavior), impulsivity, excessive emotionality, grandiosity, or "acting out" (e.g., tantrums, self-abusive behavior, angry outbursts). Cluster C consists of the anxious disorders—avoidant, dependent, and obsessive-compulsive personality disorders. They are characterized by a pervasive pattern of abnormal fears involving social relationships, separation, and need for

---

TABLE 10–1.   DSM-IV-TR personality disorders

Cluster A (the "eccentric" disorders)
  Paranoid
  Schizoid
  Schizotypal

Cluster B (the "dramatic" disorders)
  Antisocial
  Borderline
  Histrionic
  Narcissistic

Cluster C (the "anxious" disorders)
  Avoidant
  Dependent
  Obsessive-compulsive

---

control. In addition to the 10 distinct personality disorders listed in DSM-IV-TR, a residual category (personality disorder not otherwise specified) exists for individuals with mixed or atypical traits that do not fit into the better-defined categories.

Many psychiatrists and psychologists believe that the DSM approach to diagnosis has little relevance to clinical reality and is not helpful in treating patients. These clinicians generally prefer a dimensional approach in which personality traits are described along a continuum from normality to severe dysfunction. There is growing consensus among personality theorists, especially those using an evidence-based statistical approach, that the major share of differences in personality among individuals can be described by four or five major traits. In the best known scheme, the traits (or factors) are extraversion, agreeableness, conscientiousness, neuroticism, and openness to experience. The meaning of *neuroticism* is less self-evident, but persons high in this dimension are prone to worry, to feel nervous, and to be self-conscious, temperamental, and high-strung.

Another criticism of the DSM approach is that it leaves out normal personality variations and the way they shade into more dysfunctional types. In truth, few people with personality disorders show exclusively the traits of the diagnosed disorder, and they typically will have traits belonging to several of the defined types. For this reason, the residual category *personality disorder not otherwise specified* will be an appropriate diagnosis for patients who do not meet the full criteria for a particular disorder but who have traits from many different ones.

Some mental health professionals devalue the suffering of patients with personality disorders or may view their treatment as long-term, complicated, and ineffective. This situation is particularly unfortunate because it is based on misinformation and prejudice, which have no place in medical practice. In fact, most patients with personality disorders are neither difficult nor unpleasant, their treatment is not always long-term, and their treatment results are often successful and rewarding. The different personality disorders are so varied that it is rarely useful to make generalizations about all patients with personality disorders based on one's experience with a particular type.

■ Epidemiology

Epidemiological surveys confirm the high prevalence of personality disorders, with between 9% and 16% of the general population meeting criteria for one or more personality disorders. The prevalence is far greater in psychiatric samples; in some studies, 30%–50% of outpatients have a personality disorder, although the frequency and types differ among the Axis I disorders. For example, in one study, 51% of persons with major depression, 64% of persons with generalized anxiety disorder, and 56% of persons with panic disorder had a comorbid personality disorder. Incarcerated persons have an even higher frequency of personality disorder.

The frequency of specific personality disorder differs by gender. Antisocial personality disorder occurs more frequently in men, whereas borderline personality disorder, avoidant personality disorder, and dependent personality disorder are more frequent in women. Others have a fairly equal gender distribution (schizoid, schizotypal, and obsessive-compulsive personality disorders). Younger persons are at greater risk for a personality disorder than older individuals, as prevalence diminishes with advancing age. Other general risk factors for personality disorder include lower levels of education and lower socioeconomic status. Both substance misuse (alcohol and drugs) and cigarette smoking are more frequent among those with a personality disorder than those without.

Personality disorders tend to have an onset in adolescence and are established by young adulthood. Personality changes that appear later in life strongly suggest the presence of a major mental illness (e.g., early stages of schizophrenia), a brain disorder, or a disorder caused by medical illness or the effects of a substance. DSM-IV-TR requires that maladaptive personality features be present for at least 1 year if a personality disorder is to be diagnosed in a person younger than 18 years. The exception is antisocial personality disorder, in which an age requirement is specified (18 years), as is the requirement that certain childhood behaviors be present along with the adult traits. Although no other personality disorders have child or adolescent criteria, research suggests that behavioral precursors such as affective lability or impulsivity can sometimes be traced back to childhood. Furthermore, personality pathology in childhood or adolescence is predictive of adult maladjustment and of both Axis I and II disorders.

Personality disorders can cause enormous problems for individuals and society and are frequently associated with impaired social, interpersonal, and occupational adjustment. Family life, marriages, and academic and work performance suffer. Rates of unemployment, homelessness, divorce and separation, domestic violence, and substance misuse are high. These disorders also are associated with increased rates of health care utilization (e.g., emergency department visits, hospitalizations) and excessive rates of traumatic accidents. As a group, individuals with personality disorders are at risk for early death from suicide or accidents. The risk of suicide is about the same as that seen for major depression.

Personality disorders are generally thought to be stable and enduring, yet several recent follow-up studies show a more subtle and complex picture. Over varying lengths of follow-up, fewer people will meet criteria for a personality disorder, yet most remain impaired in interpersonal, occupational, and other domains of life. For example, in one large study, 668 patients at five sites were followed. By 2 years, around 40% of persons initially found to meet criteria for the schizotypal, borderline, avoidant, or obsessive-compulsive types still met criteria for the personality disorder. Persons with the poorest functioning initially tended to have the poorest functioning at follow-up. This study tends to confirm what psychiatrists have long held to be true—that is, that many persons with personality disorder become less symptomatic as they age, and although some may experience remission, most continue to have impaired functioning in important life domains. With regard to antisocial personality disorder and borderline personality disorder, this phenomenon has been called "burnout," a term implying that the disturbance diminishes over time like a light bulb dimming until its glow fades. Which symptoms lessen in severity is a matter of conjecture, but at least for borderline personality disorder, diminished impulsivity is one such symptom. Follow-up-studies also suggest that personality disorders, like other mental illnesses, tend to wax and wane in severity over time, often in response to significant life events.

Psychiatric comorbidity is the rule and not the exception. Nearly all persons with a personality disorder have comorbid Axis I disorders, with major depression being the most frequent. Other mood, anxiety, substance use, and eating disorders are all commonly diagnosed in persons with a personality disorder. Comorbidity among the personality disorders is also very common, with persons with one disorder frequently meeting criteria for another. As mentioned earlier, few persons have a "pure" case in which they meet criteria for only one personality disorder.

The presence of a personality disorder affects the course and outcome of a comorbid Axis I. For example, depressed patients with a personality disorder tend to be younger, are more likely to be female, are more likely to have a history of marital instability, are more likely to report precipitating stressors for the depression, and are more likely to have a history of nonserious suicide attempts. These findings suggest that depressed patients with personality disorder may form an important subgroup that differs biologically and perhaps genetically from depressed patients with primary depressive illness unaccompanied by a personality disorder. Importantly, the presence of a personality disorder is often associated with a poorer response to treatment, as has been shown for several Axis I disorders, including major depression, panic disorder, and obsessive-compulsive disorder.

■ Etiology

The cause of personality disorders is unknown, though various theories have focused on developmental, genetic, neurobiological, and cultural influences. Psychoanalysts have long suggested that early life events are causative factors and that personality disorders occur when a person fails to progress through appropriate stages of psychosexual development. Several of the DSM-IV-TR disorders derive from the oral, anal, and phallic character types that were described by Freud and others. Fixation at the oral stage was thought to result in a personality characterized by demanding and dependent behavior (i.e., dependent personality disorder). Fixation at the anal stage was thought to lead to a personality characterized by obsessionality, rigidity, and emotional aloofness (i.e., obsessive-compulsive personality disorder). Fixation at the phallic stage was believed to cause shallowness and an inability to engage in intimate relationships (i.e., histrionic personality). These broad character types do, in fact, show some correlation with the five-factor model of personality disorder described earlier, but little evidence shows that they are related to developmental fixations early in life.

A growing body of evidence suggests that childhood abuse or maltreatment is associated with risk for personality disorder in general and perhaps borderline and antisocial personality disorders specifically. The resulting trauma is thought to cause difficulty in developing trust and intimacy. An early home environment in which domestic abuse, divorce, separation, or parental absence is found also can contribute to the risk of developing a personality disorder.

Genetic factors help to explain some of the personality disorders. Family, twin, and adoption studies suggest that schizotypal personality disorder is genetically related to schizophrenia. Family and adoption studies also have confirmed a strong genetic factor in the etiology of antisocial and borderline personality disorders. Antisocial personality disorder, for instance, has been found more frequently in identical than in nonidentical twins, and offspring of antisocial parents adopted in childhood are more likely to develop antisocial behavior than are adoptees without an antisocial parent. Less evidence is available for the heritability of the other DSM-IV-TR personality disorders. Some evidence suggests that basic dimensions of personality (e.g., callousness, intimacy problems) are inherited along a continuum with normality.

The neurobiology of personality disorders is being actively studied. Schizotypal personality disorder has been associated with impaired smooth pursuit eye movement, impaired performance on tests of executive function, and increased ventricular-brain ratio on computed tomography. Aberrant serotonin neurotransmission has been linked to impulsive and aggressive behaviors typical of both borderline and antisocial personality disorders. As a group, antisocial persons have low resting pulse, low skin conductance, and increased amplitude on event-related potentials. These findings suggest to some that antisocial persons are chronically underaroused and that they perhaps seek out potentially dangerous or risky situations to raise their arousal to more optimal levels to satisfy their craving for excitement.

Abnormal brain structure and function have been associated with borderline personality disorder and antisocial personality disorder. With the former, positron emission tomography has shown altered metabolism in prefrontal regions, including the anterior cingulate cortex; reduced frontal and orbitofrontal volume also has been reported. One study of antisocial persons found them to have reduced prefrontal gray matter, while another identified specific abnormalities in the processing of emotions in psychopathic criminals. On functional magnetic resonance imaging scans, the criminals showed less affect-related activity in important limbic structures and increased activity in the frontotemporal cortex. Because these brain regions help regulate mood and behavior, impulsive aggression or emotional instability could stem from functional abnormalities in these areas.

Cultural factors may affect the development and expression of a personality disorder. The best evidence for this comes from cross-cultural research showing very low rates of antisocial personality disorder in Taiwan, China, and Japan. Possibly, the family structure in East Asian cultures helps to maintain high levels of cohesion. Similarly low rates of antisocial personality disorder occur in Jewish families, presumably because of their strong family structures. Yet at the same time, the repressive style seen in these same families may have an association with Cluster C disorders.

■ Diagnosis

Individuals with a personality disorder often have little insight into the difficulties their maladaptive traits create, so they are prone to view others as the source of their problems. For that reason, only rarely does the presence of a personality disorder itself lead the individual to seek help. More likely, the consequences of the person's ongoing troubles—chronic depression, poor work performance, domestic troubles—lead him or her to seek help. The clinician's task is to assist the patient to understand how the maladaptive personality traits contribute to his or her ongoing problems. The clinician can then help the patient to develop new skills to modify the maladaptive traits that contribute to the individual's difficult life situations.

The diagnosis of a personality disorder requires a thorough personal and social history and a careful mental status examination. Several structured interviews and self-report instruments are available to help with diagnosis but are mainly used in research. More typically, the clinician's inquiries will lead to the conclusion that a personality disorder may be present. When this is suspected, the clinician should inquire about the kinds of symptoms found in these patients. We have observed that one clue to the presence of a personality disorder is when the patient's immediate problem and his or her social history intertwine.

As with other psychiatric or behavioral disorders, the patient's history forms the most important basis for diagnosing a personality disorder. The clinician's initial goal is to define the extent of the disorder through relatively nonintrusive inquiries; he or she should then move on to more detailed and specific questions regarding the patient's attitudes and behaviors. For general screening purposes, a clinician might ask about problems in the following domains: interpersonal relationships, sense of self, work, affect, impulse control, and reality testing. Suggested questions include the following:

- Do you often have days when your mood is constantly changing?
- How do you feel when you are not the center of attention?
- Do you frequently insist on having what you want right now?
- Are you concerned that certain friends or co-workers are not really loyal or trustworthy?
- Are you concerned about saying the wrong things in front of other people?
- How often do you avoid getting to know someone because you are worried he or she may not like you?

Once the clinician forms his or her initial impression, detailed inquiries can be made guided by the core features of the suspected personality disorder. Because of great overlap among the different personality disorders, inquiries may need to be fairly broad.

Collateral information also is important when a personality disorder is suspected but the patient denies or seems unaware of his or her maladaptive traits. A person with antisocial personality disorder may deny criminal activity or minimize its significance ("He deserved to be mugged!"). Information from relatives, the police, or a parole officer can be helpful in confirming the severity and extent of the behavior. An informant also can be helpful in determining whether an observed behavior is characteristic of the patient's long-term functioning or whether the trait has been sufficiently severe to cause recurrent problems in how the person interacts with others. Of course, confidentiality must be preserved, so informants can only be contacted with the patient's consent.

It is important not to make a personality disorder diagnosis prematurely. Patients with major depression are often socially anxious and dependent on others, traits that tend to recede or disappear when the depression is successfully treated. For that reason, caution needs to be used in making the diagnosis, particularly when the patient has an Axis I disorder like major depression that can distort one's normal personality or exaggerate preexisting personality traits.

Long-term observation may be necessary with some patients to confirm the diagnosis of personality disorder. Sometimes the clinician will defer diagnosis of a personality disorder—even when one is suspected—until he or she has seen the patient several times and has had the opportunity to gather additional information. In this case, the word "defer" should be coded on Axis II. This word alerts other clinicians that a personality disorder is suspected but that information to confirm the diagnosis is insufficient. When a personality disorder was present before the onset of the psychotic disorder, it is coded on Axis II followed by the word "premorbid" in parentheses.

The concept of a personality disorder also needs to be separated from normal personality. Most people have minor personality quirks or idiosyncrasies, but these rarely rise to the level of a disorder. A key distinction is that the trait in question is inflexible, maladaptive, and leads to distress or impairment in one or more life domains. Most people learn to adapt to changing circumstances and learn from experience. People with a personality disorder often persist with their maladaptive behaviors regardless of the consequences. The clinician should also be aware of cultural issues that may affect a personality disorder diagnosis because certain traits may be considered normal in some societies but not others. For example, in some societies, belief in magic and sorcery is widespread and culturally accepted; in contemporary American society, such beliefs may be viewed as magical thinking associated with a schizotypal personality disorder.

■ Treatment

It is difficult to generalize about the treatment of the various personality disorders. First, few of the 10 personality disorders have been studied sufficiently to recommend specific treatments. For this reason, recommendations made below are often based on clinical experience, not empirical evidence. Second, the disorders are sufficiently different that treatment recommendations for one disorder may not apply to another. For example, the person with avoidant personality disorder has symptoms of extreme anxiety and inhibition; the person with borderline personality disorder, on the other hand, has difficulty with anger, moodiness, and impulsivity. That said, contrary to assumptions that persons with personality disorder cannot benefit from treatment, reviews of outcome studies have shown that treatment results are largely positive.

Treatment of the personality disorders can be divided into pharmacologic or psychological interventions. Although many drug treatment studies of personality disorder have been conducted over the past few decades, the pace of progress has been slow compared with the major mental disorders such as major depression or schizophrenia. There are currently no medications approved by the U.S. Food and Drug Administration for *any* personality disorder. Furthermore, some disorders have been studied extensively (e.g., borderline personality disorder) and others not at all (e.g., histrionic personality disorder). The same is true for psychotherapy (mainly involving individual and group treatments): borderline personality disorder has been actively studied, and several evidence-based psychotherapies now exist, whereas schizoid personality disorder, for example, has been virtually ignored. Other forms of psychological treatment for personality disorder, including family therapy and marital (or couples) therapy, have such a small data base that it is difficult to make sound recommendations for these forms of treatment.

■ The DSM-IV-TR Personality Disorders

Cluster A Disorders

Paranoid Personality Disorder

Paranoid personality was first described by Adolf Meyer in the early twentieth century. Early formulations of the disorder came from a psychoanalytic perspective, which emphasized the defense mechanisms of *reaction formation* and *projection*. Some researchers have hypothesized that paranoid personality disorder lies within the schizophrenic spectrum and is the product of a common genetic predisposition. A behavioral model has been suggested in which suspiciousness and mistrust are learned, leading to social withdrawal, testing of others, and ruminative suspiciousness.

These patients are chronically suspicious, distrust others, and fulfill their suspicious prophecies by leading others to be overly cautious and deceptive (see Table 10–2). Frank delusions are absent. Persons with paranoid personality disorder rarely seek treatment, most likely because of their general suspiciousness of others, including psychiatrists and therapists. The disorder has an estimated prevalence of 1%–4.5% in the general population. It is often recognized when the patient seeks treatment for a mood or anxiety disorder. Apart from diagnosing and managing the patients' main complaint, the clinician should take care to be supportive and to listen patiently to their accusations and com-

---

TABLE 10–2. DSM-IV-TR diagnostic criteria for paranoid personality disorder

---

A. A pervasive distrust and suspiciousness of others such that their motives are interpreted as malevolent, beginning by early adulthood and present in a variety of contexts, as indicated by four (or more) of the following:
   (1) suspects, without sufficient basis, that others are exploiting, harming, or deceiving him or her
   (2) is preoccupied with unjustified doubts about the loyalty or trustworthiness of friends or associates
   (3) is reluctant to confide in others because of unwarranted fear that the information will be used maliciously against him or her
   (4) reads hidden demeaning or threatening meanings into benign remarks or events
   (5) persistently bears grudges, i.e., is unforgiving of insults, injuries, or slights
   (6) perceives attacks on his or her character or reputation that are not apparent to others and is quick to react angrily or to counterattack
   (7) has recurrent suspicions, without justification, regarding fidelity of spouse or sexual partner
B. Does not occur exclusively during the course of Schizophrenia, a Mood Disorder With Psychotic Features, or another Psychotic Disorder and is not due to the direct physiological effects of a general medical condition.
Note: If criteria are met prior to the onset of Schizophrenia, add "Premorbid," e.g., "Paranoid Personality Disorder (Premorbid)."

---

plaints while being open, honest, and respectful. When rapport has been established, alternative explanations for the patients' misperceptions can be suggested. Group therapy should be avoided because patients with paranoid personality disorder tend to misinterpret statements and situations that arise in the course of the therapy. Antipsychotics may help to reduce their suspiciousness, although these drugs have not been specifically studied for this condition.

Schizoid Personality Disorder

The term *schizoid* was originally used to characterize the premorbid seclusiveness of schizophrenic patients and their eccentric relatives.

TABLE 10–3. DSM-IV-TR diagnostic criteria for schizoid personality disorder

A. A pervasive pattern of detachment from social relationships and a restricted range of expression of emotions in interpersonal settings, beginning by early adulthood and present in a variety of contexts, as indicated by four (or more) of the following:
   (1) neither desires nor enjoys close relationships, including being part of a family
   (2) almost always chooses solitary activities
   (3) has little, if any, interest in having sexual experiences with another person
   (4) takes pleasure in few, if any, activities
   (5) lacks close friends or confidants other than first-degree relatives
   (6) appears indifferent to the praise or criticism of others
   (7) shows emotional coldness, detachment, or flattened affectivity
B. Does not occur exclusively during the course of Schizophrenia, a Mood Disorder With Psychotic Features, another Psychotic Disorder, or a Pervasive Developmental Disorder and is not due to the direct physiological effects of a general medical condition.
Note: If criteria are met prior to the onset of Schizophrenia, add "Premorbid," e.g., "Schizoid Personality Disorder (Premorbid)."

Gradually, it came to be used to describe almost all persons who had difficulty achieving intimacy. The concept of schizoid personality disorder was narrowed in 1980 in DSM-III. At that time, odd, eccentric people were relegated to a new category, schizotypal personality disorder. Persons who were isolated because of an unwillingness to confront rejection were placed in another new category, avoidant personality disorder. Schizoid personality disorder became restricted to persons with a profound defect in the ability to form personal relationships and to respond to others in a meaningful way (see Table 10–3). The following case from our hospital illustrates the disorder:

> Michael, a 24-year-old man, was transferred to the psychiatric inpatient unit after receiving treatment for a self-inflicted gunshot wound to the head. The bullet grazed his scalp but did not cause a brain injury. According to his family, he had been depressed for several weeks before shooting himself. After transfer, Michael denied feeling depressed and believed that there was no reason for him to be in the hospital.
>
> Michael had always been considered shy by his relatives, he was socially isolated, and he had no friends that his family was aware of. He

had done poorly in school and had dropped out before graduating from high school. Michael had never dated and had no interest in sexual activity, apart from masturbation. Michael admitted that he was not emotionally close to any of his family members, and although he lived with his elderly father, he showed little interest or affection in describing their relationship. Despite having average intelligence, Michael had never persisted with a job and was currently unemployed. He preferred to stay home and watch television or play computer games. He had never bothered to obtain a driver's license.

Michael believed that his only problem was episodic depression. He neither complained about his social isolation and emotional aloofness nor accepted the fact that these symptoms could reflect an underlying disorder. He had no interest in changing his ways and refused referral for psychotherapy.

Like Michael, patients with schizoid personality disorder have no close relationships and choose solitary activities. They rarely experience strong emotions, express little desire for sexual experience with another person, are indifferent to praise or criticism, and display a constricted affect. The disorder is not diagnosed in persons with schizophrenia or other psychotic disorders because these conditions are typically accompanied by a schizoid lifestyle.

Schizoid personality disorder is found in less than 1% of adults in the general population. It is also uncommon in clinical settings because persons with this disturbance rarely seek psychiatric help. When schizoid persons come to clinical attention, it is generally because of a co-occurring disorder such as major depression, an anxiety disorder, or substance abuse. Schizoid persons lack the insight and motivation necessary for individual psychotherapy and would likely find the intimacy of traditional group therapy threatening. That said, these individuals may be candidates for the types of day programs or drop-in centers that are often affiliated with community mental health centers. If the patient expresses a strong desire for social contact, it may be that avoidant personality disorder may be the more appropriate diagnosis (see later discussion).

Schizotypal Personality Disorder

The diagnostic category *schizotypal personality disorder* was created during the development of DSM-III. Researchers had observed that relatives of schizophrenic patients often had a cluster of schizophrenic-like traits, a fact noted earlier by Kraepelin and Bleuler around the turn of the twentieth century. Forerunners of this disorder included Bleuler's categories of simple and latent schizophrenia, which were diagnosed in

TABLE 10–4. DSM-IV-TR diagnostic criteria for schizotypal personality disorder

A. A pervasive pattern of social and interpersonal deficits marked by acute discomfort with, and reduced capacity for, close relationships as well as by cognitive or perceptual distortions and eccentricities of behavior, beginning by early adulthood and present in a variety of contexts, as indicated by five (or more) of the following:
   (1) ideas of reference (excluding delusions of reference)
   (2) odd beliefs or magical thinking that influences behavior and is inconsistent with subcultural norms (e.g., superstitiousness, belief in clairvoyance, telepathy, or "sixth sense"; in children and adolescents, bizarre fantasies or preoccupations)
   (3) unusual perceptual experiences, including bodily illusions
   (4) odd thinking and speech (e.g., vague, circumstantial, metaphorical, overelaborate, or stereotyped)
   (5) suspiciousness or paranoid ideation
   (6) inappropriate or constricted affect
   (7) behavior or appearance that is odd, eccentric, or peculiar
   (8) lack of close friends or confidants other than first-degree relatives
   (9) excessive social anxiety that does not diminish with familiarity and tends to be associated with paranoid fears rather than negative judgments about self
B. Does not occur exclusively during the course of Schizophrenia, a Mood Disorder With Psychotic Features, another Psychotic Disorder, or a Pervasive Developmental Disorder.
Note: If criteria are met prior to the onset of Schizophrenia, add "Premorbid," e.g., "Schizotypal Personality Disorder (Premorbid)."

nonpsychotic persons who showed mild symptoms of schizophrenia such as avolition or apathy. Schizotypal personality disorder now is considered part of the schizophrenia spectrum, along with schizophreniform disorder, schizoaffective disorder, and perhaps psychotic mood disorders.

Schizotypal personality disorder is characterized by a pattern of peculiar behavior, odd speech and thinking, and unusual perceptual experiences. Schizotypal patients are frequently socially isolated and have "magical" beliefs, mild paranoia, inappropriate or constricted affect, and social anxiety (see Table 10–4).

Community surveys show that schizotypal personality disorder has a prevalence of 1%–2%. Comorbidity with mood, substance use, and anxiety disorders is common; men and women are equally likely to have the disorder.

The treatment of schizotypal personality disorder often centers on issues that led the person to seek treatment, such as feelings of alienation or isolation, paranoia, or suspiciousness. Exploratory and group psychotherapies are overly threatening to these patients, but social skills training can be helpful. The goal is to help the individual to develop an awareness of what behaviors others (e.g., coworkers, store clerks) may consider odd or eccentric and to develop a repertoire of social skills that will assist him or her in making interactions with others more productive and satisfying.

Although not well studied, antipsychotics are sometimes prescribed to patients with schizotypal personality disorder. Second-generation antipsychotics (e.g., risperidone, 1–6 mg/day; olanzapine, 5–20 mg/day) are well tolerated and may help to reduce the intense anxiety, paranoia, and unusual perceptual experiences these individuals experience.

Cluster B Disorders

Antisocial Personality Disorder

Antisocial personality disorder was first recognized in the early nineteenth century as *manie sans délire* ("mania without delirium") or *moral insanity*, phrases used to describe immoral or guiltless behavior in the absence of impaired reasoning. By the turn of the twentieth century, the disorder was known as *psychopathic personality*. In DSM-I, the disorder was called *sociopathic personality* and was renamed *antisocial personality disorder* in DSM-III in 1980. The definition recognized the continuity between childhood conduct disorder and adult antisocial behavior.

Antisocial patients typically report a history of childhood behavior problems such as fighting with peers, conflicts with adults, lying, cheating, and stealing. Fire setting and cruelty to animals and other children are particularly worrisome symptoms. As the antisocial youth reaches adulthood, other problems develop reflecting age-appropriate responsibilities, such as uneven job performance or domestic abuse. Unreliability, reckless behavior, and inappropriate aggression are frequent problems. Criminal behavior, pathological lying, and the use of aliases are also characteristic of the disorder (Table 10–5). Marriages are often marked by instability or emotional and physical abuse of the spouse; separation and divorce are common. One of the best descriptions of this

TABLE 10–5. **DSM-IV-TR diagnostic criteria for antisocial personality disorder**

A. There is a pervasive pattern of disregard for and violation of the rights of others occurring since age 15 years, as indicated by three (or more) of the following:
  (1) failure to conform to social norms with respect to lawful behaviors as indicated by repeatedly performing acts that are grounds for arrest
  (2) deceitfulness, as indicated by repeated lying, use of aliases, or conning others for personal profit or pleasure
  (3) impulsivity or failure to plan ahead
  (4) irritability and aggressiveness, as indicated by repeated physical fights or assaults
  (5) reckless disregard for safety of self or others
  (6) consistent irresponsibility, as indicated by repeated failure to sustain consistent work behavior or honor financial obligations
  (7) lack of remorse, as indicated by being indifferent to or rationalizing having hurt, mistreated, or stolen from another
B. The individual is at least age 18 years.
C. There is evidence of Conduct Disorder with onset before age 15 years.
D. The occurrence of antisocial behavior is not exclusively during the course of Schizophrenia or a Manic Episode.

disorder appears in Hervey Cleckley's *The Mask of Sanity,* originally published in 1941. Cleckley, who is better known as the coauthor of *The Three Faces of Eve,* listed 16 traits he considered characteristic of the disorder, thus creating the first operational, criteria-based definition in psychiatry.

The following case is of a patient treated at our hospital and illustrates the lifelong difficulties that arise from antisocial personality disorder:

Russell, age 18 years, was admitted for evaluation of antisocial behavior. His early childhood was chaotic and abusive. His alcoholic father had married five times and abandoned his family when Russell was 6. Because his mother had a history of incarceration and was unable to care for him, Russell was placed in foster care until he was adopted at age 8. His adoptive father was a university professor; his adoptive mother was described as compulsive and strict.

Russell had a criminal streak from early childhood. He lied, cheated at games, shoplifted, and stole money from his mother's purse. He once burglarized a church and, when older, stole an automobile. Despite an above-average IQ, Russell's school performance was poor, and he was frequently in detention for breaking rules. Because of continued law-breaking, he was sent to a juvenile reformatory at age 16 for 2 years. While in the reformatory, he slashed another boy with a razor blade in a fight. Russell had his first sexual experience before his peers and after leaving the reformatory had several different sexual partners. He chain-smoked and abused alcohol.

An electroencephalogram was normal, and his IQ was measured at 112. He was discharged after a 16-day stay and was considered to be un-improved. He was poorly cooperative with attempts at both individual and group therapy.

Russell was followed up 30 years later. He used an alias and lived in an impoverished area of a small Midwestern community. Now 48, Russell appeared ill and haggard. He admitted to more than 20 arrests and more than 5 felony convictions on charges ranging from attempted murder and armed robbery to driving while intoxicated. He had spent more than 17 years in prison. While in prison, Russell had escaped with the help of his biological mother, with whom he then had a sexual relationship. He was returned to prison 2 months later. His most recent arrest occurred within the past year and was for public intoxication and simple assault.

Russell reported at least nine hospitalizations for alcohol detoxification, the latest occurring earlier that year. He admitted to past use of marijuana, amphetamines, tranquilizers, cocaine, and heroin.

He had never held a full-time job in his life; the longest job he had held lasted 60 days. He was currently doing bodywork on cars in his own garage to earn a living but had not done any work for several months. He had lived in six different states and in the past 10 years had moved more than 20 times.

Russell reported that nine persons lived in his home, including his four children. He had met his common-law wife in a psychiatric hospital. He told us that she required tranquilizers for emotional problems and that the marriage was unsatisfactory. He reported occasionally attending Alcoholics Anonymous at a local church but otherwise did not socialize outside his family.

Russell admitted that he had not yet settled down and told us that he still spent money foolishly, was frequently reckless, and got into frequent fights and arguments. He said that he got a "charge out of doing dangerous things."

From 2% to 4% of men and 0.5% to 1% of women meet criteria for antisocial personality disorder. The percentages are much higher in psychiatric hospitals and clinics, among the homeless and the incarcerated, and among alcohol- and drug-addicted persons. The disorder is worse early in its course, and antisocial symptoms tend to recede with advancing age. In a 30-year follow-up survey of 82 subjects, 12% were in remission and another 20% had improved; the remaining subjects were considered as disturbed or more so than at the study onset. The median age for improvement in this study was 35 years. Although the most dangerous and destructive behaviors associated with antisocial personality disorder may improve or remit, other troubling symptoms continue, including domestic abuse, alcoholism or drug abuse, and general irresponsibility toward others.

Comorbid alcohol or drug use disorders, mood and anxiety disorders, attention-deficit/hyperactivity disorder, pathological gambling, and other personality disorders (e.g., borderline personality disorder) are common. Antisocial persons frequently attempt suicide, and mortality studies show high rates of death from natural causes as well as accidents, suicides, and homicides.

There is no standard treatment for antisocial personality disorder, and no medication targets the full syndrome. Several drugs have been shown to reduce aggression, the chief problem for many antisocial persons. Lithium carbonate and phenytoin, specifically, have been shown to reduce anger, threatening behavior, and assaultiveness in prisoners. Other drugs, including the second-generation antipsychotics, carbamazepine, and valproate, are sometimes used but have not been formally studied. Benzodiazepines should not be used to treat the disorder because of their abuse potential and because they may lead to behavioral dyscontrol. Medication should target comorbid mood or anxiety disorders or attention-deficit/hyperactivity disorder because treating these may help to reduce antisocial behavior.

Cognitive-behavioral therapy recently has been used to treat antisocial personality disorder and involves evaluating situations in which the patient's distorted beliefs and attitudes (e.g., "My actions have no consequences") interfere with his or her functioning. The major goal of therapy is to help patients understand how they create their own problems and how their distorted perceptions prevent them from seeing themselves as others see them. Antisocial patients can be very difficult; they tend to blame others, have a low tolerance for frustration, are impulsive, and rarely form trusting relationships. Antisocial patients with spouses (or partners) and families may benefit from couples or family counseling.

Borderline Personality Disorder

Borderline personality disorder was introduced in DSM-III, although the concept has a much longer history. As currently conceptualized, the disorder is characterized by a pervasive pattern of mood instability, unstable and intense interpersonal relationships, impulsivity, inappropriate or intense anger, lack of control of anger, recurrent suicidal threats and gestures, self-mutilating behavior, marked and persistent identity disturbance, chronic feelings of emptiness, and frantic efforts to avoid real or imagined abandonment (see Table 10–6). Patients also may experience transient paranoid ideation or dissociative symptoms. Thomas Sydenham, an English physician best known for describing Saint Vitus' dance, captures the essence of borderline personality in his quotation at the beginning of this chapter. In DSM-I, these features were recognized as *emotionally unstable personality*. Early theorists considered borderline personality disorder to be a precursor or *forme fruste* of schizophrenia, and the term *borderline schizophrenia* was coined to describe persons who experienced transient episodes of psychosis during periods of regression or during psychotherapy.

Otto Kernberg used the term *borderline personality organization* to describe a broad range of problems, including identity diffusion, reliance on primitive defense mechanisms such as splitting (e.g., exaggerated dichotomies of good and evil or black and white), and maintenance of reality testing except in the perception of self and others.

Borderline personality disorder overlaps with many other personality disorders, especially the schizotypal, histrionic, and antisocial types. It is one of the more common personality disorders among psychiatric patients; its frequency in the general population has been estimated to be as high as 6%. More than three-quarters of borderline patients engage in deliberate self-harm (e.g., cutting, burning, overdoses), and about 10% commit suicide.

Better long-term outcome is associated with higher intelligence, self-discipline, and social support from friends and relatives. Hostility, antisocial behavior, suspiciousness, and vanity are traits associated with poor outcome. These patients frequently have comorbid major depression, dysthymia, anxiety disorders, and substance abuse or dependence.

The following case example describes a patient with borderline personality disorder seen at our hospital:

> Diane, a 50-year-old divorced woman, had a history of emotional instability dating to age 10, when she made her first suicide attempt. By her early 20s, she had the onset of episodes of depression, and frequent hospitalizations that had amounted to about 3–4 months per year. From her 20s to her mid-40s, she made several serious suicide attempts, including jumping from a building (and breaking both legs in the process) and taking several drug overdoses.

TABLE 10–6. **DSM-IV-TR diagnostic criteria for borderline personality disorder**

A pervasive pattern of instability of interpersonal relationships, self-image, and affects, and marked impulsivity beginning by early adulthood and present in a variety of contexts, as indicated by five (or more) of the following:

(1) frantic efforts to avoid real or imagined abandonment. **Note:** Do not include suicidal or self-mutilating behavior covered in Criterion 5.

(2) a pattern of unstable and intense interpersonal relationships characterized by alternating between extremes of idealization and devaluation

(3) identity disturbance: markedly and persistently unstable self-image or sense of self

(4) impulsivity in at least two areas that are potentially self-damaging (e.g., spending, sex, substance abuse, reckless driving, binge eating). **Note:** Do not include suicidal or self-mutilating behavior covered in Criterion 5.

(5) recurrent suicidal behavior, gestures, or threats, or self-mutilating behavior

(6) affective instability due to a marked reactivity of mood (e.g., intense episodic dysphoria, irritability, or anxiety usually lasting a few hours and only rarely more than a few days)

(7) chronic feelings of emptiness

(8) inappropriate, intense anger or difficulty controlling anger (e.g., frequent displays of temper, constant anger, recurrent physical fights)

(9) transient, stress-related paranoid ideation or severe dissociative symptoms

Diane had a history of alcohol abuse but had been sober for nearly 25 years with the help of Alcoholics Anonymous, which she attended regularly. Diane also had a history of pathological gambling and continued to have sporadic gambling episodes. In the past, gambling behaviors had led her to steal money from her boyfriend or to write bad checks, resulting in legal charges and, on one occasion, a short jail sentence.

Anger dyscontrol and turbulent interpersonal relationships characterized by alternately overidealizing and devaluing the other person had also been problematic for her. Diane completed a significant number of college courses but failed to graduate because of her behavioral problems and her tendency to have widely fluctuating views of her academic program. In the past, her disorder had interfered with maintaining consistent employment. Abandonment issues and feelings of emptiness were also present. Her intense, frequently shifting moods often resulted in poor management of her diabetes, leading to unstable blood sugar control.

Diane was referred for group therapy, which she later credited with giving her a better understanding of the disorder. The therapy targeted her poor medication compliance, her impulsivity, and her emotional intensity. For each problem area, she learned new skills to increase her range of alternative responses and to increase her awareness of the consequences of each alternative. She was also prescribed risperidone (4 mg/day) to help stabilize her mood.

There were no suicide attempts in the subsequent 5 years, and hospital stays were limited to a few days per year. She developed a stable relationship, volunteered regularly at her church, and pursued several hobbies.

When asked about her emotional growth, she says, "I still have suicidal thoughts on a daily basis, but I know now that is the disorder talking. I also know that I do not have to act or react to my thoughts."

Some researchers have argued that borderline personality disorder is a variant of depression, as evidenced by its association with depression in family studies, follow-up studies showing that most patients with borderline personality disorder develop major depression, and a positive response to antidepressant medication. In their view, the chronic mood instability creates the personality disturbance, not vice versa. On the other hand, it can be argued that patients with borderline personality disorder develop depression because of either a psychosocial predisposition (e.g., history of verbal and sexual abuse during childhood) or a biological vulnerability.

There is no standard treatment for borderline personality disorder. In the past few decades, several evidence-based group treatment programs have been developed that appear to reduce the overall severity of the disorder and lessen the associated mood instability, impulsivity, and social disability. Several of these programs employ cognitive-behavioral techniques to help correct accompanying maladaptive thoughts, beliefs, and behaviors. Dialectical behavior therapy (DBT) is the best known and involves intensive year-long treatment that includes both individual and group therapy. The less intensive 20-week Systems Training for Emotional Predictability and Problem Solving (STEPPS) program combines psychoeducation and skills training. Through weekly sessions patients learn to recognize their symptoms, learn new skills to manage their emotions and behaviors, and make more skillful use of their social support network. Other options include schema focused therapy and mentalization therapy.

Pharmacotherapy for borderline personality disorder tends to focus on the patients' target symptoms. Selective serotonin reuptake inhibitors (SSRIs) such as fluoxetine may be helpful in reducing depressive symptoms and suicidal ideations and behaviors. Antipsychotics can help to treat perceptual distortions, anger dyscontrol, suicidal behavior, and mood instability. Because suicide attempts are frequent in these patients, physicians should be cautious about prescribing any medication that could be dangerous in overdose. Benzodiazepine tranquilizers should be avoided, except perhaps for short-term use (e.g., days to weeks), because they can cause behavioral disinhibition or may be abused.

Patients with borderline personality disorder have the potential to cause intense feelings of frustration, guilt, or anger in their caregivers. The unfortunate irony is that these individuals fear abandonment from others and yet they react to perceived signs of it in a manner that alienates those who try to be supportive. Students are well advised to seek guidance from experienced clinicians in order to set boundaries that strike an appropriate balance between being overly distant and overly involved.

Histrionic Personality Disorder

Histrionic personality disorder takes its name from *hysteria,* first described in the nineteenth century and associated with conversion, somatization, and dissociation. Self-dramatizing and attention-seeking behaviors were observed to be associated with hysteria. *Hysterical personality* was included in DSM-II and was renamed *histrionic personality* in DSM-III so as not to be confused with *hysteria* (renamed *somatization disorder*). Many persons with somatization disorder have histrionic personality disorder, but there is no one-to-one relationship.

Persons with histrionic personality disorder show a pattern of excessive emotionality and attention-seeking behavior. Typical symptoms include excessive concern with appearance and wanting to be the center of attention (see Table 10–7). Histrionic persons are often gregarious and superficially charming but can be manipulative, vain, and demanding.

The disorder has a prevalence of nearly 2% in the general population. Histrionic persons tend to seek out medical attention and to make frequent use of available health services. Some experts suggest that histrionic personality disorder is a gender-biased diagnosis that merely describes a caricature of stereotypical femininity because it is frequently diagnosed among women in clinical samples. This view contrasts with the results of research studies using structured diagnostic assessments that find virtually equal rates of histrionic personality disorder in men

TABLE 10–7.   DSM-IV-TR diagnostic criteria for histrionic personality disorder

A pervasive pattern of excessive emotionality and attention seeking, beginning by early adulthood and present in a variety of contexts, as indicated by five (or more) of the following:
(1)   is uncomfortable in situations in which he or she is not the center of attention
(2)   interaction with others is often characterized by inappropriate sexually seductive or provocative behavior
(3)   displays rapidly shifting and shallow expression of emotions
(4)   consistently uses physical appearance to draw attention to self
(5)   has a style of speech that is excessively impressionistic and lacking in detail
(6)   shows self-dramatization, theatricality, and exaggerated expression of emotion
(7)   is suggestible, i.e., easily influenced by others or circumstances
(8)   considers relationships to be more intimate than they actually are

and women. The cause of histrionic personality disorder is unknown, although it has been linked through family studies to somatization disorder and antisocial personality disorder.

The treatment of histrionic personality disorder is not well understood. Some experts recommend a supportive, problem-solving approach or cognitive-behavioral therapy to help patients counter their distorted thinking, such as the inflated self-image that many histrionic patients have. With interpersonal psychotherapy, the patient can focus on conscious (or unconscious) motivations for seeking out disappointing partners and being unable to commit oneself to a stable, meaningful relationship. Group therapy may be useful in addressing provocative and attention-seeking behavior. Patients may not be aware of their annoying behaviors, and it may be helpful to have others point them out.

Narcissistic Personality Disorder

Narcissistic personality disorder was introduced in DSM-III and is named after Narcissus from Greek mythology, who fell in love with his own reflection. Freud used the term to describe persons who were self-absorbed; it was later expanded to describe the more general concept of excessive self-love and grandiosity. Pathological narcissism became of great interest to psychoanalysts, and the concept was heavily influenced by the contributions of Heinz Kohut. In his view, narcissism develops as a response to parental failures in conveying empathy to a child's need for idealization and admiration; the child becomes self-centered and views others only in their role of satisfying his or her narcissistic needs.

The disorder is characterized by grandiosity, lack of empathy, and hypersensitivity to evaluation by others (see Table 10–8). Narcissistic persons are egotistical, inflate their accomplishments, and often manipulate or exploit those around them to achieve their own aims. They have an exaggerated sense of entitlement and believe that they deserve special treatment. They expect to receive love and admiration but have little empathy for others. Narcissistic individuals are often irritating, haughty, or difficult; although they appear outwardly charming, relationships tend to be superficial and cold. They tend to have little insight into their own narcissism. Some narcissistic individuals may view themselves as extraordinarily caring and selfless while making it clear that they believe they deserve a great deal of praise and special treatment because they are so giving to others.

The following case illustrates many of the symptoms of narcissistic personality disorder:

> Dr. Smith, a 53-year-old physician, was known for having an expansive and grandiose attitude and for belittling the accomplishments of his colleagues.
>
> While seeking the admiration and adulation of others, he rarely reciprocated, displaying superficial charm without a genuine capacity for empathy. His nurse remarked to a colleague, "When you talk to him, it's like you're not even really there as a person. It's like he can't connect."
>
> Dr. Smith's sense of entitlement led him to bill Medicare and other insurance carriers for services that he had never rendered or that were inflated on the bills. He believed that changes in the reimbursement system penalized him and that he was entitled to a higher level of payment because of his training, experience, and keen intelligence.
>
> At the urging of his colleagues in practice, and after being repeatedly caught and confronted about his billing fraud, Dr. Smith entered therapy with a well-known psychoanalyst and psychiatrist, Dr. Brown. Dr. Smith told a colleague, months into therapy: "I think Dr. Brown envies me; he knows how much money I make. I can tell the size of my practice, and my success, bothers him."
>
> Dr. Smith eventually was investigated, indicted on multiple criminal fraud counts, and tried in federal court. Many of his colleagues testified against him in federal court. "I can't believe they would *do* this to me," he was heard to say. Convicted on all counts, Dr. Smith was sentenced to 5 years in a federal penitentiary.

TABLE 10–8. DSM-IV-TR diagnostic criteria for narcissistic personality disorder

A pervasive pattern of grandiosity (in fantasy or behavior), need for admiration, and lack of empathy, beginning by early adulthood and present in a variety of contexts, as indicated by five (or more) of the following:

(1) has a grandiose sense of self-importance (e.g., exaggerates achievements and talents, expects to be recognized as superior without commensurate achievements)

(2) is preoccupied with fantasies of unlimited success, power, brilliance, beauty, or ideal love

(3) believes that he or she is "special" and unique and can only be understood by, or should associate with, other special or high-status people (or institutions)

(4) requires excessive admiration

(5) has a sense of entitlement, i.e., unreasonable expectations of especially favorable treatment or automatic compliance with his or her expectations

(6) is interpersonally exploitative, i.e., takes advantage of others to achieve his or her own ends

(7) lacks empathy: is unwilling to recognize or identify with the feelings and needs of others

(8) is often envious of others or believes that others are envious of him or her

(9) shows arrogant, haughty behaviors or attitudes

Narcissistic personality disorder has been considered uncommon, although a recent survey reported a prevalence of around 6%. Some experts argue that the disorder is not a valid syndrome because narcissistic traits are common in the general population, as well as in patients with other personality disorder types. The criteria also overlap with those of other disorders, such as borderline personality disorder, leading some to question its distinctiveness. Like other Axis II disorders, narcissistic personality disorder is generally viewed as stable over time, although research suggests that it may vary under the influence of significant life events, such as achievement and new relationships.

There are few data on the treatment of persons with narcissistic personality disorder. When they seek help, it is likely for the anger or depression they feel when deprived of something they feel entitled to, such as a promotion. This is sometimes referred to as a "narcissistic injury." Treatment recommendations have ranged from intensive psychodynamic psychotherapy to interpersonal or cognitive-behavioral psychotherapy. Narcissistic patients can be very difficult to treat because their narcissism can interfere with the process of psychotherapy. For example, their grandiosity can lead them to resist admitting personal responsibility for their problems, while their sense of entitlement can lead them to make unreasonable demands on the therapist.

Cluster C Disorders

Avoidant Personality Disorder

Avoidant personality disorder was introduced in DSM-III and represents a variant of what had previously been called *schizoid personality.* Another predecessor was *inadequate personality,* a term used to describe individuals who had experienced failure in several important life domains (e.g., interpersonal relationships, occupation).

People with avoidant personality disorder are inhibited, introverted, and anxious. They tend to have low self-esteem, are hypersensitive to rejection, are apprehensive and mistrustful, are socially awkward and timid, are uncomfortable and self-conscious, and fear being embarrassed or acting foolish in public (see Table 10–9).

Some experts have questioned the independence of the disorder, which they see as lying along a spectrum with the anxiety disorders. In fact, many features of avoidant personality disorder are indistinguishable from those of social phobia, and the two disorders frequently overlap. Avoidant personality disorder may involve a genetic predisposition to chronic anxiety.

Several psychotherapeutic strategies have been developed for the treatment of avoidant personality disorder. Group therapy may help the person to overcome his or her social anxiety and to develop interpersonal trust. Assertiveness and social skills training can be helpful, as can systematic desensitization to treat anxiety symptoms, shyness, and introversion. Cognitive-behavioral therapy can help to correct dysfunctional attitudes (e.g., "I had better not open my mouth because I'll probably say something stupid"). Benzodiazepines can be useful while the patient is attempting to enter previously avoided social situations. It is best to limit the use of these drugs to short periods (e.g., weeks to months), although some patients will benefit from long-term use. SSRIs also may be helpful because they are effective in treating social phobia (e.g., paroxetine, 20–60 mg/day; sertraline, 50–200 mg/day; escitalopram 10–20 mg/day).

TABLE 10–9.   DSM-IV-TR diagnostic criteria for avoidant personality disorder

A pervasive pattern of social inhibition, feelings of inadequacy, and hypersensitivity to negative evaluation, beginning by early adulthood and present in a variety of contexts, as indicated by four (or more) of the following:

(1) avoids occupational activities that involve significant interpersonal contact, because of fears of criticism, disapproval, or rejection

(2) is unwilling to get involved with people unless certain of being liked

(3) shows restraint within intimate relationships because of the fear of being shamed or ridiculed

(4) is preoccupied with being criticized or rejected in social situations

(5) is inhibited in new interpersonal situations because of feelings of inadequacy

(6) views self as socially inept, personally unappealing, or inferior to others

(7) is unusually reluctant to take personal risks or to engage in any new activities because they may prove embarrassing

Dependent Personality Disorder

Dependent personality disorder was listed as a subtype of the DSM-I passive-aggressive personality, was omitted from DSM-II, and was reintroduced in DSM-III. The disorder is characterized by a pattern of relying excessively on others for emotional support (see Table 10–10). Psychoanalysts have linked dependency to fixation at the oral stage of development, which focuses on the biological gratification that arises from feeding. Other theorists have tied dependent personality to the disruption of attachments early in life. Others view dependency as stemming from overprotectiveness and parental authoritarianism experienced in childhood.

The following patient, in whom dependency issues were important, was seen at our hospital:

> Bob, a 45-year-old farm laborer, presented for evaluation of major depression, which had been chronic for several years. He also reported a long-standing eating disorder, which had resulted in significant weight loss. For 10 years, Bob had feared becoming fat like his father, who had died unexpectedly of a myocardial infarction.

TABLE 10–10. DSM-IV-TR diagnostic criteria for dependent personality disorder

A pervasive and excessive need to be taken care of that leads to submissive and clinging behavior and fears of separation, beginning by early adulthood and present in a variety of contexts, as indicated by five (or more) of the following:

(1) has difficulty making everyday decisions without an excessive amount of advice and reassurance from others

(2) needs others to assume responsibility for most major areas of his or her life

(3) has difficulty expressing disagreement with others because of fear of loss of support or approval. **Note:** Do not include realistic fears of retribution.

(4) has difficulty initiating projects or doing things on his or her own (because of a lack of self-confidence in judgment or abilities rather than a lack of motivation or energy)

(5) goes to excessive lengths to obtain nurturance and support from others, to the point of volunteering to do things that are unpleasant

(6) feels uncomfortable or helpless when alone because of exaggerated fears of being unable to care for himself or herself

(7) urgently seeks another relationship as a source of care and support when a close relationship ends

(8) is unrealistically preoccupied with fears of being left to take care of himself or herself

In addition to these problems, Bob described a dull and passive lifestyle. The third of eight children, Bob had left school after eighth grade to work on the family farm, as had his siblings. The family remained close because there were few opportunities for outside friendships. Bob reported that he had rarely dated, although he had once been "sweet on a girl." He denied any current interest in developing a relationship.

Bob lived with his mother until she insisted he move out at age 44, which he did reluctantly. Although he lived alone, he remained in close contact with his mother, eating meals with her twice daily and phoning her 10–20 times a day. He relied on her to make decisions for him, even minor ones about day-to-day activities.

Bob had no interests or hobbies apart from his farm chores. He admitted that he was uncomfortable being alone in his mobile home, which prompted him to telephone his mother. He cried when he was asked how he would handle his mother's eventual death. (She was then in her 80s.)

Although Bob gained weight steadily on a refeeding protocol, it became clear that he would need supervision outside the hospital. Because his mother was too old to help (and it was felt that her supervision would only worsen his dependency on her), a decision was made by his family to place Bob in a residential care facility.

There has been considerable research on the psychology of dependency, yet there have been few empirical studies of dependent personality disorder. One criticism of the disorder is that it is not sufficiently distinctive to stand alone and that dependency on others commonly occurs in people with other personality disorder types; it is also common in persons with chronic medical or psychiatric disorders. One study showed that persons with dependent personality disorder are more likely to be female and to be older than patients with other types of personality disorders. Comorbid mood and anxiety disorders are common. Persons with dependent personality have poor social and family ties, in part because their dependency on others accentuates and promotes interpersonal conflicts.

There is little consensus on the treatment of dependent personality disorder. Cognitive-behavioral therapy is recommended as a way to encourage emotional growth, assertiveness, effective decision making, and independence. The therapist might have the patient set goals for each session and challenge his or her assumptions related to dependency (e.g., "I won't be able to make up my mind without Mother's input"). Some patients benefit from more focused assertiveness training or social skills training. Marital counseling is indicated when the patient's dependence on his or her spouse is adversely affecting their relationship.

Obsessive-Compulsive Personality Disorder

Obsessive-compulsive personality disorder is thought by psychoanalysts to represent a fixation at the anal stage of development, characterized by obstinacy, parsimony, and orderliness. Originally termed *compulsive personality* in DSM-I, this disorder was long thought to lead to the development of obsessive-compulsive disorder (OCD). Although early research showed that some patients with OCD are likely to have a premorbid obsessional personality, it became clear that obsessive-compulsive personality disorder and OCD do not have a one-to-one relationship. Individuals with OCD are generally more willing to identify their symptoms as pathological, whereas individuals with obsessive-compulsive personality disorder tend to view many of their symptoms (e.g., collecting, perfectionism) as desirable.

Obsessive-compulsive personality disorder is characterized by perfectionism and inflexibility associated with overconscientiousness and

TABLE 10–11. DSM-IV-TR diagnostic criteria for obsessive-compulsive personality disorder

A pervasive pattern of preoccupation with orderliness, perfectionism, and mental and interpersonal control, at the expense of flexibility, openness, and efficiency, beginning by early adulthood and present in a variety of contexts, as indicated by four (or more) of the following:

(1) is preoccupied with details, rules, lists, order, organization, or schedules to the extent that the major point of the activity is lost

(2) shows perfectionism that interferes with task completion (e.g., is unable to complete a project because his or her own overly strict standards are not met)

(3) is excessively devoted to work and productivity to the exclusion of leisure activities and friendships (not accounted for by obvious economic necessity)

(4) is overconscientious, scrupulous, and inflexible about matters of morality, ethics, or values (not accounted for by cultural or religious identification)

(5) is unable to discard worn-out or worthless objects even when they have no sentimental value

(6) is reluctant to delegate tasks or to work with others unless they submit to exactly his or her way of doing things

(7) adopts a miserly spending style toward both self and others; money is viewed as something to be hoarded for future catastrophes

(8) shows rigidity and stubbornness

constricted emotions (see Table 10–11). It has an estimated prevalence of 1%–2% in the general population. Unlike other personality disorders, this disorder appears to be more common in those with higher levels of education and those in higher income brackets. Comorbidity with mood and anxiety disorders is frequent.

Obsessive-compulsive personality disorder is relatively difficult to treat. Some experts recommend psychodynamic psychotherapy; however, although these patients tend to intellectualize and may be insightful, they develop little feeling or emotion. Cognitive-behavioral therapy may help these individuals understand that the world is not made up of clearly defined black and white lines of rigidly held beliefs. SSRIs (e.g., fluoxetine, 20 mg/day; paroxetine, 20–60 mg/day; citalopram, 20–40 mg/day) may be helpful in reducing the need for perfectionism and the unnecessary ritualizing that sometimes develops.

Key points to remember about personality disorders

1. Patients have enduring, long-term problems, and therapy may be long-term as well. Decades of maladaptive behavior cannot be easily understood or reversed.

2. Have a positive attitude! Personality disorders cause a great deal of pain and suffering to patients and those in their lives. Have empathy for them.

3. Avoid becoming overinvolved, such as giving out your home telephone number or relating your personal problems to the patient. These behaviors are called "boundary" issues, which indicate that the lines separating the relationship between doctor and patient have become blurred.

4. Ground rules for therapy must be established (e.g., that the therapist is willing to see the person regularly, at a specified time).

    *   Spell out what the patient should do or whom the patient should call when he or she is in a crisis.

    *   Spell out the consequences of self-damaging acts (e.g., hospitalization, referral to another therapist).

5. Seek support for yourself from peers or supervisors. Some patients with personality disorders are a handful, and the therapist may need advice or consultation now and then.

6. Support groups can be enormously helpful to the patient, and referral to community-based organizations is essential.

■ Self-Assessment Questions

1. What are the Greek temperaments, and why are they still useful descriptively?

2. How are the personality disorders defined?

3. Why is the term *personality disorder* sometimes considered pejorative?

4. How common are the personality disorders? Which ones are more common in men? Which ones are more common in women? Are the disorders stable over time?

5. What evidence is there for genetic or biological origin for the personality disorders? Which personality disorders?

6. Describe the three personality disorder clusters.

7. How do schizoid and schizotypal personality disorders differ? How do these two categories differ from avoidant personality disorder?

8. Are medications useful in treating Cluster A disorders? Which medications?

9. For which disorders might social skills training or assertiveness training be useful?

10. What is the childhood precursor of antisocial personality disorder? What biological abnormalities have been found in these patients? Are medications of any value?

11. What features characterize the Cluster C disorders? What are the general treatment recommendations for these disorders? How does obsessive-compulsive personality disorder differ from OCD?

12. What are "boundary" issues and how might they interfere with treatment?

CHAPTER 11

Sexual Dysfunction, Paraphilias, and Gender Identity Disorders

Lolita, light of my life, fire of my loins. My sin, my soul. Lo-lee-ta.

Vladimir Nabokov, Lolita

SEXUAL DISORDERS or dysfunctions are surprisingly common. The recent Global Study on Sexual Attitudes and Behaviors (GSSAB) found that among persons in North America, the prevalence of sexual dysfunctions occurring either periodically or frequently was 38% for women and 29% for men. Yet these conditions remain "off the radar screen" because few patients report them to their physicians, and fewer still seek treatment for them. Typical examples seen in everyday practice include the man with diabetes who is no longer able to maintain an erection, the postmenopausal woman who finds intercourse painful, and the man taking antidepressants who is unable to ejaculate. Paraphilias are less common but are more problematic because they may lead to behavior that at a minimum annoys nonconsenting adults and at its most extreme endangers vulnerable children. Gender identity disorders (e.g., transsexualism) are relatively rare yet remain of interest to psychiatrists and other mental health professionals because of the distress and dysfunction they may potentially cause.

Because the sexual disorders are common and problematic, students and residents should learn to take sexual histories without embarrassment. They also should learn to diagnose these conditions and understand their treatment. The DSM-IV-TR sexual disorders are listed in Table 11–1.

■ Human Sexual Response Cycle

Any discussion of the sexual disorders should begin with a description of the normal human sexual response cycle, originally proposed by William Masters and Virginia Johnson in the 1960s. The cycle consists of four phases, as described in DSM-IV-TR:

1. The *desire phase* lasts minutes to hours. In this stage, sexual fantasies and the desire for sexual intimacy occur.
2. The *excitement phase* ("foreplay") consists of a subjective sense of pleasure and accompanying physiological changes that include penile tumescence and erection in men and vasocongestion of the pelvis, vaginal lubrication and expansion, and swelling of the external genitalia in women.
3. The *orgasmic phase* consists of a peaking of sexual pleasure, with release of sexual tension and rhythmic contractions of the perineal muscles and reproductive organs. In men, there is a sensation of ejaculatory inevitability, which is followed by ejaculation of semen, In women, there are contractions (not always subjectively experienced as such) in the outer one-third of the vagina. In both men and women, the anal sphincter rhythmically contracts.
4. The *resolution phase* consists of a sense of muscular relaxation and general well-being. During this phase, men are physiologically refractory to further erection and orgasm for a variable period of time. In contrast, women may be able to respond to additional stimulation almost immediately.

TABLE 11–1. DSM-IV-TR sexual and gender identity disorders

Sexual dysfunctions	Paraphilias
Sexual desire disorders	Exhibitionism
Hypoactive sexual desire disorder	Fetishism
	Frotteurism
Sexual aversion disorder	Pedophilia
Sexual arousal disorders	Sexual masochism
Female sexual arousal disorder	Sexual sadism
	Transvestic fetishism
Male erectile disorder	Voyeurism
Orgasmic disorders	Paraphilia not otherwise specified
Female orgasmic disorder	
Male orgasmic disorder	**Gender identity disorders**
Premature ejaculation	Gender identity disorder
Sexual pain disorders	Gender identity disorder not otherwise specified
Dyspareunia	
Vaginismus	**Sexual disorder not otherwise specified**
Sexual dysfunction due to a general medical condition	
Substance-induced sexual dysfunction	
Sexual dysfunction not otherwise specified	

■ Sexual Dysfunctions

DSM-IV-TR identifies four major categories of sexual dysfunction: sexual desire disorders, sexual arousal disorders, orgasmic disorders, and sexual pain disorders. Each category tends to correspond with a different phase of the sexual response cycle. Two residual categories, sexual dysfunction not otherwise specified and sexual disorder not otherwise specified, may be used to diagnose sexual disorders that do not meet the criteria for a more specific disorder. All of the sexual dysfunctions can be classified as due to either psychological factors or a combination of psychological factors and a general medical condition.

Sexual Desire Disorders

Hypoactive sexual desire disorder and sexual aversion disorder correspond to the desire phase of the sexual response cycle.

Persons with *hypoactive sexual desire disorder* have a persistent or recurrent deficiency in or absence of sexual fantasies and desire for sexual activity that does not result from major depression or another Axis I disorder that may be associated with low sex drive. The direct effects of a substance or a general medical condition (e.g., diabetes mellitus) also must be ruled out as causing the disturbance. Many persons with this disorder have significant trouble with social uneasiness, lack self-confidence, and avoid social situations.

The disorder is common in the general population. In the GSSAB survey of North American adults ages 40–80 years, 33% of women and 18% of men reported that they had experienced lack of sexual interest. Lack of interest was more common among women and among older persons. (See Table 11–2 for additional findings from this study.)

Low sexual interest sometimes temporarily results from stressful situations such as overwork, lack of privacy, or lack of opportunity for sexual activity. Many persons with this disorder are poorly educated about sexual matters or are unduly inhibited for reasons of religion or culture. Before making a diagnosis of hypoactive sexual desire disorder, a clinician should take into account factors that affect sexual functioning, including age, gender, and cultural background.

Sexual aversion disorder represents a persistent and recurrent aversion to and avoidance of genital contact with a sexual partner. The disorder is not due to obsessive-compulsive disorder, major depression, or another serious Axis I condition. Some persons with this disorder have been sexually victimized in the past and harbor unpleasant memories or beliefs about sexual activity.

Sexual Arousal Disorders

The sexual arousal disorders include male erectile disorder (impotence) and female sexual arousal disorder.

Primary impotence occurs when a man has never been able to achieve an erection sufficient for vaginal insertion. With *secondary impotence*, the man has successfully achieved an erection sufficient for vaginal penetration in the past but is currently unable to do so. Primary impotence is rare, but secondary impotence is reported to occur in about 25% of men. Prevalence is age dependent; erectile difficulties are uncommon in young men but frequent in older men.

TABLE 11–2. Frequency of self-reported sexual problems in North American men and women ages 40–80 years

Sexual dysfunction	%
Women	
Lack of sexual interest	33
Lubrication difficulties	27
Inability to reach orgasm	25
Pain during sex	14
Men	
Early ejaculation	27
Erectile difficulties	21
Lack of sexual interest	18
Inability to reach orgasm	15

Source. Adapted from Laumann et al. 2005.

Female sexual arousal disorder occurs in up to one-third of all married women and is defined as the partial or complete failure to attain or maintain the lubrication-swelling response characteristic of the excitement stage or the complete lack of sexual excitement and pleasure. The disorder may result in painful intercourse, sexual avoidance, and disturbance of marital or sexual relationships. It is often associated with lack of sexual desire and anorgasmia.

Orgasmic Disorders

The orgasmic disorders include female orgasmic disorder (anorgasmia), male orgasmic disorder, and premature ejaculation. *Female orgasmic disorder* is manifested by the delay in or absence of orgasm following a normal sexual excitement stage. Also, the clinician judges the woman's orgasmic capability to be less than expected for her age, sexual experience, and amount of sexual stimulation received. *Male orgasmic disorder* occurs when a man achieves ejaculation during sexual activity only with great difficulty, if at all. Again, the clinician must take into account the man's age, sexual experience, and amount of sexual stimulation received.

Premature ejaculation is reported by more than 25% of adult men and is a common complaint among men seeking help for a sexual disorder.

The disorder is diagnosed when the man has persistent or recurrent ejaculation with minimal sexual stimulation before, on, or shortly after vaginal penetration and before the man wants to ejaculate. There is no corresponding disorder in women.

Sexual Pain Disorders

Dyspareunia is genital pain associated with sexual intercourse in men or women. This condition should not be diagnosed when it is better accounted for by an Axis I disorder, such as somatization disorder, or when it is thought to be due to the direct effects of a substance or a general medical condition. Furthermore, it is not diagnosed when caused exclusively by vaginismus or lack of lubrication. Women who have undergone pelvic surgery or recently given birth may experience dyspareunia temporarily. The disorder is rare in men.

Vaginismus is a condition in which there are recurrent or persistent involuntary muscle contractions of the perineal muscles surrounding the vagina when penetration by a penis, finger, tampon, or speculum is attempted. The diagnosis of vaginismus is not better accounted for by another Axis I disorder and is not due exclusively to the direct physiological effects of a general medical condition. In some women, even the anticipation of vaginal penetration results in a muscle spasm. Sexual desire and orgasmic potential may be unimpaired unless penetration is attempted or anticipated. The disorder is more common in younger than older women and may be a reason for an unconsummated marriage or for infertility.

Etiology of Sexual Dysfunctions

Sexual dysfunction may be caused by psychological or physical factors or sometimes a combination of the two. For example, lack of sexual desire can result from chronic stress, anxiety, or depression or can result from medications that either depress the central nervous system or decrease testosterone production. Prolonged sexual abstinence itself may suppress desire. Major physical stresses, such as illness or surgery, especially when they alter body image (e.g., mastectomy, ileostomy), also may depress sexual desire.

Anorgasmia may result from physical factors, such as the effects of medication or surgery, or psychological factors, such as fears of impregnation, rejection by the sexual partner, or major depression. Cultural factors also may contribute. For example, in Victorian times, young women often were told by their mothers that sexual intercourse was a marital duty. In many cultures today, women still receive similar messages.

TABLE 11–3.   Causes of male erectile disorder (impotence)

Medical illness	Psychiatric illness
Acromegaly	Anxiety disorders
Addison's disease	Dementia
Diabetes	Major depression
Hyperthyroidism	Schizophrenia
Hypothyroidism	**Drugs**
Klinefelter's syndrome	Alcohol
Multiple sclerosis	Antiandrogens
Parkinson's disease	Anticholinergics
Pelvic surgery or irradiation	Antidepressants
Peripheral vascular disease	Antihypertensives (especially
Pituitary adenoma	centrally acting ones)
Spinal cord injury	Antipsychotics
Syphilis	Barbiturates
Temporal lobe epilepsy	Finasteride
	Marijuana
	Opioids
	Stimulants

Erectile dysfunction (impotence) may be caused by both physical and psychological conditions (Table 11–3). Research shows that up to 75% of the men evaluated for erectile dysfunction have a physical cause for the disorder, such as cardiovascular disease (e.g., atherosclerotic disease), renal disorders (e.g., chronic renal failure), liver disease (e.g., cirrhosis), malnutrition, diabetes mellitus, multiple sclerosis, traumatic spinal cord injury, abuse of alcohol or other drugs, psychotropic medication, prostate surgery, or pelvic irradiation.

In assessing the cause of erectile problems, it is important to determine whether spontaneous erections occur at times when the man does not plan to have intercourse (e.g., morning erections, erections with masturbation). A psychological cause is likely if erections occur at these times. Because medications (see below) are so effective for male erectile disorder, there is little reason for an extensive workup. A limited investigation should include fasting blood glucose to rule out diabetes, and a fasting lipid screen because erectile dysfunction is a known marker for cardiovascular disease. Some experts also recommend thyroid function tests to rule out hypo- or hyperthyroidism. Measuring serum testosterone may be indicated in some patients to rule out hypogonadism associated with testosterone deficiency. If the assay is low, follow-up should include further endocrine testing such as luteinizing hormone, follicle-stimulating hormone, and prolactin levels.

Specialized procedures may be helpful in assessing the cause of erectile dysfunction when treatment fails. This can begin with an injection of a vasoactive drug, such as alprostadil, into the corpus cavernosum to assess erectile potential. Obtaining an erection confirms the integrity of the penile vascular system. If the patient is unable to obtain an erection, additional investigations may include color Doppler ultrasonography of the penile vasculature, dynamic infusion cavernosumetry, and bulbocavernosus reflex latency times and somatosensory evoked potentials to assess the integrity of penile innervation. Penile angiography can be used to further explore the possibility of an isolated arterial occlusion if suggested by Doppler scanning. The latter procedure is for the rare patient who is a candidate for vascular reconstructive surgery.

Male orgasmic disorder is relatively uncommon and must be differentiated from retrograde ejaculation, in which ejaculation occurs but the seminal fluid passes backward into the bladder. Both male orgasmic disorder and retrograde ejaculation most likely have a physiological cause, such as the effects of medication, genitourinary surgery (e.g., prostatectomy), or neurological disorders involving the lumbosacral section of the spinal cord. Centrally acting antihypertensives (e.g., guanethidine, α-methyldopa), tricyclic antidepressants (e.g., amitriptyline), or antipsychotics, particularly the phenothiazines (e.g., chlorpromazine, thioridazine), can be responsible for the disorder.

Antidepressants are a frequent cause of sexual dysfunction and may be responsible for low libido, ejaculation disorders, and orgasm disorders. Up to 65% of persons taking one of the selective serotonin reuptake inhibitor (SSRI) antidepressants (e.g., fluoxetine, paroxetine, sertraline) report some degree of sexual dysfunction when carefully queried. In men, SSRIs often cause ejaculatory delay or failure. This is probably a common yet underrecognized cause for treatment noncompliance.

Age itself must be taken into account as a cause of sexual dysfunction. Older persons are more likely to report lack of sexual desire, as well as other forms of sexual dysfunction itself. For example, older men may not ejaculate at every sexual encounter but perhaps only every second or third time.

Clinical Management of Sexual Dysfunctions

Modern sex therapy for the treatment of sexual dysfunction is rooted in the nonmedical approach pioneered by Masters and Johnson in the 1970s. Their brief sex therapy (e.g., 8–12 sessions) was behaviorally oriented and represented a clear break from the mainstream traditional therapy common at the time. Although Masters and Johnson focused on treating couples, their approach also can apply to individuals. Their "dual" sex therapy can be used equally well with heterosexual and gay/lesbian couples.

In this approach, therapy begins by educating the couple on the psychological and physiological aspects of sexual functioning, and evaluating their attitudes about sexual behavior and their ability to communicate. Once the sexual problem has been identified, a series of graded assignments are given for specific sexual activities that the couple is expected to carry out in private. Sexual intimacy is emphasized as a natural and healthy part of life. Cognitive-behavioral methods are used to challenge dysfunctional thoughts and beliefs (e.g., "both partners must reach orgasm simultaneously"). These methods can be used for many of the sexual dysfunctions and are modified depending on whether the problem represents a disorder of the desire, excitement, or orgasmic phase of the sexual response cycle.

As an example of sex therapy for male erectile disorder, the couple is prohibited from engaging in sexual activity other than that prescribed by the therapist. Exercises focus on increasing sensory awareness of erogenous zones, so that couples can learn to give and receive bodily pleasure. *Sensate focus* exercises are a technique in which the patient engages initially in nongenital, nondemanding caressing with his or her partner, with the focus on the patient's own pleasure and feelings. At this point, intercourse is prohibited. Couples are encouraged to separate sexual pleasure from intercourse.

Genital stimulation is gradually included in the exercises; couples are instructed to try various positions for sexual intercourse but not to concern themselves with completing the act. In time, the couple gains confidence and learns to communicate better. They also learn to give and receive pleasure without experiencing sexual intercourse. Without the pressure to perform, the man is eventually able to have erections and successfully complete vaginal intercourse.

Specific behavioral instructions depend on the presenting complaint. In cases of male orgasmic disorder, the woman may be instructed to insert her partner's penis herself. With anorgasmia, therapy may involve training the woman to first have an orgasm by masturbation before treating the couple. Vaginismus may require individual therapy, meditation or other relaxation techniques, or the use of Hegar dilators, which are inserted into the vagina. (The size of the dilators is slowly increased over 3–5 days to gradually enlarge the vaginal opening.) The "squeeze method" is used to treat premature ejaculation. The woman is instructed that when her partner feels he is about to ejaculate, she is to squeeze his penis (for up to 5 seconds) by placing her thumb on the frenulum and her first and second fingers on the opposite side. This action effectively halts ejaculation so that the couple may prolong foreplay.

SSRIs can be used to treat premature ejaculation because a common side effect is delayed ejaculation (e.g., paroxetine, 20 mg/day). Alternatively, men may benefit from 1% dibucaine (Nupercaine) ointment applied to the coronal ridge and frenulum of the penis to reduce stimulation.

A case of male orgasmic disorder and its treatment follows:

> Robert, a 34-year-old bank officer, had been happily married for 6 months but reported that he was now having trouble achieving orgasm. Although he had had no sexual experience before marriage, he and his more experienced wife had quickly developed a satisfying sexual relationship. They both had versatile sexual interests and were both able to achieve orgasm with adequate stimulation.
>
> Robert reported that for the past month he had been having difficulty achieving orgasm, even with adequate foreplay. Although he was able to reach orgasm through masturbation, he was unable to achieve orgasm with vaginal intercourse, despite trying a variety of positions.
>
> An evaluation showed no evidence of an anxiety disorder or major depression or a physical disorder. Robert had denied any recent change in his marital relationship but had disclosed to the therapist a deep-seated fear that he was unworthy of his new mate and felt that he could not satisfy her sexually. The therapist met with the couple, recommended that Robert abstain from masturbation, prescribed sensate focus exercises to be tried initially without intercourse, and suggested that as intercourse was attempted, the wife take a dominant role. Learning that he could give and receive pleasure without the pressure of sexual intercourse apparently allowed Robert and his wife to experience intercourse and each to achieve a satisfactory orgasm.

Testosterone has been used to treat both men and women with hypoactive sexual desire disorder, although research on its use for this indication is inconsistent. Furthermore, it has the potential to induce masculinizing side effects (e.g., hirsutism), which is problematic in women.

Three oral medications have been approved by the U.S. Food and Drug Administration (FDA) for the treatment of male erectile dysfunction. Sildenafil, vardenafil, and tadalafil are all classified as phosphodiesterase-5 inhibitors. They enhance the effect of nitric oxide, which relaxes smooth muscles in the penis, increasing blood flow and allowing an erection to develop in response to sexual stimulation. They differ in dosage, duration of effect, and adverse effects. Sildenafil (Viagra) works relatively quickly to produce an erection and is taken as needed in doses ranging from 25 to 100 mg. Vardenafil (Levitra), which lasts up to a day, is taken as needed at doses ranging from 5 to 20 mg. Tadalafil (Cialis) lasts up to 3 days and is taken in doses ranging from 5 to 20 mg/ day. All of these drugs can cause headaches, upset stomach, nausea, and muscle aches. These drugs have also been used to treat female orgasmic disorder.

Alprostadil, a synthetic version of the hormone prostaglandin E, is another drug approved for the treatment of impotence. The drug either is injected directly into the base or side of the penis or is placed directly into the urethra with a special syringe. Either method of administration results in increased penile blood flow within minutes. The main drawback to this drug is the inconvenience and discomfort involved with its use.

Surgical treatments for impotence are also available, but these are indicated only when medication is ineffective. The most common technique involves the insertion of a penile prosthesis. These devices are generally either semirigid or inflatable; each has advantages and disadvantages. As an alternative, vacuum pump devices can be used to produce an erection by increasing blood flow to the penis. Once an erection is achieved, a metal ring is placed around the base of the penis to maintain the erection for about 30 minutes.

Key points to remember about sexual dysfunction

1. The clinician must learn to take a sexual history without shame or embarrassment. Patients will detect the clinician's anxiety, which will only serve to increase their own.

2. The clinician should not apologize for asking intimate questions. How a person behaves sexually is important to assess.

   - Most people will be surprisingly forthcoming in describing their sex lives.

Key points to remember about sexual dysfunction *(continued)*
3. Both couples and individuals can engage in sex therapy. The therapy may be used with equal success in heterosexual and gay/lesbian couples.
4. The principles of sex therapy are relatively simple to learn and emphasize education about sexual functioning, helping couples to communicate better, and correcting dysfunctional attitudes about sex that one or both partners may hold.
5. Therapy involves homework assignments, which assist the couple in learning to increase sensory awareness. Techniques may include masturbation, sensate focus experiences, special coital techniques, and learning to separate pleasure from physiological response (e.g., penile erection).
6. Male erectile disorders can be effectively treated pharmacologically, whether the disorder is primarily psychologically motivated or medically based. Oral medications include sildenafil, vardenafil, and tadalafil. Another drug, alprostadil, is placed into the urethra with a special applicator or is injected directly into the penis.
• Surgical techniques are available and involve the placement of a semirigid or an inflatable device.
• Vacuum pump devices that draw blood into the penis also are available.

■ Paraphilias (Sexual Deviations)

DSM-IV-TR defines paraphilias as recurrent, intense sexually arousing fantasies, sexual urges, or behaviors generally involving 1) nonhuman objects, 2) the suffering or humiliation of oneself or one's partner, or 3) children or other nonconsenting persons that occur over a period of at least 6 months. For some, paraphilic fantasies or stimuli are obligatory for erotic arousal and are always included in sexual activity. In others, the paraphilic preferences occur only episodically, such as during periods of stress, where at other times the person is able to function sexually without paraphilic fantasies or stimuli. Importantly, the paraphilia must cause marked distress, result in interpersonal difficulties, or impair social, occupational, or other important areas of functioning. (See Table 11–4 for a list of the paraphilias.)

TABLE 11–4. Paraphilias (sexual deviations)

Preferential sexual act	Behaviors/objects of gratification
Exhibitionism	Exposing self to others
Fetishism	Using inanimate object (e.g., shoe)
Frotteurism	Rubbing against nonconsenting persons
Pedophilia	Preferring prepubertal children
Sexual masochism	Enjoying pain and humiliation
Sexual sadism	Inflicting pain on others
Transvestic fetishism	Cross-dressing
Voyeurism	Window peeping
Paraphilia not otherwise specified	
Coprophilia	Feces
Hypoxyphilia	Desire to achieve altered state of consciousness secondary to hypoxia
Infantilism	Behaving as though one is an infant
Klismania	Enemas
Necrophilia	Dead persons
Oralism	Focusing on oral-genital contact to the exclusion of intercourse
Partialism	Focusing on one part of the body (e.g., feet) to the exclusion of all else
Telephone scatologia	Obscene telephone calls
Urophilia	Urine
Zoophilia (bestiality)	Animal contacts

DSM-IV-TR provides specific criteria for eight paraphilias and includes a residual category, *paraphilia not otherwise specified,* for other disorders that fail to meet criteria for any of the specific paraphilias. One of the more unusual paraphilias is *infantilism,* in which the person obtains sexual gratification by behaving like an infant. In one such case seen at our hospital, a 30-year-old former fighter pilot reported that he could function sexually only while wearing a diaper and sucking on a pacifier. He enjoyed having his partner change the diaper, apply baby powder, and bottle-feed him. Although the role-play initially was used for sexual gratification, he later found it comforting and generally wore a diaper under his clothing at all times.

The paraphilias are seen as having three aspects. First, the behavior does not conform to the generally accepted views of what constitutes normal sexual activity. (The accepted view of normal sexual behavior varies from society to society and has changed over time.) Second, the behavior may cause emotional or physical harm to another person involved in the sexual behavior, such as sex with children or extreme forms of sexual sadism. Third, the behavior causes subjective distress or interferes with social, occupational, or other important areas of functioning. For example, these persons may experience distress because they see their sexual urges as being at odds with their personal moral standards or societal standards.

A patient with exhibitionism and compulsive masturbation is described in the following case:

> Frank, a 38-year-old mechanic, presented to the emergency department requesting help. He had left his wife 3 days earlier, fearing that another arrest for indecent exposure would humiliate his family and friends. His story soon unfolded.
>
> At age 10, Frank had lost a testicle in an accident—a fact that was known to his classmates. He was teased endlessly, leading to feelings of insecurity and inadequacy. He began to masturbate at age 12 and was soon masturbating up to five times daily. Although he could not remember when it first occurred, he began to masturbate in public settings where he might be discovered. He found the challenge of avoiding detection sexually exciting. His masturbation had a compulsive quality, and he felt powerless to stop.
>
> The behavior continued over a 25-year period, leading to several arrests for indecent exposure. Feeling guilty and wanting to make amends, Frank sought psychotherapy after each arrest, but he would soon drop out. He denied other paraphilic behaviors and thought that pedophilia was "disgusting." He admitted to only two episodes of exhibitionism, first at age 18 to a girl sitting next to him in class and once during his honeymoon. Frank had married at age 23 and described the marriage as stable and his sexual relationship with his wife as satisfying.
>
> Frank was admitted to the hospital for further evaluation. Physical examination confirmed the absence of the right testicle, but results of the examination were otherwise normal. His serum testosterone level was 288 ng/dL (normal serum level is 200–800 ng/dL). Treatment was begun with medroxyprogesterone. At a follow-up visit 1 month later, his serum testosterone had fallen to 41 ng/dL. He had been able to resist masturbating in public places and no longer had spontaneous erections. He was back with his wife, who was happy with his progress. Six months later, he chose to discontinue the medication and within 1 month had relapsed.
>
> Frank presented for follow-up 10 years later after an arrest for soliciting a prostitute. He had continued to compulsively masturbate and to expose himself to unsuspecting women. He had divorced in the meantime and had not sought treatment. Paroxetine (40 mg/day) was prescribed, and over the next year, Frank reported that the drug helped him to control his sexual urges and behaviors. He also had become involved in a support group for "sex addicts."

Etiology

For centuries, variations of the sexual act were regarded as offenses against nature, God, or the law rather than as disorders that physicians should study and treat. The systematic study of the paraphilias began in the 1870s with the work of Krafft-Ebing, Hirschfeld, Ellis, and others. In 1886, Richard Krafft-Ebing, a Viennese psychiatrist, compiled the first systematic account of paraphilias in his book *Psychopathia Sexualis*. He considered sexual deviations to be hereditary and believed that they could be modified by social and psychological factors. Freud, also active at this time, explained sexual deviations as resulting from failures of the developmental processes during childhood.

Learning theory has also informed our understanding of the paraphilias and suggests that sexual behavior is reinforced through sexual fantasies and masturbation. With the paraphilias, deviant patterns of arousal (including inappropriate fantasies and urges) become paired with masturbation. For example, an adolescent boy experiments with wearing his mother's shoes and in the process becomes sexually aroused. This links the deviant fantasy with the positive experience of orgasm. Once this process becomes established, it is likely to reoccur because orgasm is such a powerful reinforcement. In this example, the behavior leads to a fetish involving women's shoes.

Paraphilic acts also may result from poor impulse control that occurs in the context of psychosis or a brain disorder such as dementia. brain injury). Patients with antisocial personality disorder occasionally commit deviant sexual acts to gratify their immediate urges, although a true paraphilia may not exist.

Some sexually deviant behavior may have a biological basis. Evidence supporting this view includes the finding of an increased frequency of abnormal results on neurocognitive tests and electroencephalograms (EEGs) in sex offenders. Abnormal brain computed tomography scans have been reported in pedophiles and other sexually aggressive men; dilation of the temporal horns, especially the right horn, is one finding. Familial transmission and hypothalamic-pituitary-gonadal axis dysfunction have been reported in pedophilia.

Epidemiology

The prevalence of the paraphilias is unknown. They are relatively uncommon in psychiatric practice, and most cases come to attention only if treatment is sought (like Frank in the vignette above) or if there are forensic issues following an arrest. Many paraphilias would scarcely be reported at all because the activity takes place between consenting adults or by a lone individual. For example, the man who cross-dresses, is comfortable with his preference, and experiences no subjective distress is unlikely to come to clinical attention. Thus, people who are comfortable with their paraphilias are completely underrepresented in all samples.

The best statistics regarding prevalence are legal. In 2007, nearly 84,000 persons were arrested on sexually related charges in the United States, excluding forcible rape and prostitution; perpetrators are overwhelmingly male. These figures are biased toward impulsive individuals and persons with paraphilias that are considered either dangerous or a public nuisance. Among the legally identified cases, pedophilia is the most common paraphilia, probably because of the great effort made to apprehend persons with this condition. Exhibitionism is commonly reported, possibly because it involves repeated public displays that may inadvertently help police to identify the perpetrator. Sexual masochism and sexual sadism are underrepresented in crime statistics because it is unlikely that these disorders would come to public attention unless a tragedy occurred (e.g., autoerotic suffocation, in which a person dies accidentally after tying a rope around his or her neck to reduce blood flow in an effort to heighten masturbatory pleasure).

Clinical Findings, Course, and Outcome

Paraphilias are generally established in adolescence, usually before age 18 years. They occur almost exclusively among men, although cases are described in women. Most people with paraphilias are heterosexual, not homosexual, contrary to widely held views. These demographic features appear to hold true for fetishists, pedophiles, exhibitionists, and voyeurs. People with one paraphilia often meet criteria for others and thus have multiple paraphilias. Co-occurring psychiatric disorders are common and include substance misuse, mood disorders, and personality disorders. These disorders are chronic but tend to vary in frequency of expression and severity depending on the individual's level of stress, opportunity for sexual activity, and sexual drive. Many people with paraphilias have relatively normal sexual lives with their partner or spouse apart from the paraphilia; some partners may be unaware of the individual's paraphilic behavior.

Exhibitionism involves the exposure of one's genitals to a stranger. This disorder accounts for about one-third of the sexual offenders referred for treatment. The person (usually a man) will often masturbate when exposing his genitals. There is generally no attempt at having sexual activity with the stranger. When exhibitionism begins in older adults, the behavior may indicate the presence of a brain disorder, such as Alzheimer's disease. Fewer arrests are made for exhibitionism in older age groups suggesting that the condition becomes less severe with age, or that the individual has better control.

The person with *fetishism* may use rubber garments, women's underclothing, and high-heeled shoes as objects of gratification. The diagnosis is not made if the fetish objects are limited to articles of female clothing used in cross-dressing or devices such as a vibrator designed for the purpose of tactile genital stimulation. Typically, contact with the object produces sexual arousal, which is followed by masturbation. Some fetishists spend considerable time seeking their desired objects. The following vignette describes a man with fetishism who was seen in our clinic:

> Daniel, a 41-year-old attorney, had his law license suspended after admitting to breaking into and entering more than 100 homes to obtain women's underwear for sexual gratification. He entered the houses through unlocked doors or would sometimes jimmy a lock with a credit card or knife. Once inside the house, he would seek undergarments to use later in solitary acts of masturbation. He was finally caught after he entered a neighbor's home, where he was found searching for the woman's underwear. He was apprehended and charged with criminal trespass. Daniel was later convicted and placed on probation. He denied subsequent episodes of pilfering undergarments at a follow-up 5 years later, but he admitted that the urges remained. He believed that a renewed interest in religion was responsible for improved self-control.

Frotteurism involves touching or rubbing against a nonconsenting person. This tends to occur in crowded places from which the person can readily escape, such as a busy sidewalk or a subway car. The behavior may include rubbing his genitals against a victim's thighs or buttocks, or touching her genitals or breasts with his hands. Frotteurism is most common in the 15- to 25-year age group.

Pedophilia involves sexual activity with a prepubescent child, generally age 13 or younger. The individual with pedophilia must be 16 years or older and at least 5 years older than the child. People with pedophilia generally report an attraction to children of a particular age range. Some individuals prefer boys, some prefer girls, and some are aroused by both boys and girls. Activity may be limited to undressing the child and looking, or exposing one's genitals and masturbating in front of the child. Others will have oral, anal, or vaginal sex with the child. Importantly, experiencing distress about having sexual fantasies, urges, or behaviors involving children is not required for the diagnosis mainly because many people with pedophilia are comfortable with their behavior. They may justify their sexual activity with children by claiming that the behavior is educational, or that the child enjoyed (or wanted) the experience. The disorder tends to begin in adolescence and is chronic, more so among those who have a preference for boys.

Transvestic fetishism involves cross-dressing by a man in women's clothing. The disorder often begins at puberty. Persons may start by putting on only a few women's garments. In time, the individual may dress entirely in female clothing. Early on, the person experiences the cross-dressing as sexually stimulating. As the person gains confidence, the clothes may be worn in public, and the individual may become part of a transvestic subculture. The disorder tends to be chronic, although the urge to cross-dress may decline as the sexual drive lessens.

Voyeurism involves the act of observing unsuspecting persons, usually strangers, who are naked, in the act of disrobing, or engaging in sexual activity. The act of looking ("peeping") is for the purpose of achieving sexual excitement, and generally no sexual activity with the observed person is sought. Voyeurism is often an expression of sexual curiosity in adolescents and typically has an onset before age 15 years. The course tends to be chronic. The following case of voyeurism was reported in a local paper:

> A 27-year-old law student pleaded guilty to five counts of criminal trespass after admitting that he had repeatedly spied on women in dormitory showers. He was arrested near the dormitory one morning after students had caught him lying on the floor outside the women's shower and looking through the ventilation grate. He was chased out of the dormitory by the women who had found him there.
>
> Residents of the dormitory had banded together and would watch for him daily from 5:00 A.M. to 9:00 A.M., believing that he would repeat his act. The "peeper" was well known at the dorm for his voyeurism and for making a nuisance of himself.

Sexual masochism and *sexual sadism* are also listed in DSM-IV-TR but are less common. Sexual masochism involves sexual fantasies, urges, or behaviors of being humiliated, bound or otherwise made to suffer that cause clinically significant distress or impairment in social, occupational, or other important areas of functioning. Sexual sadism involves sexual fantasies, urges, or behaviors in which the psychological or physical suffering (including humiliation) of a victim is sexually exciting to the person. In addition, the person has acted on the urges with a nonconsenting person, or the urges or fantasies cause marked distress or interpersonal difficulty.

Clinical Management

Behavioral interventions have become the mainstay of treatment of the paraphilias and are widely incorporated into programs for sex offenders. Methods to reduce deviant arousal patterns include *masturbatory satiation* (satiating or boring the patient with his own deviant fantasies) and *covert sensitization* (replacing fantasies with unpleasant images). *Masturbatory conditioning* is used to generate arousal to nondeviant themes. Social skills training is used to help the patient learn to communicate more effectively with appropriate adult partners. Cognitive-behavioral methods are used to help restructure the faulty cognitions that people with paraphilias use to justify their behavior (e.g., erroneously interpreting a child's docility as an expression of sexual desire). Relaxation training may help reduce the anxiety and stress that frequently precede paraphilic behavior. A follow-up study of 194 child molesters treated with behavior modification showed an 82% success rate (defined as no recidivism) at 12 months posttreatment. Although these results are encouraging, it is not known whether they can be generalized to the other paraphilias or to persons not motivated by threats of arrest or incarceration.

There are no FDA-approved medications for the treatment of paraphilias. Research has mainly focused on testosterone-lowering drugs, the SSRIs, and naltrexone.

Both medroxyprogesterone and leuprolide act peripherally to reduce serum testosterone levels and centrally to reduce sexual drive. The aim is to decrease paraphilic fantasies and their associated behaviors while avoiding erectile dysfunction. Medroxyprogesterone is given orally at dosages ranging from 100 to 400 mg/day. A long-acting preparation (Depo-Provera) may be given intramuscularly at dosages of 200–400 mg every 7–10 days. Leuprolide, a luteinizing hormone–releasing hormone agonist, has been used at a dose of 7.5 mg/month by depot injection. The long-term risks of these medications have not been adequately studied, and for that reason they should be used with caution. The gonadotropin-releasing hormone analogue triptorelin was found effective in a controlled trial, but the drug is unavailable in the United States.

SSRIs have also been used to reduce paraphilic fantasies and behavioral impulsivity. An open-label study with sertraline showed that individuals with various paraphilias seemed to benefit. Naltrexone, an opioid receptor blocker, may be effective in curbing paraphilic fantasies and behavior as well.

Testosterone-lowering drugs should be reserved for patients whose symptoms do not respond to SSRIs or naltrexone or for those whose hypersexuality is uncontrolled or dangerous. Other drug therapy, including antipsychotic or antidepressant medication, is indicated when the paraphilia is associated with schizophrenia, major depression, or an anxiety disorder.

Key points to remember about paraphilias

1. The history is of utmost importance in treating paraphilias. The therapist must learn where and when the behavior occurs and whether the focus of desire is a person or an object.

   • Most persons with paraphilias have a variety of deviant sexual interests and behaviors, and the therapist is safe in assuming that more is present than initially meets the eye.

2. Paraphilias are difficult to treat, but behavior therapy may offer the best hope for success. The purpose of treatment is to reduce deviant arousal patterns and to generate new arousal in response to nondeviant themes.

   • Methods may include masturbatory satiation and conditioning, social skills training, and cognitive restructuring.

3. Medications may help to reduce paraphilic fantasies and inappropriate sexual behaviors but none are FDA approved.

   • SSRIs and naltrexone have been used with some success.

   • Testosterone-lowering agents are generally reserved for repeat offenders whose actions are uncontrolled or potentially dangerous.

4. Difficult cases should be referred to clinicians experienced in treating these disorders.

■ Gender Identity Disorders

The essential feature of gender identity disorders ("transsexualism") is a strong and persistent cross-gender identification and, for many, the desire to become a member of the opposite sex. Individuals with this disorder typically have a sense of inappropriateness about their assigned gender. This may lead them to become preoccupied with getting rid of their primary and secondary sex characteristics and acquiring the sex characteristics of the opposite gender. A residual category, gender identity disorder not otherwise specified, exists for disorders that do not meet the full syndromal criteria (e.g., a person preoccupied with castration but having no desire to acquire the sex characteristics of the opposite gender).

The following case describes a patient with gender identity disorder evaluated in our clinic:

> Will, a 25-year-old felon, was referred for evaluation of gender dysphoria. He had recently filed a lawsuit requesting that the state pay for his gender reassignment surgery and allow him to wear women's clothing in prison. He sought transfer to a women's unit and asked for hormone injections. Corrections officials had refused these requests.
>
> Will reported that he had never felt comfortable with his gender. He was effeminate as a child and enjoyed playing house, in which he would assume feminine roles such as playing the mother or sister. He also liked games associated with girls, such as hopscotch and jump rope, and was not very good at team sports. He began to cross-dress at age 9 and said that he felt more comfortable and natural when dressed as a girl.
>
> Will began to cross-dress full-time in his early 20s and for a 5-month period lived as a woman, calling himself Julie. Although he never had a desire for heterosexual relationships, he was able to perform sexually with a woman and achieve orgasm, but "didn't like it." During sexual intercourse, Will would fantasize about being made love to as a woman. He reported homosexual experiences with more than 100 partners and had several relationships lasting as long as 6 months' duration. He had attempted to mutilate his genitals on three occasions and several months before his evaluation had managed to lacerate his penis with a shard of glass.
>
> In addition to gender dysphoria, Will had a lifelong history of disciplinary and behavior problems and as a young boy had been placed in detention. He had a history of misusing alcohol and marijuana and had run-ins with the law for shoplifting, theft, and forgery. He also had had several psychiatric hospitalizations, mostly for depression or suicidal behavior.
>
> There was no evidence of a mood disorder, a formal thought disorder, hallucinations, or delusions. Will ended his personal history with the comment, "It's all a confused mess."
>
> Although he clearly met criteria for gender identity disorder, Will's lawsuit ultimately failed, and he remained at the men's prison.

In making the diagnosis of transsexualism, it is important to rule out other potential causes of gender dysphoria, including schizophrenia and transvestic fetishism. With schizophrenia, a desire to change one's anatomical gender may be part of a complex delusion (e.g., the belief that the Federal Bureau of Investigation is conspiring to change the patient's sex). People with transvestic fetishism who cross-dress occasionally may come to feel that sex change surgery is a natural extension of their cross-dressing.

Gender identity disorder usually begins in childhood. In boys, early features include overidentification with the mother, overtly feminine behavior (e.g., playing with dolls), little interest in typical male pursuits (e.g., disliking sports), and peer relationships primarily with girls. Tomboyishness is found in young transsexual girls, but the behavior is more acceptable in our society than is feminine behavior in boys and tends to draw less attention. The prevalence of the disorder is estimated at 1 in 30,000 men and 1 in 100,000 women.

DSM-IV-TR subtypes transsexuals according to their attraction to males or females. Those not attracted to either gender generally have a history of either no sexual activity or of deriving little pleasure from the genitals. Transsexual persons often deny any interest in homosexuality because they believe themselves to be members of the opposite sex.

Depression, substance abuse, and personality disorders are frequently comorbid in persons with gender identity disorders. Borderline personality traits are relatively frequent because many transsexuals have persistent identity problems, engage in self-mutilation, or have angry outbursts. Some of this could be explained as the outward expression of their frustration with being trapped in the wrong body. The self-mutilation may involve damage to their genitals, including autocastration in extreme cases. These acts are generally not suicide attempts because they are designed to force the physician to deal with the patient's transsexualism.

Many transsexual persons seek hormonal therapy and request sex reassignment surgery. Clinics in the United States and elsewhere offering sex reassignment surgery often require that the patient live as a member of the opposite sex for more than 1 year before considering him or her for surgery.

In the transition from male to female, the individual is prescribed hormones (e.g., estradiol, progesterone) to promote breast development; laser treatment and electrolysis are used to remove hair. Finally, surgery is performed to remove the testes and penis and to create an artificial vagina (vaginoplasty). The female-to-male transsexual patient undergoes mastectomy, hysterectomy, and oophorectomy. Testosterone is prescribed to help develop muscle mass and deepen the voice. Some transsexual persons will choose to have an artificial penis constructed.

Transsexual patients who adjust well after surgery tend to have had a lifelong cross-gender identification, were able to "pass" convincingly as a member of the opposite sex before surgery, have good social support, have a college education, and have a steady job. The overwhelming majority are satisfied with the outcome of surgery. Many patients will continue to benefit from psychotherapy following surgery to assist them in adjusting to their new gender role.

Individual or group psychotherapy may be useful for patients who do not seek surgery. Psychotherapy may help the patient to accept his or her anatomical sex; to develop an ability to experience pleasure from his or her genitals; and make a successful adjustment in other important areas of life.

■ Self-Assessment Questions

1. What are the three major types of sexual disorders?
2. What are the stages of the sexual response cycle?
3. What are the disorders of the appetitive stage?
4. What are the causes of male erectile disorder (impotence)?
5. Describe "dual" sex therapy. What are "sensate focus" exercises?
6. What medications are used to treat male impotence?
7. How common are paraphilias?
8. How can learning theory help explain paraphilic behavior?
9. How are paraphilias treated? Describe cognitive-behavioral therapy for a person with a paraphilia. What medications can be used to dampen unwanted sexual behaviors?
10. What are the antecedent behavioral characteristics of transsexual persons?
11. What are the treatments for gender identity disorder? What factors predict a good outcome to gender reassignment surgery?

CHAPTER 12

Eating Disorders

O! that this too, too solid flesh would melt.

William Shakespeare, Hamlet

ANOREXIA NERVOSA and bulimia nervosa, the two major eating disorders, are each characterized by the presence of disturbed eating behaviors combined with an intense preoccupation with body weight and shape. Many persons believe that these syndromes have developed relatively recently, perhaps reflecting contemporary society's obsession with youth, beauty, and slimness. In fact, the disorders have been recognized for centuries. Richard Morton, an English physician, is generally credited with describing the syndrome of anorexia nervosa in 1694, although it was Sir William Gull who coined the term in 1873. Gull's patients were mostly emaciated young women with amenorrhea, constipation, and an abnormally slow pulse who were nonetheless remarkably overactive. His account of anorexia nervosa as a disorder of starvation motivated by the pursuit of thinness is still noteworthy for its attention to detail.

■ Definition

Anorexia nervosa is diagnosed when a person induces weight loss leading to a body weight of less than 85% of a healthy norm or refuses to

---

TABLE 12–1.   **DSM-IV-TR diagnostic criteria for anorexia nervosa**

A. Refusal to maintain body weight at or above a minimally normal weight for age and height (e.g., weight loss leading to maintenance of body weight less than 85% of that expected; or failure to make expected weight gain during period of growth, leading to body weight less than 85% of that expected).
B. Intense fear of gaining weight or becoming fat, even though underweight.
C. Disturbance in the way in which one's body weight or shape is experienced, undue influence of body weight or shape on self-evaluation, or denial of the seriousness of the current low body weight.
D. In postmenarcheal females, amenorrhea, i.e., the absence of at least three consecutive menstrual cycles. (A woman is considered to have amenorrhea if her periods occur only following hormone, e.g., estrogen, administration.)

Specify type:

>   **Restricting Type:**   during the current episode of Anorexia Nervosa, the person has not regularly engaged in binge-eating or purging behavior (i.e., self-induced vomiting or the misuse of laxatives, diuretics, or enemas)

>   **Binge-Eating/Purging Type:**   during the current episode of Anorexia Nervosa, the person has regularly engaged in binge-eating or purging behavior (i.e., self-induced vomiting or the misuse of laxatives, diuretics, or enemas)

---

gain appropriate weight while growing taller; has an intense fear of gaining weight or becoming fat even though underweight; has a disturbance in the perception of his or her body shape; and (in women) has missed three consecutive menstrual cycles (see Table 12–1). The patient's body mass index (BMI; weight in kilograms/height in meters^2) is generally less than 17.5 (25 is considered healthy). The requirement that the person with anorexia be 15% underweight for body height emphasizes severity, and the requirement for amenorrhea adds to the specificity of the diagnosis. (In men, there is no comparable requirement for reproductive hormone abnormality.) The clinician should further specify whether the disorder is the restricting type (i.e., no bingeing or purging) or the binge-eating/purging type.

Bulimia nervosa consists of recurrent episodes of binge eating; a feeling of lack of control over eating during the binges; recurrent use of inappropriate compensatory behaviors to prevent weight gain, such as vomiting, use of laxatives or diuretics, strict dieting or fasting, or vigorous exercise; an average of two binge episodes weekly for 3 months; and

---

TABLE 12–2. DSM-IV-TR diagnostic criteria for bulimia nervosa

A. Recurrent episodes of binge eating. An episode of binge eating is characterized by both of the following:
(1) eating, in a discrete period of time (e.g., within any 2-hour period), an amount of food that is definitely larger than most people would eat during a similar period of time and under similar circumstances
(2) a sense of lack of control over eating during the episode (e.g., a feeling that one cannot stop eating or control what or how much one is eating)
B. Recurrent inappropriate compensatory behavior in order to prevent weight gain, such as self-induced vomiting; misuse of laxatives, diuretics, enemas, or other medications; fasting; or excessive exercise.
C. The binge eating and inappropriate compensatory behaviors both occur, on average, at least twice a week for 3 months.
D. Self-evaluation is unduly influenced by body shape and weight.
E. The disturbance does not occur exclusively during episodes of Anorexia Nervosa.

Specify type:
Purging Type: during the current episode of Bulimia Nervosa, the person has regularly engaged in self-induced vomiting or the misuse of laxatives, diuretics, or enemas
Nonpurging Type: during the current episode of Bulimia Nervosa, the person has used other inappropriate compensatory behaviors, such as fasting or excessive exercise, but has not regularly engaged in self-induced vomiting or the misuse of laxatives, diuretics, or enemas

---

persistent overconcern with body shape and weight (see Table 12–2). Furthermore, the disturbance does not occur exclusively in the course of anorexia nervosa. The clinician should specify whether the disorder is of the purging type (e.g., self-induced vomiting) or the nonpurging type.

The discrepancy between weight and perceived body image is key to the diagnosis of anorexia nervosa. Most underweight persons are concerned about their weight. They recognize when it is too low and express a desire to gain weight. By contrast, people with anorexia nervosa take delight in their weight loss and fear gaining weight. Bulimic persons often successfully hide their binge-eating and purging behaviors and often have normal weight. In practice, the two syndromes tend to overlap, so that patients often have a mixture of symptoms.

Another category, *eating disorder not otherwise specified*, is used for symptoms that do not meet the criteria for a more specific eating disorder. A woman who has features of anorexia nervosa but who still menstruates would fit this category. Another example is the person with eating binges but no compensatory purging behavior; this person would receive a diagnosis of *binge-eating disorder*, which tends to occur in older persons and is found in about one-quarter of morbidly obese individuals.

■ Epidemiology

There has been some concern that eating disorders are increasing in prevalence, and several investigators have suggested that anorexia nervosa is more common than it was decades ago. It seems more likely that increasing public awareness has simply led to increased recognition of the disorder. Also, because treatments have become available, patients may be more likely to seek help. Estimates from high school– and college-age populations yield a prevalence among women of approximately 1% for anorexia nervosa and up to 4% for bulimia nervosa. For either disorder, the frequency in men is about one-tenth that for women. Isolated symptoms, such as binge eating, purging (e.g., self-induced vomiting), or fasting, are far more common than the disorders themselves. The gender difference is probably not artifactual, because population surveys confirm what clinicians have noted.

Eating disorders have an onset during adolescence or young adulthood. Studies comparing anorexia and bulimia generally find an earlier age at onset for anorexia (early teens) than for bulimia (late teens, early 20s). These disorders are found in all social strata, although in the past they were thought to be more common in the higher socioeconomic groups. Anorexia nervosa, however, is uncommon in nonindustrialized countries and is less frequent among African Americans in the United States. Eating disorders are overrepresented in occupations that require rigorous control of body shape (e.g., modeling, ballet). Male athletes—particularly wrestlers and jockeys—often develop eating disorders because they must meet strict weight criteria.

The following case example illustrates a patient who developed anorexia nervosa first and later achieved normal weight complicated by bulimia nervosa:

Mary, a 36-year-old registered nurse, had a 16-year history of abnormal eating behaviors. Although she now maintained a normal weight and had regular periods, she had frequent binge/purge episodes.

Mary grew up in a competitive, upper-middle-class family. The middle of five children, Mary felt unloved and ignored by her parents, who she believed favored the other children. Apart from occasional temper outbursts during her childhood and teen years, Mary was well adjusted, performed well in school, was active in clubs, and had many friends, yet she felt insecure and unattractive.

At age 20, she and a friend toured Europe together and would skip meals to save money. Both felt that they could afford to lose some weight. Indeed, she lost about 25 pounds, and upon her return, her family became concerned with Mary's scarecrow-like appearance. Mary was happy with her weight loss and felt more attractive. In fact, she expressed a desire to lose more weight.

Over the next 5 years, her weight fluctuated, but she remained underweight. Family members were concerned with her eating habits. She refused to eat meals with her family, adopted a vegetarian diet, and was often observed preparing high-calorie snacks. Her mother noted that cakes, cookies, and other desserts prepared for the family would mysteriously disappear or a cake might be found with all of the frosting eaten. Mary eventually moved into her own apartment. Her brother remembers running into her at a grocery store and finding only diet soda, a single head of lettuce, and several bags of candy in the shopping cart.

Early on Mary had learned to induce vomiting, which later occurred spontaneously. She would keep empty jars in her room to hold her emesis. After she had moved out of the family home, several filled jars were found under her bed.

Always active, Mary became obsessed with exercise. She jogged 10 miles each day and entered several marathons. She eventually cut back on her jogging when bone spurs and an old back injury flared up. Instead, she developed a new routine consisting of a 10-mile bicycle ride followed by a 45-minute swim. Mary was so busy with exercise that she had little time for friends and lost interest in dating. Nonetheless, she lived independently, maintained a full-time job, and attended school part-time.

When Mary was 25, her mother talked her into seeing a physician for evaluation of her thinness, but the physician was not familiar with eating disorders and explained that Mary's thinness and abnormal eating behaviors were a harmless idiosyncrasy. Mary later sought help from a counselor for relationship problems but never sought help for her eating disorder.

Nine years later, Mary continued to engage in occasional bingeing and purging but maintained a normal weight. She continued to work full-time, had married, and had two healthy children.

■ Clinical Findings

Anorexia nervosa is accompanied by a repertoire of behaviors designed to promote weight loss. Examples include extreme dieting, adoption of special diets (or vegetarianism), and refusal to eat meals with family members or to eat in restaurants. Anorexic persons often show an unusual interest in food that belies their fear of gaining weight. The individual may clip and collect recipes or prepare elaborate meals for friends and relatives; some persons develop an interest in nutrition. At mealtime, the anorexic person may play with the food on his or her plate or cut meat into tiny pieces. Despite the concern of friends and family, persons with anorexia will insist that their weight is normal and, in fact, that they are overweight. Like Mary in the vignette, many anorexic persons develop an intense, obsessive interest in fitness and develop elaborate exercise routines. Abuse of laxatives, diuretics, or stimulants in an effort to enhance weight loss is relatively common.

Anorexic persons with bulimic behavior and persons with bulimia nervosa carry out their binge eating and purging in private. Enormous amounts of food can be consumed during a binge (e.g., an entire cake, a quart of ice cream, and a package of cookies). Although parents and other family members may be unaware of the binge eating, they might notice that the family food bill is increasing or that certain foods, particularly those high in calories or carbohydrates, seem to disappear. Binge eating may initially provide tension relief for the patient, but this relief is short-lived and generally leads to feelings of guilt and disgust. The person then induces vomiting, typically by placing the fingers in the throat; later, she or he may be able to vomit at will. Ipecac or other emetics are sometimes used to facilitate vomiting. Many bulimic persons, perhaps more than 10%, steal food by shoplifting or other means.

Profound weight loss can occur in anorexic persons. In addition to appearing emaciated, they may develop hypothermia, dependent edema, bradycardia, and hypotension. Some persons with anorexia develop sensitivity to temperature and report feeling cold much of the time. Near-chronic constipation leads many to become dependent on laxatives. Hormonal abnormalities can develop, including elevated growth hormone levels, increased plasma cortisol, and reduced gonadotropin levels. Thyroxin and thyroid-stimulating hormone may be normal even when triiodothyronine (T_3) is reduced. Men with anorexia nervosa generally have low levels of circulating testosterone and may show clinical signs of hypogonadism. For these reasons, many young people with anorexia have delayed sexual development and a diminished interest in sex. Amenorrhea precedes the onset of obvious weight loss in one-fifth of female patients.

Bulimic persons sometimes develop calluses on the dorsal surface of the hands (resulting from the irritation caused by placing fingers down the throat), dental erosion, and multiple caries. Rarely, esophageal erosion or tears occur. All are complications of frequent vomiting.

Medical complications caused by bulimic behavior include hypocalcemia or hypokalemic alkalosis (in those who engage in self-induced vomiting or who abuse laxatives and diuretics); electrolyte disturbances resulting in weakness, lethargy, or electrocardiographic changes such as depressed T waves; elevated serum transaminases, reflecting fatty degeneration of the liver; elevated serum cholesterol and carotenemia, reflecting malnutrition; and parotid gland enlargement and elevated serum amylase. The medical complications of the eating disorders are summarized in Table 12–3.

■ Course and Outcome

The long-term course of the eating disorders ranges from full recovery to malignant weight loss and rapid death. One study of patients with anorexia showed a death rate of 11% during a 12-year follow-up, a rate significantly higher than expected. From 25% to 40% of eating disorder patients have a good outcome, meaning that they eat normally, do not binge or purge, and are emotionally well adjusted. In the remaining patients, the characteristic symptoms of the illness (e.g., distorted body image, abnormal eating behaviors) persist. Poor outcome is associated with longer duration of illness, older age at onset, prior psychiatric hospitalizations, poor premorbid adjustment, and the presence of a comorbid personality disorder.

■ Etiology and Pathophysiology

The cause of eating disorders is unknown but likely involves a combination of biological vulnerability, psychological predisposition, and societal influences. Genetic factors are probably important in anorexia nervosa, which has a concordance rate of nearly 70% for identical twins and only about 20% for nonidentical twins. Several studies have shown an increased frequency of bulimia nervosa among the relatives of bulimic persons.

TABLE 12–3. Medical complications of the eating disorders

Physical manifestations	Laboratory abnormalities
Amenorrhea	Dehydration[a]
Sensitivity to cold	Hypokalemia[a]
Constipation	Hypochloremia[a]
Low blood pressure	Alkalosis
Bradycardia	Leukopenia
Hypothermia	Elevated transaminases
Lanugo hair	Elevated serum cholesterol
Hair loss	Carotenemia
Petechia	Elevated BUN[a]
Carotenemic skin	Elevated amylase levels[a]
Parotid gland enlargement[a]	
Dental erosion, caries[a]	
Pedal edema	
Dry skin	

Endocrine abnormalities

Increased growth hormone levels

Increased plasma cortisol and loss of diurnal variation

Reduced gonadotropin levels (LH, FSH, impaired response to LHRH)

Low T_3, high T_3RU impaired TRH responsiveness[a]

Abnormal glucose tolerance test results

Abnormal dexamethasone suppression test results[a]

Note. BUN=blood urea nitrogen; FSH=follicle-stimulating hormone; LH=luteinizing hormone; LHRH=luteinizing hormone–releasing hormone; T_3=triiodothyronine; T_3RU= triiodothyronine reuptake; TRH=thyrotropin-releasing hormone.
[a]Seen in patients who binge and purge.

Another factor may be a disturbance in serotonergic neurotransmission in the central nervous system (CNS). In the hypothalamus, serotonin helps to modulate feeding behavior by producing feelings of fullness and satiety. Patients with anorexia frequently report feeling "too full" after eating. Another effect of the CNS serotonin pathways involves regulation of mood, impulses, and obsessionality. Patients with anorexia nervosa are often rigid, inhibited, and perfectionistic. One study showing high levels of central nervous system 5-hydroxyindoleacetic acid (5-HIAA)—a metabolite of serotonin—in recovered anorectic patients suggested that an overactive serotonin system could contribute to behavioral restraint, obsessionality, and an inhibited appetite.

Once dieting begins, psychological and physiological changes occur that perpetuate abnormal eating behavior. Anorexia nervosa often serves a positive function in the person's life by providing a refuge from upsetting life events or developmental issues involving relationships and sexuality. Some clinicians believe that anorexia nervosa represents an attempt to prolong childhood and escape the responsibilities of adulthood. Patients cling to their disorder and take comfort in their success with dieting. The tension relief gained from the avoidance of food or purging behavior is strongly reinforcing.

Physiological changes that occur in anorexia nervosa also reinforce the disorder. Corticotropin-releasing hormone secretion is enhanced in anorexia nervosa and may act to maintain abnormal eating behavior. Levels of vasopressin are high and oxytocin levels are low in the cerebrospinal fluid of underweight persons with anorexia. One hypothesis is that both hormones work together to promote distorted thinking patterns and obsessional concerns about food.

■ Diagnosis and Assessment

The diagnosis of an eating disorder is based on the patient's history and a careful mental status examination. In addition, a thorough physical examination should be part of the workup. Particular attention should be given to vital signs, weight, skin quality and turgor, and the cardiovascular system. The patient's weight and height should be measured, and the appropriateness of weight for height, age, and gender should be determined according to his or her expected body weight or the BMI (see Figure 12–1). This information can help guide decisions with respect to medical and nutritional management.

Laboratory studies can help to rule out alternative diagnoses. The workup should include a complete blood count, urinalysis, blood urea nitrogen, and serum electrolytes. For malnourished and severely symptomatic patients, other tests are indicated, including serum cholesterol and lipids; serum calcium, magnesium, phosphorus, and amylase; liver

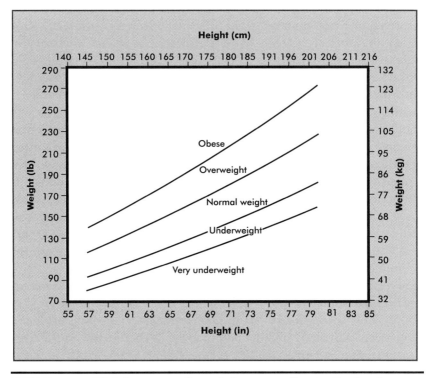

FIGURE 12–1. **Weight ranges for adults according to the body mass index (BMI).**

Anorexia nervosa is characterized by a BMI of 17.5 or lower.

Source. Reprinted from Becker et al. 1999. Used with permission of the Harris Center for Education and Advocacy in Eating Disorders.

enzymes; and an electrocardiogram. Brain imaging with magnetic resonance or computed tomography is indicated in some patients to rule out a mass lesion. Thyroid function tests are indicated when hyperthyroidism is suspected as a cause of weight loss. Bone mineral densitometry is helpful in assessing and monitoring osteoporosis; bone-density measurements are more than two standard deviations below normal in about half of women with anorexia nervosa.

Other major mental illnesses must be excluded before a diagnosis of anorexia nervosa or bulimia nervosa is made. Schizophrenia is sometimes accompanied by bizarre eating habits, but they are usually related to the patient's delusions. Major depression is frequently accompanied by poor appetite and significant weight loss, but this weight loss is not associated with a distorted body image and is unwanted. Ritualistic eating behaviors resulting in weight loss sometimes occur in patients with obsessive-compulsive disorder, but the weight loss is not accompanied by a distorted body image or fears of gaining weight.

Co-occurring mental illnesses are common. Many patients with anorexia nervosa or bulimia nervosa fulfill criteria for another psychiatric disorder, such as major depression, an anxiety disorder, or a personality disorder. Obsessive-compulsive disorder, specific phobias, and agoraphobia are the most frequent anxiety disorders diagnosed in patients with anorexia nervosa. Bulimic persons are at high risk for substance misuse and "acting out" personality disorders such as borderline personality disorder.

Medical illnesses also need to be ruled out as a cause of the eating disorder and weight loss. Conditions associated with severe weight loss include gastrointestinal disorders (e.g., a malabsorption syndrome) and endocrine disorders (e.g., hyperthyroidism). Midline tumors in the brain can be associated with anorexia and weight loss in the absence of localizing neurological abnormalities. Nevertheless, when the core features of an eating disorder are present—morbid fear of fatness and self-induced starvation—a medical cause is highly unlikely.

■ Clinical Management

The treatment of eating disorders has three main goals. The first and most important goal is to restore the patient's nutritional state. In patients with anorexia nervosa, this means restoring weight to within a normal range. In bulimic persons, this means ensuring that metabolic balance is achieved. The second goal is to modify the patients' distorted eating behaviors. This will help the patient maintain his or her weight within a normal range and reverse (or lessen) binge eating, purging, and other abnormal eating behaviors. The third goal is to help change the patient's distorted and erroneous beliefs about the benefits of weight loss.

Treatment usually occurs on an outpatient basis, but many patients will need to be hospitalized. Severe starvation and weight loss, hypotension or hypothermia, and electrolyte imbalance are the main indications for hospitalization. Depressed patients with eating disorders who have suicidal ideations or psychosis also require hospitalization. Failure of outpatient treatment, as indicated by the inability to gain weight or the inability to reverse severe binge/purge cycles, is another reason to hospitalize the patient. Partial hospital (or day treatment) programs are helpful to patients who need more supervision and support than can be obtained in an outpatient clinic but who do not require inpatient care. In these programs, patients attend the hospital during the day but live at home.

The psychological treatment of anorexia nervosa or bulimia nervosa generally involves behavioral modification combined with individual and group psychotherapy. The purpose of behavior therapy is to restore normal eating behavior. In the hospital, this goal is accomplished by setting goals for both eating and weight gain and by targeting certain abnormal behaviors for correction (e.g., reducing the number of vomiting episodes for bulimic patients). Positive reinforcement is used to help patients achieve the goals outlined in a treatment contract that is agreed to by the patient. For example, patients who are able to achieve their weight goals are rewarded with special privileges, such as a pass with a family member. An example of a behavioral modification program is presented in Chapter 19.

The patient should be weighed regularly, early in the morning after emptying the bladder and while wearing only a hospital gown. Daily fluid intake and output should be recorded. Patients should be observed for at least 2 hours after meals to prevent vomiting, even if attendants must accompany them to the bathroom. Patients are typically started on a diet providing about 500 calories more than the amount required to maintain their present weight; the caloric intake is gradually increased. At first, to prevent discomfort, it may be advisable to spread meals out over six feedings throughout the day. Patients who are significantly underweight or are having trouble gaining weight may need tube feedings.

An electrocardiogram is essential for assessing palpitations or for evaluating changes consistent with hypokalemia. Prolongation of the QT interval contraindicates the use of tricyclic antidepressants and should lead to immediate medical intervention because it may increase the risk of ventricular tachycardia and sudden death. Gastric motility agents rarely relieve bloating sensations associated with refeeding. Stool softeners or bulk laxatives can help to alleviate the severe constipation associated with long-term use of stimulant laxatives or their withdrawal. The use of estrogen supplementation usually is not necessary, but patients should receive vitamins, including calcium, at a dosage of 1,000–1,500 mg/day and a multivitamin to ensure that vitamin D intake is adequate (400 IU/day).

Psychotropic medication can be helpful in some patients, particularly those with bulimic behaviors. Several classes of antidepressant medications have been shown to decrease binge eating and purging behaviors, but they have no specific role in treating anorexia nervosa. The selective serotonin reuptake inhibitor (SSRI) fluoxetine (60 mg/day) is the only medication approved by the U.S. Food and Drug Administration for the treatment of bulimia nervosa. Other SSRIs are routinely prescribed and may be as effective. Tricyclic antidepressants and monoamine oxidase inhibitors are probably effective as well in reducing binge and purge cycles, but they are not considered first-line agents. Bupropion is contraindicated because it can lower seizure threshold in eating disorder patients with electrolyte disturbances. Antidepressants appear effective in the short term and may reduce binge/purge cycles by up to 70%. Less is known about their long-term effectiveness, as most studies have been of short duration. One study suggests that patients who respond in the short term should be treated for a minimum of 6 months. Second-generation antipsychotics (e.g., olanzapine) have been used in patients with anorexia nervosa and may be effective in helping to promote weight gain and reduce cognitive distortions. Other drug therapy, including mood stabilizers, antidepressants, or anxiolytics, is indicated when the eating disorder is accompanied by psychosis, major depression, bipolar disorder, or an anxiety disorder.

Antidepressants often have little effect in relieving depression in emaciated patients with anorexia nervosa. In these patients, weight gain itself may have an antidepressant effect.

Many patients with eating disorders will not seek treatment on their own and will deny their illness. They are sometimes brought unwillingly to a physician by their family or friends and may resist treatment; if hospitalized, they may leave against medical advice. For these reasons, the physician must use tact and skill to enlist the patient's cooperation. Once the patient is in treatment, the physician and patient should agree on a behavioral contract. The contract often becomes a focus of criticism, and the patient may make repeated requests of the physician to change it. The best approach is to stand firm with the contract so as to avoid repeated battles with the patient over additional changes that are sure to be requested.

Individual psychotherapy should be practical and goal oriented. The therapy should focus on educating the patient about the illness, helping the patient to understand her or his symptoms, and explaining the need for treatment. Later, approaches that aim to promote insight can be used to help the patient resolve problems and conflicts that may have contributed to (or reinforced) the abnormal eating behavior. Family therapy is often helpful, especially when the patient is living at home and the disturbed eating behavior has been prompted by family interactions or when the disturbed eating behavior has created problems within the family. Intensive programs that emphasize a behavioral approach, such as nutritional education, cognitive restructuring techniques, and psychosocial support, seem to be the most effective.

Cognitive-behavioral therapy and interpersonal psychotherapy have both been shown to be effective in patients with bulimia nervosa. Cognitive-behavioral therapy has as its goal correcting inappropriate thoughts and beliefs that bulimic patients have about themselves and their disorder. With interpersonal psychotherapy, interpersonal sources of stress thought to precede or contribute to the person's disturbed eating behavior are addressed. Both therapies help to normalize eating behavior by reducing the number of binge/purge episodes. These therapies also are effective in patients with binge-eating disorder.

Key points to remember about eating disorders

1. An empathic relationship should be encouraged. This goal may be hard to achieve because patients with anorexia can be oppositional and not sufficiently motivated to make the needed changes. Some will lack insight and refuse treatment.

2. The clinician should assess the patient carefully for psychiatric comorbidity.

    •   The presence of psychiatric comorbidity complicates treatment and must be addressed. Eating disorder patients are highly likely to have comorbid major depression, anxiety disorders, substance abuse, or a personality disorder.

    •   The presence of a personality disorder, particularly from Cluster B (e.g., borderline personality disorder), is common in bulimic persons and is associated with poor treatment outcome.

3. Clinicians should set a firm but nonpunitive behavioral contract with patients and have them sign it.

    •   Reasonable targets for behavioral modification should be developed.

    •   The goals should be set and the clinician should stand firm against changes. Minor changes in the protocol can open a Pandora's box.

4. Medication is of limited value in treating anorexia nervosa.

5. Medication is an important treatment adjunct in patients with bulimia nervosa.

> **Key points to remember about eating disorders** *(continued)*
>
> - SSRIs are the drugs of first choice; fluoxetine (20–60 mg/day) is the best researched, but others are likely to be effective as well (e.g., sertraline, 50–200 mg/day; paroxetine, 20–60 mg/day; escitalopram, 10–20 mg/day).
> - Tricyclic antidepressants and monoamine oxidase inhibitors are effective but are considered second-line choices because of their potential side effects and dangerousness in overdose.
> - Bupropion should be avoided because of its tendency to lower the seizure threshold.
>
> 6. Family therapy can be especially helpful with patients who still live at home or whose behavior has created problems within the family. Marital therapy will be helpful to those whose eating disorder has disrupted their marriage.

■ Self-Assessment Questions

1. How do bulimia nervosa and anorexia nervosa differ? How do they overlap?

2. What are the social and demographic characteristics of eating disorder patients? Is the prevalence of eating disorders increasing?

3. What are some of the physiological and psychological theories about the cause of anorexia nervosa?

4. Describe typical clinical symptoms in anorexia nervosa and bulimia nervosa.

5. What potential medical complications may result from anorexia nervosa? From bulimia nervosa?

6. What is the natural history of the eating disorders? Can patients die from eating disorders?

7. What are the major goals in the treatment of eating disorders?

8. Which medications are used in treating eating disorder patients?

CHAPTER 13

Adjustment Disorders

Whether 'tis nobler in the mind to suffer
The slings and arrows of outrageous fortune...

William Shakespeare, Hamlet

A STUDENT learns he has failed an important exam and may lose a scholarship; a physician discovers her husband has been unfaithful; a CEO must deal with an impending bankruptcy and staff lay-offs. These are examples of everyday stressful events that, while unpleasant, most persons adjust to and cope with. Some people, however, feel overwhelmed by these situations and develop symptoms of emotional distress, such as depression, anxiety, or impaired work ability. These symptoms may be sufficiently severe to require brief periods of psychiatric care, usually on an outpatient basis. The term *adjustment disorder* acknowledges the fact that some people develop symptoms as a direct consequence of a stressful situation that they have difficulty adjusting to.

■ Definition

Specific criteria for adjustment disorders were introduced in DSM-III in 1980. DSM-IV-TR criteria for adjustment disorder specify that the emotional or behavioral symptoms must arise within 3 months of the stressor and must be clinically significant. The symptoms cannot merely represent an exacerbation of a preexisting disorder, and they cannot be accounted for by bereavement. Furthermore, the maladaptive reaction cannot persist for more than 6 months after the termination of the stressor or its consequences (see Table 13–1).

Five subtypes of adjustment disorder are listed. The specific diagnosis depends on the predominant symptoms that develop in response to the stressor, such as depressed mood, anxiety, mixed anxiety and depressed mood, disturbance of conduct, or mixed disturbance of emotions and conduct. An unspecified subtype also exists for reactions that do not fit into any specific categories (e.g., a patient who responds to a new diagnosis of AIDS with denial and noncompliance with his or her treatment regimen).

■ Epidemiology

Adjustment disorders are undoubtedly common, but there are no good prevalence estimates. The frequency of these disorders in psychiatric clinics and hospitals is estimated to range from 5% to 10%, and adjustment disorders are even more common on psychiatric consultation-liaison services at general hospitals. For example, in one study, 51% of cardiac surgery patients were diagnosed with an adjustment disorder, whereas a study of newly hospitalized cancer patients reported a rate of 32%. Among adolescents recently diagnosed with diabetes mellitus, the rate of adjustment disorders was 36%.

One study found that medical illness was the identified stressor for more than two-thirds of patients with adjustment disorders seen on a consultation service. These patients were largely free of preexisting psychiatric illness and had endured prolonged hospitalizations for serious physical illnesses such as cancer or diabetes. Those in whom medical illness was not the stressor were more likely to have established psychiatric histories and recurrent problems with relationships or finances.

The diagnosis appears to be more common in women, unmarried persons, and younger people. Common symptoms in adolescents include behavioral changes or acting out. Adults typically develop mood or anxiety symptoms. Adjustment disorders can occur at any age from childhood through senescence, but the mean age at diagnosis tends to be in the mid-20s to early 30s.

TABLE 13–1. **DSM-IV-TR diagnostic criteria for adjustment disorders**

A. The development of emotional or behavioral symptoms in response to an identifiable stressor(s) occurring within 3 months of the onset of the stressor(s).
B. These symptoms or behaviors are clinically significant as evidenced by either of the following:
  (1) marked distress that is in excess of what would be expected from exposure to the stressor
  (2) significant impairment in social or occupational (academic) functioning
C. The stress-related disturbance does not meet the criteria for another specific Axis I disorder and is not merely an exacerbation of a preexisting Axis I or Axis II disorder.
D. The symptoms do not represent Bereavement.
E. Once the stressor (or its consequences) has terminated, the symptoms do not persist for more than an additional 6 months.
Specify if:
  Acute: if the disturbance lasts less than 6 months
  Chronic: if the disturbance lasts for 6 months or longer
Adjustment Disorders are coded based on the subtype, which is selected according to the predominant symptoms. The specific stressor(s) can be specified on Axis IV.
  With Depressed Mood
  With Anxiety
  With Mixed Anxiety and Depressed Mood
  With Disturbance of Conduct
  With Mixed Disturbance of Emotions and Conduct
  Unspecified

■ Clinical Findings

Different subtypes of adjustment disorder reflect the varied symptoms that can occur in response to a stressor:

• Depressed mood: dysphoria, tearfulness, hopelessness
• Anxiety: psychic anxiety, palpitations, jitteriness, hyperventilation
• Conduct disturbance: violating the rights of others or disregarding age-appropriate societal norms and rules (e.g., vandalism, reckless driving, fighting)

- Mixed disturbance of emotions and conduct: emotional symptoms, such as depression or anxiety, in addition to a behavioral disturbance
- Unspecified: for example, a person who has developed difficulty functioning at work

Table 13–2 presents the frequency of psychosocial stressors thought to have contributed to an adjustment disorder in a study of adults and adolescents. Many of these people had multiple, recurrent, or continuous stressors. School problems were the most frequently cited stressor in adolescents. Parental rejection, alcohol and/or drug problems, and parental separation or divorce also were common. In adults, the most common stressors were marital problems, separation or divorce, moving, and financial problems. Stressors were sometimes chronic. For example, among adolescents, nearly 60% of the stressors had been present for a year or more, and only 9% had been present for 3 months or less. Among adults, stressors showed more variation, but 36% had been present for a year or more, and nearly 40% had been present for 3 months or less. Another study suggests that stressors are gender specific in adolescents. School and legal problems were common stressors for boys as was parental illness for girls.

The following case is of a patient seen at our hospital who developed an adjustment disorder with depressed mood:

Joanne, a 34-year-old homemaker, was admitted to the hospital following a tricyclic antidepressant overdose. She had felt well until earlier that day until learning she had lost custody of her 13-year-old daughter to her ex-husband; she became upset, anxious, and tearful. That evening, feeling desperate, Joanne took a handful of nortriptyline tablets she had in her medicine chest (prescribed months earlier for migraine) because she felt life was no longer worth living. When her current husband returned home from work, Joanne told him what she had done. An ambulance was called, and Joanne was taken to the hospital emergency department, where she underwent charcoal lavage. There was no prior psychiatric history.

After calming sufficiently, Joanne explained that her current husband had been accused of sexually molesting her daughter, an allegation reported to local social service agencies. This led to her daughter's placement in foster care. Although she denied her husband had ever touched the girl inappropriately, she conceded that such an allegation was serious and would be taken into account by a judge in determining custody. After considering her situation, Joanne reported she was no longer depressed or suicidal and was now in an appropriate frame of mind to work with her lawyer to regain custody of her child.

TABLE 13–2. Stressors occurring in adolescents and adults with adjustment disorders

Adolescents		Adults	
Stressor	%	Stressor	%
School problems	60	Marital problems	25
Parental rejection	27	Separation or divorce	23
Alcohol and/or drug problems	26	Move	17
Parental separation or divorce	25	Financial problems	14
Girlfriend or boyfriend problems	20	School problems	14
Marital problems in parents	18	Work problems	9
Move	16	Alcohol and/or drug problems	8
Legal problems	12	Illness	6
Work problems	8	Legal problems	6
Other	60	Other	81

Source. Adapted from Andreasen and Wasek 1980.

■ Course and Outcome

Adjustment disorders are generally transient, typically lasting only days or weeks, although some are more chronic, particularly when there is an ongoing stressor (e.g., a woman with an alcoholic husband). By definition, adjustment disorders last no longer than 6 months after *termination* of the stressor (or its consequences). When a disturbance lasts longer, it will presumably meet criteria for another disorder, such as generalized anxiety disorder, major depression, or dysthymia.

Adjustment disorders in adults usually have a good outcome. In a 5-year follow-up of 48 adults with this diagnosis, 79% were well at follow-up, with 8% having an intervening problem. In another study, adults with an adjustment disorder had shorter psychiatric hospital stays and fewer re-admissions during a 2-year follow-up than comparison subjects with other psychiatric diagnoses. These data are consistent with a more recent study in which patients with adjustment disorders were compared with patients with depression. The former were less symptomatic and had better functioning at a 6-month follow-up than the latter. Together, these data suggest that for adults, the diagnosis identifies persons with acute-onset disorders who recover quickly and tend not to have preexisting mental illness.

The data are somewhat mixed for adolescents who receive the diagnosis. In a 5-year follow-up of 52 adolescents with adjustment disorders, 57% were well at follow-up, but 43% had a current mental disorder, including schizophrenia, major depression, alcohol or drug abuse, and antisocial personality disorder. Adolescents were also more likely to be suicidal at admission and had readmission rates similar to those of comparison subjects. These findings suggest that the diagnosis may be less useful in adolescents because they tend to have more varied outcomes. However, some clinicians consider the diagnosis of adjustment disorder appealing for younger patients because it is relatively nonpejorative. They believe the diagnosis avoids stereotyping patients with a harsher, more severe diagnosis that may lead to self-fulfilling prophecies.

■ Etiology

According to DSM-IV-TR, adjustment disorders must occur in reaction to identifiable psychosocial stressors within 3 months of their onset. As a result of this definition, adjustment disorder is one of the few psychiatric diagnoses in which a cause-and-effect relationship is presumed. Most people are remarkably resilient and do not develop psychiatric symptoms in response to stressful situations, which suggests that individuals who develop an adjustment disorder may have an underlying psychological vulnerability.

One way to conceptualize this is to recognize that each person has his or her own "breaking point," depending on the amount of stress applied, underlying constitution, personality structure, and temperament. To draw an analogy, if enough pressure is applied to a bone, it will fracture; however, the amount of pressure required will differ from person to person, depending on age, gender, and physical well-being. To carry the analogy a bit further, adjustment disorders can occur in psychiatrically "normal" people, just as healthy bones will break if subjected to sufficient stress. At the other end of the continuum, people with fragile personalities, like bones with osteoporosis, will "break" more readily.

■ Differential Diagnosis

In making the diagnosis of adjustment disorder, the crucial question is: "What is the patient having trouble adjusting to?" Without a stressor to cause maladjustment, an adjustment disorder cannot be diagnosed. Yet even when a stressor exists, other major mental disorders must be ruled out as causing the symptoms, and the stressor cannot represent bereavement. Another Axis I diagnosis takes precedence over—or preempts—a diagnosis of adjustment disorder. A person who experiences an important stressor (e.g., recent marital separation) and develops depressed mood receives a diagnosis of adjustment disorder *only* when his or her symptoms fail to meet criteria for major depression.

The differential diagnosis reflects the broad range of symptoms seen in adjustment disorders. The differential diagnosis includes mood disorders (such as major depression), anxiety disorders (such as panic disorder or generalized anxiety disorder), and conduct disorders in the child or adolescent. Personality disorders should be considered because they are frequently associated with mood instability and behavior problems. For example, patients with borderline personality disorder often react to stressful situations in maladaptive ways (e.g., verbal outbursts, anger fits, suicide threats), so an additional diagnosis of adjustment disorder usually is unnecessary, unless the new reaction differs from their usual maladaptive pattern. Psychotic disorders are often preceded by the development of social withdrawal, work or academic inhibition, or dysphoria and need to be differentiated from adjustment disorders. Other psychiatric disorders that are believed to occur in reaction to a stressor also must be considered, including brief psychotic disorder, in which a person develops psychotic symptoms in response to a stressor, and acute stress disorder or posttraumatic stress disorder, which develops after a traumatic event that involves actual or threatened death or serious injury (e.g., wartime experiences).

As with the assessment of any mental disorder, the patient being evaluated for an adjustment disorder should undergo a thorough physical examination and mental status examination to rule out alternative diagnoses.

■ Clinical Management

The management of adjustment disorders has not been systematically evaluated, but supportive psychotherapy is probably the most widely used intervention. Individual psychotherapy may give the patient an opportunity to review the meaning and significance of the psychosocial stressor that led to the disturbance. The therapist can help the patient to adapt to the stressor when it is ongoing or to better understand the stressor once it has passed. Group psychotherapy can provide a supportive atmosphere for persons who have experienced similar stressors, such as patients who have received a diagnosis of breast cancer.

Medications also may be beneficial and should be prescribed based on the patient's predominant symptoms. For example, a patient with initial insomnia may benefit from a hypnotic (e.g., zolpidem, 5–10 mg at bedtime) for a few days. A patient experiencing anxiety may benefit from a brief course (e.g., days to weeks) of a benzodiazepine (e.g., lorazepam, 0.5–2.0 mg twice daily). If the disorder persists, the clinician should reconsider the diagnosis. At some point, an adjustment disorder with depressed mood, for example, may develop into major depression, which would respond best to antidepressant medication.

Key points to remember about adjustment disorders

1. The key question is: "What is the patient having trouble adjusting to?" When there is no stressor, there is no adjustment disorder.

    • Even with an identified stressor, if the patient fits full criteria for another Axis I disorder such as major depression, that diagnosis preempts adjustment disorder.

2. Adjustment disorders can evolve into other, better-defined disorders, such as major depression.

    • Be alert to changes in mental status and to both the evolution and duration of symptoms.

3. Most adjustment disorders are transient. Tincture of time and supportive psychotherapy are usually all that is necessary.

4. Patients with common psychosocial stressors (e.g., diagnosis of cancer or AIDS, chronic back pain, breakup of a relationship) can benefit from attending support groups with others who have experienced the same stressor.

5. Psychotropic medication taken short-term (i.e., days to weeks) should be targeted to the predominant symptoms:

    • Hypnotics (e.g., zolpidem, 5–10 mg at bedtime) for those with insomnia.

    • Benzodiazepines (e.g., lorazepam, 0.5–2.0 mg twice daily) for those with anxiety.

6. If long-term treatment is needed, the patient may have another disorder (e.g., major depression, generalized anxiety disorder), which will need to be diagnosed and treated.

■ Self-Assessment Questions

1. How common are adjustment disorders, and what are their typical precipitants and manifestations?

2. Describe how to distinguish between an adjustment disorder and a major syndrome, such as major depression or generalized anxiety disorder.

3. What is the differential diagnosis for adjustment disorders?

4. What is the "cause" of adjustment disorders, and why do they affect some persons and not others?

5. How do the stressors differ between adolescents and adults?

6. How are adjustment disorders managed clinically?

CHAPTER 14

Impulse-Control Disorders

Even on my way to the gambling hall, as soon as I hear...the clink of scattered money, I almost go into convulsions.

Fyodor Dostoevsky, The Gambler

FIVE TYPES of impulse-control disorders (ICDs) are listed in DSM-IV-TR: intermittent explosive disorder, kleptomania, pyromania, pathological gambling, and trichotillomania. The category *impulse-control disorder not otherwise specified* (NOS) exists for ICDs that do not meet criteria for a more specific disorder; examples include compulsive buying and Internet addiction (see Table 14–1 for a list of ICDs).

Disorders of impulse control are common yet frequently underdiagnosed and underappreciated. All can cause considerable emotional distress and social and/or occupational impairment. Some can lead to financial or legal problems. All are characterized by the presence of irresistible urges or impulses to carry out potentially harmful or self-destructive behaviors.

■ Intermittent Explosive Disorder

Intermittent explosive disorder (IED) is diagnosed when a person has several discrete episodes of losing control over his or her aggressive

TABLE 14-1. DSM-IV-TR impulse-control disorders

Disorder	Uncontrolled behavior
Intermittent explosive disorder	Aggression
Kleptomania	Stealing
Pyromania	Fire setting
Pathological gambling	Gambling
Trichotillomania	Hairpulling
Impulse-control disorder not otherwise specified	
Compulsive buying	Shopping
Internet addiction	Computer use

impulses that are out of proportion to any stressor; these episodes may involve assaultive acts or destruction of property. The diagnosis is used for persons in whom the loss of control is out of character and not merely part of a pattern of overreacting to life's problems. Therefore, psychiatric conditions in which assaultive behaviors occur as a matter of course need to be ruled out, such as antisocial or borderline personality disorder, psychotic disorders, mania, or alcohol or drug intoxication. A sudden behavioral change accompanied by outbursts in an otherwise healthy person suggests a brain disorder, which also needs to be ruled out.

IED was first included in DSM-III in 1980. Patients who receive the diagnosis are predominantly young men with relatively low frustration tolerance. A recent study suggested a 7% lifetime prevalence. Some investigators suggest that "pure" cases of IED—that is, cases unaccompanied by any indication of a brain disorder (e.g., abnormal electroencephalographic findings, neurological soft signs, presence of abnormal personality traits)—are rare. Comorbid mood and anxiety disorders are common in IED.

There is little consensus on the proper management of IED because treatments have not been well studied. A recent study showed that cognitive-behavioral therapy (CBT) was superior to a wait list in reducing anger and hostility in persons with IED. With CBT, patients can learn to recognize when they are becoming angry and to identify and defuse the triggers that lead to outbursts.

Medication to reduce or eliminate aggressive impulses may be helpful. Both the selective serotonin reuptake inhibitor (SSRI) fluoxetine and the antiepileptic drug oxcarbazepine have been found superior to placebo in reducing impulsive aggression in people with IED. Other SSRIs (sertraline, citalopram), mood stabilizers (e.g., lithium carbonate, carbamazepine), and β-blockers (e.g., propranolol) have been used to treat IED, but their use is supported mainly by case studies or small case series. Second-generation antipsychotics (e.g., risperidone) have been used to dampen aggressive impulses in other clinical populations (e.g., dementia patients, patients with borderline personality disorder) and may be helpful in treating IED. Benzodiazepines may be helpful in treating the unbearable tension that leads to outbursts in some patients. These drugs should be used with caution because of their potential to cause behavioral disinhibition.

■ Kleptomania

Kleptomania involves the recurrent failure to resist impulses to steal objects not needed for personal use or for their monetary value; an increasing sense of tension immediately before committing the theft; and pleasure, gratification, or relief at the time of the theft. The stealing is not committed to express anger or vengeance, is not in response to hallucinations or delusions, and is not better accounted for by antisocial personality disorder, conduct disorder, or a manic episode.

A study of psychiatric inpatients showed kleptomania to have a lifetime prevalence of around 9%. A recent survey of the U.S. general population showed shoplifting to have a lifetime prevalence of 11%. While most shoplifters do not have kleptomania, the data suggest that kleptomania may be more common than once thought.

Kleptomania begins in adolescence or early adulthood and tends to be chronic. Nearly three-quarters of persons with kleptomania are women. One of us (D.W.B.) followed an 88-year-old woman with a history of impulsive stealing since age 16. Only the humiliation of an arrest at age 78, and the resultant publicity, kept her from stealing again, despite her nearly continuous urges.

Mood disorders frequently co-occur with kleptomania. Stealing impulses and behaviors often change along with the patient's mood alterations. Anxiety disorders, including obsessive-compulsive disorder, panic disorder, and social phobia, also are common, as are substance use and eating disorders.

Various forms of behavioral treatment, including aversive therapy and covert sensitization, have been used to treat kleptomania. In covert sensitization, patients are instructed to pair images of nausea and vomiting with the urge to steal. Psychodynamic approaches in which kleptomania is conceptualized as a symptom of an underlying emotional conflict have also been used. None of these treatments has been carefully studied.

A randomized controlled trial found that the opioid antagonist naltrexone (50–150 mg/day) led to significant reductions in stealing urges and behaviors compared with placebo. A similar trial of the SSRI escitalopram showed that the drug was no better than placebo. In a case series of 20 patients with kleptomania, 10 of the 18 patients receiving various antidepressants and/or mood stabilizers improved after several weeks of treatment. In 2 of the patients, stealing behavior resumed when the medication was discontinued.

As with the elderly woman described earlier, many persons with kleptomania are arrested for shoplifting and are processed through the legal system. The embarrassment and shame they experience may keep some from acting on their urges, but this tends not to last. Probation may help some by providing a regular reminder of what might occur if the person is caught stealing again. A self-imposed ban on shopping in an attempt to head off potential thefts is probably the most common approach to managing the urges, but this is seldom sustainable in the long run.

■ Pyromania

Pyromania is defined in DSM-IV-TR as deliberate and purposeful fire setting on more than one occasion; tension or affective arousal before the act; fascination with, interest in, curiosity about, or attraction to fire and its contents and characteristics; and pleasure, gratification, or relief when setting fires or when witnessing or participating in their aftermath. Based on this definition, the arsonist who sets fires for monetary gain or for political or criminal purposes does not qualify for the diagnosis. Persons with antisocial personality disorder, conduct disorder, or mania sometimes set fires but do not have a sense of fascination with fire, nor do they experience the tension and relief with fire setting that people with pyromania describe. Deliberate fire setting is probably motivated most frequently by anger or revenge.

There are few data on prevalence, but a study of psychiatric inpatients found that about 6% had a lifetime history of pyromania. Although pyromania was once thought to occur primarily in boys or men, a recent report suggests that gender distribution may be equal. Onset tends to be in the late teens or early 20s. Mood, substance use, and other ICDs are common in people with pyromania. Fire setting is considered a poor prognostic sign for children with conduct disorders and correlates with adult aggression.

Clinicians should begin by identifying other comorbid psychiatric disorders that can be a focus of treatment (e.g., major depression). Treatment of the coexisting disorder may itself reduce fire-setting behavior. There is no clear role for medication in the treatment of pyromania itself. If the patient is a child or adolescent, the parents should be taught consistent but nonpunitive methods of discipline. Family therapy may help in dealing with the broader issue of family dysfunction often found in patients with pyromania. The patient needs to understand the dangerousness and significance of the fire setting. A visit to a burn unit or scene of a fire may help to make patients aware of the consequences of their behavior. Patients also need to learn alternative ways of coping with stressful situations to decrease reliance on fire setting as an outlet.

■ Pathological Gambling

Pathological gambling is characterized in DSM-IV-TR by a continuous or periodic loss of control over gambling. The diagnostic criteria are patterned after those used for substance dependencies because many superficial similarities exist (e.g., preoccupation with gambling, repeated efforts to stop gambling). Many experts consider gambling an addiction. The disorder is easily diagnosed, particularly in advanced cases, despite the patient's denial. This characteristic is also typical of the substance abuser.

Pathological gambling affects 0.4%–2% of the general population. The prevalence is lower in areas with limited gambling opportunities. About one-third of pathological gamblers are women; they generally start gambling later in life than do men. In men, the disorder typically begins in adolescence, and some become "hooked" almost from their first bet. Men who seek help will typically have had the problem for decades, whereas women will have been ill for only a few years. Some will have an insidious onset following years of social gambling. Mood, anxiety, and substance use disorders are common in people with pathological gambling. There is no "gambling personality," yet research suggests that pathological gamblers tend to be impulsive and have difficulty delaying gratification.

The following case example shows how damaging pathological gambling can be:

Mary, a 42-year-old accountant, had gambled recreationally for years. At age 38, for reasons she could not explain, she became hooked on casino slot machines. Her interest in gambling gradually escalated, and within a year Mary was gambling during most business days. She also gambled most weekends, telling her husband she was at work. To acquire money for gambling, Mary created a fake company to which she transferred nearly $300,000 from her accounting firm. The embezzlement was eventually detected and Mary was arrested. Following her arrest, and the associated public humiliation, Mary became severely depressed and attempted suicide by drug overdose. After a brief hospital stay, Mary entered counseling and was prescribed paroxetine. In the plea bargain, she agreed to perform 400 hours of community service.

Pathological gambling has been the most actively researched of the ICDs. Data show that it runs in families and may be genetically related to substance misuse and antisocial personality disorder. Brain imaging research in pathological gamblers shows that gambling activates the brain's "reward" circuitry, but also that reduced activity occurs in areas mediating planning and decision-making.

The use of medications to treat pathological gambling is being actively researched. The opioid antagonist naltrexone (50–200 mg/day) has been shown to be more effective than placebo. Nalmefene, another opioid antagonist, has also been shown to reduce gambling urges and behaviors, but it is unavailable in the United States. The SSRIs are being studied and may be helpful, particularly in depressed or anxious patients.

Referral to Gamblers Anonymous, a 12-step program similar to Alcoholics Anonymous, may be helpful, although dropout rates are high. Inpatient treatment and rehabilitation programs similar to those for substance use disorders may be helpful for selected patients.

Other patients will benefit from individual psychotherapy geared toward helping them understand why they gamble and assisting them in dealing with feelings of hopelessness, depression, and guilt. CBT can be used to address the irrational thoughts and beliefs associated with pathological gambling ("I'll win big with the next bet!"). CBT is often combined with motivational interviewing (MI) techniques that were pioneered in the treatment of alcohol and drug use disorders. MI is a nonjudgmental approach in which therapists encourage the patient to make needed changes in his or her behavior. Relapse prevention methods can help patients identify the triggers that promote gambling and teach them how to deal more effectively with these triggers. Family therapy offers the gambler an opportunity to make amends, to learn better communication skills, and to repair the rifts that gambling inevitably creates in families.

■ Trichotillomania

Trichotillomania is characterized by recurrent pulling out of one's hair that results in noticeable hair loss. This is usually associated with an increasing sense of tension before pulling out the hair and pleasure, gratification, or relief when pulling out the hair. Persons with trichotillomania usually report substantial subjective distress or develop other evidence of impairment.

The disorder is generally chronic, although it tends to wax and wane in symptom severity. It can affect any site where hair grows, including the scalp, eyelids, eyebrows, body, and axillary and pubic regions. In clinic samples, 70%–90% of hairpullers are female, and most report a childhood onset. Surveys show that it affects 1%–4% of adolescents and college students. Compulsive hairpullers frequently have comorbid mood and anxiety disorders, other ICDs, or personality disorders.

The diagnosis is easily made once alternative diagnoses and medical conditions have been ruled out. Most patients have no obvious balding, but they may have small, easily disguised bald spots or patches or missing eyebrows and eyelashes. The following case example describes a patient seen in our clinic:

> Shirley, a 42-year-old married homemaker, presented for evaluation of compulsive hairpulling. She had recently learned that clomipramine might be helpful and wanted to try it.
>
> Shirley grew up in a small Midwestern farming community. Her childhood was relatively happy, and her family life was harmonious. As a young girl, she began to twist and twirl her hair and later, before age 10, began to pull out scalp, eyebrow, and eyelash hair.
>
> The amount of hairpulling had fluctuated over the years, but she had never been free of it. The pulling was sometimes automatic, such as when she was reading or watching television, but at other times, it was more deliberate. Shirley reported that she was unable to stop pulling her hair.
>
> During the interview, Shirley removed her wig, revealing an essentially bald scalp except for a fringe around the top. She had no eyebrows or eyelashes, which she disguised with makeup and eyeglasses. She was embarrassed by and ashamed of her hairpulling and tearfully recalled how classmates had made fun of her as a child. Over the years, she had received many medical and dermatological evaluations. Ointments and solutions had been prescribed, all without benefit.
>
> A trial of clomipramine (up to 150 mg/day) boosted her mood but had no effect on the hairpulling. Supportive psychotherapy helped boost Shirley's low self-esteem. On follow-up 13 years later, Shirley's hairpulling behavior was unchanged, but she reported being happy and feeling fulfilled.

Treatment for trichotillomania consists of medication and behavioral therapy, often in combination, although few patients seek help. With behavior therapy, patients learn to identify when their hairpulling occurs (it is often automatic) and to substitute other, more benign behaviors (e.g., squeezing a ball). Some patients also benefit from learning to apply barriers to prevent hairpulling, such as wearing gloves or a hat. These techniques are often referred to as *habit reversal.* In a controlled trial, habit reversal was more effective than negative practice (in which a patient is taught to go through the motions of hairpulling but to stop short of pulling it), and the benefits persisted during a 4-month follow-up. Several additional studies have since confirmed that behavior therapy is effective in reducing hairpulling.

Medication studies have shown mixed results. An early study using clomipramine showed benefit, but other drugs have not shown consistent benefit. SSRIs are probably the most frequently prescribed medications for trichotillomania. One promising alternative is the glutamate modulator *N*-acetylcysteine, which was associated with significant reductions in hairpulling in a recent controlled trial.

Some patients also will benefit from cognitive-behavioral psychotherapy that aims at upgrading their often low self-esteem, addressing relationship and family issues, and helping to correct faulty cognitions (e.g., "No one likes me because my eyebrows are missing"). Topical steroids may be helpful to patients who describe localized itching that prompts hairpulling. Hypnosis also has been used and is reported to benefit some persons.

■ Other Disorders

Both compulsive buying and Internet addiction are examples of impulsive disorders that, while not specifically listed in DSM-IV-TR, would fall within the category *impulse-control disorder not otherwise specified.*

Compulsive Buying

Compulsive buying was originally described by Emil Kraepelin, a German psychiatrist best known for his work with schizophrenia and manic-depressive (bipolar) illness. Compulsive buying is characterized by an irresistible urge to buy items that are either unneeded or unwanted. The person usually has a feeling of tension before buying, followed by a sense of gratification or relief with buying. Feelings of guilt or remorse may follow. Compulsive shopping behavior can lead to serious financial problems, including bankruptcy, and can contribute to marital and family strife.

The disorder is chronic and typically has an onset in the late teens or early 20s, corresponding to the age when most persons become emancipated from their families and first obtain credit cards. Most compulsive buyers are young women who spend excessive amounts on clothing, shoes, and makeup. Many have co-occurring psychiatric disorders, including major depression or an anxiety, substance use, or eating disorder. Many have other ICDs, such as pathological gambling.

Treatment of this condition has not been established, although individual psychotherapy may be helpful in exploring the significance of the compulsive buying and in helping the patient to recognize and learn how to avoid situations that lead to shopping episodes. Group CBT programs have been developed and appear effective, but may not be available. SSRIs may be helpful in reducing the behavior, particularly in depressed or anxious patients. Two small controlled trials with fluvoxamine showed no difference from placebo, but a larger study that used citalopram showed it to be helpful. Referral to Debtors Anonymous, a 12-step program, or to a consumer credit counseling service may be helpful.

Internet Addiction

Internet addiction, or *problematic Internet use,* involves excessive or poorly controlled computer use that leads to impairment or distress. The condition has attracted increasing attention in the popular media— attention that has paralleled the growth in computer use and Internet access. The disorder has been described to occur worldwide, but mainly in countries where computer access and technology are widespread. Persons with this disorder are preoccupied with computer use, often losing all sense of time when online. Internet "addicts" describe urges to use the computer when offline, to have a sense of tension or arousal before logging on, and to feel guilty or depressed when spending too much time online. Because this condition has been relatively recently described, there is no consensus regarding its treatment. If the Internet addict lives at home, parents may want to consider limiting computer access or canceling their Internet service.

Key points to remember about impulse-control disorders

1. IED may respond to the SSRI fluoxetine, a mood stabilizer (e.g., oxcarbazepine), propranolol, or a second-generation antipsychotic.

    *   CBT may help patients learn to identify stressors that trigger outbursts, which patients can then defuse.

    *   Patients must know that they are responsible for the consequences of their behavior.

2. Persons with kleptomania may benefit from naltrexone or one of the SSRIs (e.g., fluoxetine, paroxetine).

    *   A self-imposed shopping ban may be the best short-term strategy to forestall stealing.

3. Pathological gambling may respond to naltrexone or one of the SSRIs.

    *   Persons with pathological gambling may benefit from CBT to help counter the distorted thinking that often develops ("I'll win the next time!").

    *   Patients should be referred to a local Gamblers Anonymous chapter.

    *   Because pathological gambling can affect the individual's marriage and family life, marriage and/or family therapy may be important.

4. Trichotillomania probably responds best to behavior therapy.

    *   Habit reversal methods have been shown to be beneficial.

    *   SSRIs or clomipramine may reduce the urge to pull, but response to these drugs is inconsistent.

    *   For patients with extensive hair loss, wigs and other forms of hair replacement may be the most sensible solution to restore self-esteem and boost morale.

5. Patients with compulsive buying or spending may benefit from SSRIs but also need to be counseled to give up credit cards and other means of gaining easy credit access.

    *   Patients should be encouraged to find other meaningful ways to spend their time.

    *   Patients may benefit by attending Debtors Anonymous, a 12-step program for overspenders.

    *   Consumer credit counseling may be beneficial.

Key points to remember about impulse-control disorders *(continued)*
6. The Internet addict who lives at home should have his or her computer access monitored.   • Parents should consider canceling Internet service or limiting computer use.

■ Self-Assessment Questions

1. What are the five DSM-IV-TR impulse-control disorders?

2. Define *intermittent explosive disorder*. Which disorders exclude a diagnosis of intermittent explosive disorder?

3. How does the person with kleptomania differ from the ordinary shoplifter?

4. What kinds of problems do pathological gamblers develop? How is pathological gambling treated?

5. What is trichotillomania, and how is it treated? Describe habit reversal therapy.

6. Describe two examples of an impulse control disorder not otherwise specified.

PART III

SPECIAL TOPICS

CHAPTER 15

Psychiatric Emergencies

The thought of suicide is a great consolation; by means of it one gets successfully through many a bad night.

Friedrich Nietzsche

PSYCHIATRIC EMERGENCIES involving violent or dangerous
situations are relatively common in busy emergency departments,
psychiatric units, and even general medical wards. Examples include
the manic patient who is agitated and out of control and requires sedation; the patient with borderline personality disorder who has just
cut her wrists and says she has no reason to live; and the intoxicated
alcoholic patient who is threatening bodily harm to emergency personnel. These scenarios involve relatively common situations that
physicians encounter in the course of their clinical duties, particularly psychiatrists and those who work in emergency departments.
For this reason, students and residents should understand how to assess and clinically manage situations that involve assaultive, violent,
or suicidal patients.

■ Assaultive and Violent Behavior

Violence is all too common. News stories about senseless killings and assaults, drive-by shootings, and domestic violence document these events. People fear the possibility of becoming victims of violent crime, even as crime rates have steadily dropped in the past decade. Too often, the media have exaggerated the link between violence and mental illness, contributing to the fear felt by the public and the stigma experienced by psychiatric patients.

Most mentally ill persons are law-abiding and nonviolent. Nonetheless, research shows that patients with schizophrenia, mania, cognitive disorders (e.g., dementia, delirium), or drug or alcohol intoxication are more likely to become violent than are patients with other diagnoses or persons who are not mentally ill. Psychotic persons are more likely to commit violent acts than are nonpsychotic individuals. Brain-injured and mentally retarded persons also are at higher risk for committing violent acts.

The public (and often the courts) expect psychiatrists and other mental health professionals to be especially skilled in predicting violent behavior. In truth, they are no more skilled than laypersons in making long-term predictions about violence. That said, mental health professionals *are* in a position to predict violence in clinical settings. Certain elements of the clinical situation, including the patient's diagnosis and past behavior, can give an indication of the patient's potential for imminent violence, thereby allowing appropriate interventions to be made. A patient's history of violent behavior is probably the single best predictor of future dangerousness. Clinical wisdom suggests that past behavior predicts future behavior. The accuracy of predictions is improved in clinical populations that have high base rates for violence, such as patients on a locked psychiatric inpatient unit.

The following vignette describes the unfortunate but rather typical case of an aggressive patient with dementia seen in our hospital:

> Donald, a 71-year-old man with advanced Alzheimer's disease, was admitted for evaluation of violent and unpredictable behavior. His wife and family had cared for him at home during the 7-year illness. As the illness progressed, Donald became more confused and made more frequent misinterpretations of external stimuli. For example, his wife had a deep voice, which led him at times to conclude that a strange man was in the house. This was especially frightening to him and led him to threaten his wife with a knife.
>
> Donald was observed to be disoriented and confused. He did not know the date, his location, or the situation. He required considerable assistance with his grooming and dress. At times, without apparent

provocation, he would strike his nurses or would make threatening gestures, such as karate chops. This behavior was frightening because of its unpredictability.

He was given a high-potency antipsychotic (haloperidol, 2 mg/day) to reduce his paranoia and agitation. He was placed in a nursing home familiar with the care of patients with Alzheimer's disease.

Etiology and Pathophysiology

Many factors contribute to violent behavior. One of the most common factors in clinical settings is the presence of substance abuse. Alcohol is strongly associated with violence because of its well-known tendency to cause disinhibition, to decrease perceptual and cognitive alertness, and to impair judgment. Other substances of abuse, including amphetamines, cocaine, hallucinogens, phencyclidine (PCP), and sedative-hypnotics, also have been associated with violent behavior. Sadly, much of the violence in society is related to the misuse of alcohol and other drugs, either indirectly through activities involved in obtaining these substances or directly through their misuse.

One of the strongest predictors of adult violence is childhood aggression. This may be evident from a history of childhood behavioral problems or delinquent behavior, or a past diagnosis of conduct disorder. Of special concern is a history of fire setting or animal cruelty during childhood. Many violent persons have experienced abuse (emotional, physical, or sexual) in childhood, a sad fact noted in many adult perpetrators of abuse. For some, violence has its roots in a chaotic home environment, but for others there may be a biological predisposition toward violence. Antisocial behavior is well known to run in families.

Other factors also contribute to violence. Both antisocial and borderline personality disorders are associated with violent behavior, a fact that is reflected by their high prevalence among incarcerated persons. With advancing age and maturity, persons with these disorders are less likely to act out. Low-income persons are more likely to be both perpetrators and victims of violence, perhaps because of the alienation, discrimination, family breakdown, and general sense of frustration that the poor experience. The presence of readily available firearms in our society also has contributed to the general level of violence because they can turn what would be an assault into a murder.

At a neurophysiological level, aggressive behavior has been associated with disturbed central nervous system serotonin function. Low cerebrospinal fluid (CSF) 5-hydroxyindoleacetic acid (5-HIAA) levels are correlated with impulsive violence, one of the best-replicated laboratory findings in psychiatry. (5-HIAA is a metabolite of serotonin.) Serotonin has been hypothesized to act as the central nervous system's natural policing mechanism, helping to keep impulsive and violent behavior in check.

Violence is sometimes related to a brain injury or disorder (e.g., tumors, strokes) or to a seizure disorder (e.g., partial complex seizures). Whereas persons with traumatic brain injuries are more likely than noninjured persons to become violent or aggressive, aggressive acts by patients with epilepsy are relatively uncommon.

Assessing Risk for Violence

Risk assessment for violent behavior involves a review of pertinent clinical variables and requires a thorough psychiatric history and careful mental status examination. Even in routine assessments, patients should be asked the following questions:

1. Have you ever thought of harming someone else?
2. Have you ever seriously injured another person?
3. What is the most violent thing you have ever done?

The prediction of violence can be compared to weather forecasting. Like weather forecasting, assessment of violence risk becomes less accurate beyond the short term (i.e., 24–48 hours). Furthermore, like weather forecasts, risk assessments should be updated frequently. Clinical variables associated with violence are summarized in Table 15–1.

A careful differential diagnosis should be made using the history, mental status examination, and in some cases, laboratory findings, because interventions are generally based on the diagnosis. A violent schizophrenic patient will need treatment with antipsychotic medication. A violent manic patient will probably require a combination of a mood stabilizer and an antipsychotic.

When interviewing the violent or threatening patient, the clinician should remain calm and speak softly. Comments or questions should appear nonjudgmental, such as "You seem upset; maybe you can tell me why you feel that way." The interviewer should always have an easy escape route in case the patient becomes aggressive and should avoid towering over the patient. If possible, both patient and clinician should be seated, allowing personal distance between the two. Direct eye contact should be avoided, and the interviewer should try to project a sense of empathy and concern. Family members, friends, police, and others who have pertinent information on the patient should be interviewed.

TABLE 15–1.   Clinical variables associated with violence

A history of violent acts

Inability to control anger

History of impulsive behavior (e.g., recklessness)

Paranoid ideation or frank psychosis

Lack of insight in psychotic patients

Command hallucinations in psychotic patients

The stated desire to hurt or kill another person

Presence of an acting-out personality disorder (e.g., antisocial or borderline personality disorder)

Presence of a dementia, delirium, or alcohol or drug intoxication

Managing the Violent Patient

In the hospital or clinic setting, the violent patient presents an emergency. To ensure the safety of the patient and others, it is important that staff be sufficient in number and well trained in seclusion and restraint techniques. Students and residents should remember that seclusion or restraint is considered an emergency safety measure that aims to prevent injury to the patient and others and is never used as punishment or for the convenience of the staff.

Once a decision has been made to restrain or to seclude the patient, a staff member—backed up by at least four other team members—should approach the patient after first clearing the area of other patients. The patient should be told that he or she is being secluded or restrained because of uncontrolled behavior and should be asked to walk quietly to the seclusion area with or without underarm support. If the patient does not cooperate, staff members should each take a limb in a plan agreed to beforehand. The patient is brought to the ground, with his or her head controlled to avoid biting. Restraints should be applied. If the patient is taken to the seclusion room, staff members should grasp the patient's legs at the knee and the patient's arms around the elbow with underarm support. Specific techniques will vary by institution.

Once secluded, the patient should be thoroughly searched. Belts, pins, and other potentially dangerous items should be removed, and the patient should be dressed in a hospital gown. If tranquilizing medication is needed, it can be injected (or taken orally if the patient is cooperative). With agitated patients, the best strategy is to combine a high-potency antipsychotic with a benzodiazepine (e.g., haloperidol, 2–5 mg; lorazepam, 1–2 mg). The dose of both agents can be repeated every 30 minutes until the patient has calmed down. One-on-one observation by nursing staff is generally mandatory for secluded or restrained patients.

Although rules differ from hospital to hospital, the clinician needs to carefully document the reasons for seclusion or restraint (e.g., harm to self or others, threatening gestures), the condition of the patient, any laboratory investigations being pursued (e.g., urine drug screen), medication being administered, type of restraint to be used, and the criteria for discontinuation of restraints.

Key points to remember about violent patients

1. Predicting violent behavior is difficult, even under the best of circumstances, but is often associated with the following:
   - Alcohol or other drug intoxication.
   - Cognitive disorders, such as Alzheimer's disease, delirium, or traumatic brain injury.
   - Psychotic disorders.
   - "Acting out" personality disorders (e.g., antisocial personality disorder, borderline personality disorder).

2. The patient should be approached in a slow and tactful manner.
   - The clinician should not appear threatening or provocative.
   - The clinician should use a soft voice, appear passive, and maintain interpersonal distance.
   - Allow for ready escape: never let the patient get between you and the door.

3. The clinician should ask the patient what is wrong or why he or she feels angry.
   - Most patients are willing to disclose their feelings.

4. Violent psychiatric patients need to be in the hospital, where their safety and the safety of others can be assured.

5. Orders for violence precautions and seclusion or restraint orders should be written, when applicable.
   - The risk of violence and the presence of assaultive behaviors should be carefully monitored.

> **Key points to remember about violent patients** *(continued)*
>
> - The clinician should document the assessment and plan and review them frequently.
> 6. The underlying condition should be vigorously treated.
> 7. For outpatients, the risk of violent behaviors should be monitored at each contact; the patient (or family) should remove all firearms from the home.
>   - Family members should be instructed to contact the local police (i.e., call 911) if violence erupts.

■ Suicide and Suicidal Behavior

Suicide is the eleventh most frequent cause of death for adults and the third leading cause of death for persons between ages 15 and 24. About 33,000 suicides occur each year in the United States—about one every 18 minutes. A suicide affects not only surviving friends and family members but also the victim's physician, because most people who commit suicide communicate their suicidal intentions to and see physicians before they die. For this reason, clinicians must familiarize themselves with suicide and be prepared to educate patients and family members about risk for suicide, assess risk for suicide in their patients, and intervene when appropriate to prevent a suicide.

Epidemiology

Nearly 1% of the United States general population ultimately commits suicide, a rate of nearly 12.5 suicides per 100,000 persons. Suicide rates are specific for age, gender, and race. Rates for men tend to increase steadily with age and reach a peak after age 75 years. Rates for women are curvilinear and tend to peak in the late 40s or early 50s (see Figure 15–1). Nearly three times as many men take their lives as women, and whites are more likely than blacks to kill themselves. An alarming trend has been the rise in the suicide rate among young men and women, possibly as a result of increasing rates of drug abuse or perhaps attributable to the cohort effect (discussed later in this chapter).

About two-thirds of suicide completers are men. Most tend to be older than 45, white, and separated, widowed, or divorced. Psychiatric diagnosis tends to vary with age. Suicide completers younger than 30 years are more likely to have an alcohol or drug use disorder or antisocial personality disorder; suicide completers older than 30 years are more likely to have a mood disorder.

Suicide rates differ by geographic region as well. In the United States, rates are highest in the western states and lowest in the mid-Atlantic states. In Europe, rates are highest in the former Eastern bloc countries and in Scandinavia; for example, in Hungary, the rate hovers around 40 suicides per 100,000 persons. Rates are particularly low in countries with large Catholic or Muslim populations.

Suicide rates tend to peak during the late spring and have a smaller secondary peak in the fall. Rates are affected by economic conditions and were very high during the Great Depression of the 1930s; they are typically low during times of war. Certain occupations are associated with a high risk for suicide. Professionals, especially physicians, are at high risk; in contrast to suicide statistics in general, female physicians are at higher risk for suicide than are male physicians.

Etiology and Pathophysiology

More than 90% of suicide completers had a major psychiatric illness, and more than half were clinically depressed at the time of the act. Nearly one-third of suicides occur in persons with an alcohol use disorder; schizophrenia, anxiety disorders, and other mental illnesses are less common among suicide completers. One study found drug abuse in 45% and alcoholism in 54% of the suicide completers. These findings may reflect the growing drug and alcohol abuse problem in the United States.

The risk for suicide is much higher among psychiatric patients than in the general population. Research shows that certain psychiatric disorders are associated with high rates of suicide. For example, 10%–15% of the persons hospitalized with mood disorders, 10% of the patients with schizophrenia, and 2%–4% of the patients with chronic alcoholism will commit suicide. Risk for suicide is further increased by the presence of a personality disorder, particularly in persons with a mood or substance use disorder. Thus, although psychiatric and/or medical illnesses usually are necessary for suicide to occur, their presence is not a sufficient explanation, because most mentally ill persons do not kill themselves.

About 5% of suicide completers have serious physical illnesses at the time of suicide. Suicide rates are reported to be high in persons who

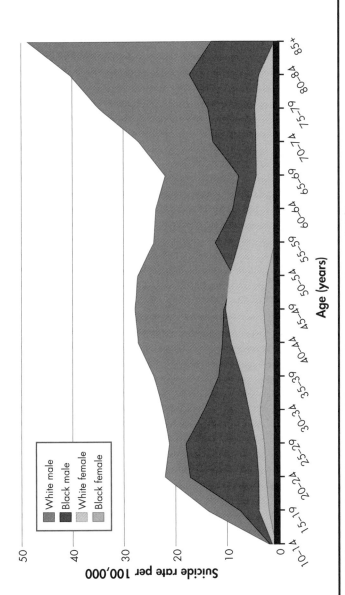

FIGURE 15–1. Suicide rates in U.S. men and women by race and age: 2004.

Suicide rates are highest among those over age 60. A growing body of research indicates that suicide is a serious health problem among older Americans—especially white males—that calls for a national response, according to suicide-prevention advocates. The graph uses data from 2004, the most recent year of available data as of this writing.

Source. National Center for Health Statistics.

have traumatic brain injuries, epilepsy, multiple sclerosis, Huntington's disease, Parkinson's disease, cancer, and AIDS. The suicide rate in patients with AIDS in the United States is nearly seven times that in the general population.

A small number of persons committing suicide appear to have no evidence of mental or physical illness. Many have argued that these suicides are rational—that is, they are based on a logical appraisal of the need for death. An example is an elderly widower with terminal cancer who is not clinically depressed but has no hope for the future and wishes to end his physical pain. Many of these apparently rational suicides are probably irrational, but information was simply unavailable to confirm the presence of a mental illness because the person who died was socially isolated and informants were not available for interview.

Suicide runs in families. Examination of large kindreds, such as the Old Order Amish in Pennsylvania, showed that suicide tends to cluster in certain pedigrees—pedigrees that are also filled with mood disorders. Twin studies have reported higher concordance for suicide among identical twins than nonidentical twins, suggesting that suicide may be genetic as well as familial. One large adoption study found a higher prevalence of suicide among biological relatives of probands who had killed themselves than among the relatives of control probands, providing further evidence of a hereditary contribution to suicide.

At a physiological level, suicide—like impulsive violence—has also been associated with low levels of CSF 5-HIAA and with other findings that suggest disturbed serotonin neurotransmission. Follow-up studies have shown that many suicide completers had abnormal dexamethasone suppression test results, suggesting the presence of hypothalamic-pituitary-adrenal axis hyperactivity. Suicide completers also have been found to have high levels of urinary metabolites of cortisol and to have enlarged adrenal glands. All of these measures are abnormal in severe depression; therefore, they may indicate depression rather than risk for suicide.

Suicide Methods

Firearms are the most common method used to commit suicide in the United States, perhaps because firearms are readily available and are immediately lethal. Firearms are followed in frequency by poisoning (i.e., a drug overdose), hanging, cutting, jumping, and other methods. Men are more likely than women to use violent methods, such as firearms or hanging, a tendency that may explain why men are more successful in killing themselves. Women tend to use less violent means, such as poisoning by overdose. Women are beginning to choose more lethal methods, a trend that may ultimately lead to higher suicide rates.

Clinical Findings

Suicide is an act of desperation. Suicidal persons frequently convey their distress to others, and nearly two-thirds communicate their suicidal intentions to others. Their communication may be as direct as reporting their plan and the date they intend to carry it out. Other communications are less obvious; for instance, the patient may say to his relatives, "You won't have to put up with me much longer!"

Suicide can occur during all phases of a depressive episode. It is commonly believed that suicide risk is highest during the recovery phase, when a patient has regained sufficient energy to carry out the suicide. Because the suicidal urge waxes and wanes during the course of a depressive episode, the clinician should not be lulled into a false sense of security based on the phase of a patient's illness.

Suicide completers tend to be socially isolated. Nearly 30% of suicide completers have a history of suicide attempts, and about one in six leaves a suicide note. Clinicians should be alert to behaviors that suggest suicidal intent: preparing a will, giving away possessions, or purchasing a burial plot. One of the strongest correlates of suicidal behavior is hopelessness, a finding independent of psychiatric diagnosis.

In one study, about 40% of suicide completers had alcohol in their bloodstream at the time of death, suggesting that alcohol may have disinhibited them sufficiently to give them the courage to carry out the act. Of alcoholic persons who kill themselves, the figure rises to about 90% with alcohol in their bloodstream at the time of death.

Patients remain at high risk for suicide after hospital discharge. Although depressed patients may appear to be significantly improved at the time of discharge, relapse can occur quickly. In a follow-up of unipolar and bipolar depressed patients, nearly 42% of 36 suicides occurred within 6 months of hospital discharge, 58% by 1 year, and 70% by 2 years. Therefore, recently discharged patients need close follow-up.

Events that appear to trigger suicide differ by age and diagnostic group. Triggering events in adolescents or young adults often include academic problems or troubled relationships with parents. In older persons, the event may be poor finances or health. More than 50% of alcoholic persons who commit suicide have a history of relationship loss (usually of an intimate relationship) within the year before suicide. This is not the case among persons with major depressive disorder.

Youth Suicide

Suicide rates have been increasing in both males and females between ages 15 and 24 years. In fact, studies have shown that recent cohorts (i.e., groups of persons in the population with similar characteristics, such as being born in the same decade) have higher suicide rates than older cohorts. Why rates are increasing in younger age groups is a mystery, but other data seem to show that the prevalence of depression also is increasing in each successive cohort. Drug abuse has become a serious problem for society, especially young persons, and may be contributing to the higher rates of suicide.

Teenagers are more prone to the effects of peer pressure than are adults, and this may be reflected in suicide clusters. It has been suggested that media portrayals of suicide, such as those in television movies or documentaries, are followed by an increased rate of both suicide attempts and suicides, often by the method depicted.

Suicide Attempters Versus Suicide Completers

Suicide attempts are intentional acts of self-injury that do not result in death. They are 5–20 times as frequent as suicides—perhaps more so, because most suicide attempts go unreported and many persons who attempt suicide do not seek medical attention. Although suicide completers usually have a diagnosis of major depression or alcoholism, suicide attempters are less likely to have these disorders and frequently have other conditions, including personality disorders.

Suicide completers carefully plan their act, use effective means (e.g., firearms, hanging), and carry out the suicide in private or make provisions to avoid discovery. They are serious about ending their lives. In contrast, suicide attempters, who are three times more likely to be women and usually younger than 35 years, act impulsively, make provisions for rescue, and use ineffective means such as drug overdoses. Suicide attempters are at risk for future attempts, and each year thereafter an estimated 1%–2% of those who have attempted suicide will complete the act—up to a total of about 10%. The differences between suicide attempters and completers are highlighted in Table 15–2.

Assessing the Suicidal Patient

The assessment of suicide risk involves obtaining a thorough psychiatric history and mental status examination as well as an understanding

TABLE 15–2. **Differences between suicide completers and attempters**

Variable	Completers	Attempters
Gender	Male	Female
Age	Older	Younger
Diagnosis	Depression, alcoholism, schizophrenia	Depression, alcoholism, personality disorder
Planning	Careful	Impulsive
Lethality	High (e.g., firearms)	Low (e.g., poisoning)
Availability of help	Low	High

of common risk factors. The clinician should be alert to the possibility of suicide in any psychiatric patient, especially a patient who is depressed or has a depressed affect. In these patients, the assessment will focus on vegetative signs and cognitive symptoms of depression, death wishes, suicidal ideation, and suicidal plans. Common risk factors associated with suicide are summarized in Table 15–3. Remembering these risk factors can be facilitated through the use of a simple mnemonic: SAD PERSONS. The initials stand for **S**ex (male gender), **A**ge (older), **D**epression, **P**revious (suicide) attempt, **E**thanol abuse, **R**ational thinking loss, **S**ocial support lacking, **O**rganized plan, **N**o spouse, **S**ickness.

Suicidal patients are generally willing to discuss their thoughts with a physician if asked, but research shows that only one in six clinicians asks his or her patients about suicide. A common myth is that asking a patient about suicide will give the patient ideas that he or she has not already had. Yet because suicidal thoughts are common in depression, most depressed patients will have had these thoughts. Patients are often fearful and even feel guilty about having suicidal thoughts. Giving the patient an opportunity to discuss them may itself provide relief. Specific questions that should be asked of the patient include the following:

• Are you having any thoughts that life isn't worth living?
• Are you having any thoughts about harming yourself?
• Are you having any thoughts about taking your life?
• Have you developed a plan for committing suicide? If so, what is your plan?

TABLE 15–3. Clinical variables associated with suicide

Being a psychiatric patient

Being male, although the gender distinction is less important among psychiatric patients than in the general population

Age: risk increases as men age but peaks in the middle years for women

Being divorced, widowed, or single

Race: whites are at higher risk than nonwhites

Diagnosis: depression, alcoholism, schizophrenia

History of suicide attempts

Expressing suicidal thoughts or developing plans for suicide

Recent interpersonal loss (especially among alcoholic patients)

Feelings of hopelessness and low self-esteem

Timing: early in the post–hospital discharge period

Adolescents: a history of drug abuse and behavior problems

The physician also should assess the patient's history of suicidal behavior by asking the following questions:

- Have you ever had thoughts of killing yourself?
- Have you ever attempted suicide? If so, would you tell me about the attempt?

The physician should approach the topic of suicide in a slow and tactful manner, after having developed rapport with the patient. Because suicidal thoughts may fluctuate, physicians should reassess suicide risk at each contact with the patient. Patients who have developed well thought-out plans and have the means to carry them out require protection, usually in a hospital on a locked psychiatric unit. When the suicidal patient refuses admission, it may be necessary to obtain a court order requiring hospitalization. Suicidal patients may plead with the doctor, family, or friends to be kept out of the hospital, but family members and friends are neither sufficiently prepared nor sufficiently educated to handle a suicidal person. Hospitalization is the best way for a physician to ensure the safety of the patient.

Managing the Suicidal Patient

In the hospital, the nursing staff will take sharp objects, belts, and other potentially lethal items from the patient. Patients at risk for elopement are carefully watched. The physician should fully document the patient's signs and symptoms of depression, along with the physician's assessment of suicide risk and protective measures taken.

Once the patient's safety has been ensured, treatment of the underlying illness can begin. Treatment will depend on the diagnosis. Antidepressant medication or electroconvulsive therapy (ECT) can be used for the treatment of depression; mood stabilizers and antipsychotics are appropriate additions to the treatment of bipolar disorder and psychotic depression, respectively. Antipsychotic medications are helpful in the suicidal schizophrenic patient. Among the antipsychotics, only clozapine has been associated with lower rates of suicide. Lithium is also reported to lower suicide risk in bipolar patients. ECT is often specifically recommended for the treatment of major depression in suicidal individuals because it tends to have a quicker onset of action than medication.

When the patient receives treatment as an outpatient, close follow-up is mandatory. Follow-up must include frequent physician visits (or telephone contacts) for assessment of mood and suicide risk and for psychotherapeutic support. The physician should consider prescribing antidepressants with a high therapeutic index that are unlikely to be fatal in overdose, such as one of the serotonin reuptake inhibitors. Family members can help monitor the patient's medication use. They should also be instructed to remove all firearms from the home.

Key points to remember about suicidal patients

1. Depressed patients should always be asked about suicidal thoughts and plans. The clinician will not plant ideas that were not there merely by asking.

    • Suicidality should be reassessed and documented at every visit with depressed patients.

2. Some suicidal patients should be hospitalized, even when it is against their will. Patients without suicidal plans can probably be managed at home provided that they have supportive families who are willing to watch them carefully.

> **Key points to remember about suicidal patients** *(continued)*
>
> 3. In the hospital, "suicide precautions" should be written in the doctors' orders; one-to-one protection should be ordered if needed.
>   - Signs and symptoms must be carefully documented.
> 4. Suicidality should be frequently monitored in outpatients. Antidepressants with a high therapeutic index are preferred, such as SSRIs or one of the newer antidepressants (e.g., bupropion, mirtazapine, duloxetine, venlafaxine).
>   - The family should be told to remove all firearms from the home.
> 5. Even though the risk factors are known, it is not possible to predict who will commit suicide.
>   - One should use good clinical judgment, provide close follow-up, and prescribe effective treatments.

■ Self-Assessment Questions

1. What are the risk factors for violent behavior? What is the pathophysiology underlying violent behavior?

2. How is the violent or potentially violent patient assessed and managed?

3. What are the indications for seclusion and restraint? How are seclusion and restraint orders implemented?

4. Why is suicide a major health problem?

5. What is a helpful mnemonic for common suicide risk factors?

6. How do completed suicides differ from attempted suicides?

7. What is a rational suicide?

8. Are there different risk factors for suicide among youth?

9. How should the suicidal patient be managed in the hospital? In an outpatient setting?

CHAPTER 16

Child Psychiatry

Children sweeten labors, but they make misfortunes more bitter. They increase the cares of life, but they mitigate the remembrance of death.

Francis Bacon

AS ANY 17-YEAR-OLD will testify, the distinction between childhood and adulthood is arbitrary and frequently fluctuates in response to the needs of the person invoking the distinction. Psychiatric classification is no exception, and many of the disorders described in other chapters occur frequently in children, such as the mood and anxiety disorders. Schizophrenia often arises during adolescence and occasionally during childhood. Furthermore, "childhood" disorders such as mental retardation or autism may be diagnosed in adults. Nevertheless, DSM-IV-TR has specified a group of disorders that are considered to be relatively specific to children and adolescents, in that these disorders typically *arise* during that period of life rather than simply *occur* during childhood and adolescence (see Table 16–1).

Childhood mental disorders are quite common. Estimates of prevalence vary depending on breadth or narrowness of definition, but it is probably a reasonable estimate that 5%–15% of children will experience a psychiatric disturbance that is sufficiently severe to require treatment or to impair their functioning during the course of a

TABLE 16–1.   DSM-IV-TR disorders usually first diagnosed in infancy, childhood, or adolescence

Mental retardation	Attention-deficit and disruptive
Mild	behavior disorders
Moderate	Attention-deficit/hyperactivity
Severe	disorder
Profound	Conduct disorder
Learning disorders	Oppositional defiant disorder
Reading	Feeding and eating disorders of
Mathematics	infancy or early childhood
Written expression	Tic disorders
Motor skills	Tourette's disorder
Communication disorders	Other disorders
Pervasive developmental	Separation anxiety disorder
disorders	

year. Unfortunately, many childhood disorders will go unrecognized and untreated.

To permit more complete coverage of the most important disorders, we selectively review only some of them in this chapter, focusing on those that are most frequently seen in child psychiatry clinics or in a family practice setting. These include mental retardation, learning disorder, autistic disorder, attention-deficit/hyperactivity disorder (ADHD), conduct disorder, oppositional defiant disorder (ODD), Tourette's disorder, and separation anxiety disorder. In addition, a brief overview is provided of those adult disorders that are commonly seen in children, including major depression, bipolar disorder, and schizophrenia.

Child psychiatry is one of the most challenging and interesting areas of specialization within psychiatry. Because the child psychiatrist must know a great deal about other childhood illnesses, maturational processes, and developmental disorders, the field is closely allied with pediatrics and requires a good knowledge of general medicine. Furthermore, the clinician working in child psychiatry has an opportunity to catch disorders at their earliest; because children are adaptable, fresh in outlook, and pleasantly unpredictable, working with them and helping them overcome their problems can be particularly rewarding.

■ Special Aspects of the Assessment of Children

There are many continuities between adult and child psychiatry, but there are also important differences in emphasis and approach. These differences include techniques of assessment, the importance of flexible norms or criteria, an involvement of family or significant others, an increased role of nonphysicians in the health care team, and the frequent occurrence of psychiatric comorbidity.

Trajectories of Development

The pace of growth and development and the effect of life events is much greater in children than in adults. For that reason, when working with children it is important to emphasize a longitudinal and developmental approach. This approach must take into account the growth and maturational processes that all children undergo, assessing them in the light of each particular child's life situation and strengths and weaknesses. Each child has a natural trajectory of development that will be completed through the process of passing from infancy to adulthood. As each child is evaluated, the clinician must ask him- or herself the following questions:

- What level of emotional and intellectual maturity does this child have?
- What are his or her particular strengths?
- How do they provide a protective and healing element?
- What particular weaknesses are present?
- What stresses are affecting the child?
- How do those stresses affect him or her at this particular stage of life?
- How do gender-specific challenges affect the expression of illness and its treatment?

For example, maternal death would have a very different effect on each child in a family of five children, the oldest of whom is a 16-year-old girl (who is likely to assume the maternal role) and the youngest of whom is 2 years old. The effect would be different for the children whose surviving father is unemployed and alcoholic than it would be for the children whose surviving father is a high-functioning blue- or white-collar worker. The effect also would be different depending on whether the eldest child is herself highly functional or has some mental illness, such as autism or conduct disorder. The effect on each child would vary depending on the availability of other social supports, such as an extended family with grandparents, a good or a weak school system, and a safe environment or one characterized by crime, violence, and drug use. All things being constant, a 2-year-old will have a very different understanding of parental loss or abandonment than will an older child, because the younger child will have had little time to build either a self-image incorporating that parent or a conceptual structure that can be used to comprehend parental loss.

Who Is the Patient?

Children rarely pick up the telephone and make an appointment to see a child psychiatrist. Usually they are brought in at someone else's request. The child may be unwilling, noncompliant, distrusting, or resentful. In this instance, the assessment is likely to be particularly challenging because the clinician must win the child's trust. Even when the child is the identified patient, the parents usually are interviewed and evaluated as well. Not infrequently, it becomes clear that the parents themselves have serious problems that can complicate the situation further. In this instance, it may be necessary to reassess and to suggest treatment of the parents in addition to (or even instead of) the child. This can be especially challenging, because such recommendations need to be made in a tactful and noncritical manner to avoid alienating the parents. Furthermore, in child psychiatry, as in few other medical specialties, the clinician is likely to feel ambivalent and confused from time to time about the appropriate role to play. The child usually will be the identified patient, even though others may be in greater need of intervention and yet do not seek or accept it.

The Assessment of Children

Childhood disorders can be diagnosed in individuals ranging from infants through people in their late teens or early 20s. Obviously, standard approaches to interviewing and assessment, described in Chapter 2, do not apply well to infants, children, or young teenagers. Standard techniques for the psychiatric assessment of adults, which may be applicable to patients in their late teens and are applicable to patients in their early 20s, require verbal and cognitive skills not yet achieved in the maturational process of children. For example, young children may not be able to respond to questions about concepts such as depression, loneliness, or anger. The interviewer often needs to talk to children at a much more concrete level, asking questions such as

- Do you feel like crying?
- What kinds of things make you feel like crying?
- Do you ever want to hit people?
- Whom do you feel like hitting?
- Who are your best friends?
- How often do you see them?
- What kinds of things do you do together?
- Do they like you?

In addition to interviewing, playing games with the child often gives the clinician some insight into the child's ability to function interpersonally, to tolerate frustration, or to focus his or her attention. Imaginative play, using dolls that can represent important figures in the child's life, also may give some sense as to his or her feelings toward and relationships with others. Taking turns in telling stories also may elicit interesting information. For example, if the clinician suspects that the child may be feeling anxious about something, he or she may tell a story about "how Jimmy is afraid of going to school because the other children make fun of him." When the child then tells his or her own story, he or she may be able to describe his or her own fears in this indirect manner. Direct observation of activity level, motor skills, verbal expression, and vocabulary is also a fundamental component of assessment. Observing the child's behavior may help compensate for the limited reliability of any symptom reporting in very young children. For that reason, it is important to interview parents to fill in historical details and to elicit their observations of their child. Schoolteachers also are in a unique position to provide additional behavioral observations about the child.

Application of Norms and Criteria

When assessing children, the clinician must have a good sense of what is normal for a given child at a given age, as well as an awareness that norms may vary widely. Younger clinicians who are completing medical school or a residency usually have not had the experience of rearing their own children or of watching a large number of younger siblings develop. Thus they must get their sense of norms from reading textbooks, from observing large numbers of children, or from recalling their own experiences in the process of growing up.

Having a sense of what is normal or abnormal for a given child, in a given family, and in a given social and intellectual environment can be extremely difficult. For example, a typical normal 10-year-old has an IQ of 100, is able to read at a fourth-grade level, is able to perform addition and subtraction and some multiplication, and is able to throw, catch, and kick a ball with at least some accuracy. Some normal children have an IQ of only 85, however, whereas some have an IQ of 160. These children will clearly differ from one another a great deal in their school performance. Boys and girls also have quite different levels of maturation both physically and mentally, and these differences are especially pronounced in younger children. Boys and girls also have different maturational tasks as they go through puberty and enter adolescence, and consequently they experience different stresses. Success and failure also mean different things to an inner-city child than to a child from an affluent background.

Involvement of Family and Significant Others

Clinicians who work with children usually need to work with their families and significant others as well. The degree of family involvement varies, of course, depending on the age of the child. In the case of very young children, the parents are likely to be the primary informants and important recipients of treatment as well because they will probably need both psychological support and assistance in learning behavioral techniques to manage their child's behavior. For grade school children, involvement of family members is essential, but the child becomes an increasingly important protagonist in both assessment and treatment. Teenagers, who are going through important maturational changes as they move into adulthood, usually are brought to the forefront of the assessment and treatment process, although the family also will provide resources much of the time.

Deciding whether to maintain complete confidentiality or to share information becomes a critical issue in the assessment of teenagers. In general, teenagers should be assured that what they tell the clinician will end there, unless the teenager gives permission to share the information or can be encouraged to bring it out in a family or group setting. The assurance of confidentiality is important in establishing a bond of trust between teenager and clinician, because the patient otherwise is likely to see the therapist as a potentially antagonistic authority figure.

Only in situations dangerous to the child, such as a clear risk of suicide, should the rule of confidentiality be broken. This rule should be explained to the parents in a tactful manner so that they do not feel excluded. Depending on circumstances, the clinician also may choose to see the parents independently. Alternatively, he or she may refer the parents to another psychiatrist, psychologist, or social worker with whom he or she has a good working relationship.

Involvement of Nonphysicians in the Health Care Team

Because of the diversity of the domains involved, many clinicians working in the area of child psychiatry like to operate within the context of a health care team. This team may be relatively small, involving a psychologist or social worker in addition to the psychiatrist. In larger settings, however, it includes a psychiatrist (who works primarily with the child in psychotherapy and the prescription of medication), a social worker (who works primarily with the family), an educational specialist (who assesses the child's educational achievement and assists in designing a nonfrustrating remedial program as needed), and a psychologist (who develops programs for behavioral management, may do psychotherapy as needed, and may work with child, family, and school system as needed).

Psychological and Educational Testing in Child Psychiatry

Psychological and educational testing often play a central role in the evaluation of children. Several tests that are commonly used in child psychiatry are listed in Table 16–2.

General Intelligence

General intelligence may be assessed with the Stanford-Binet Intelligence Scale, the fourth edition of the Wechsler Intelligence Scale for Children (WISC-IV), and other well-validated instruments. The Stanford-Binet Intelligence Scale was one of the earliest IQ tests to be developed, and it is still appropriate for relatively young children because its

TABLE 16-2. Cognitive, psychological, and educational tests used in child psychiatry

Factor	Test
Intelligence	Stanford-Binet Intelligence Scale, Wechsler Intelligence Scale for Children (WISC-IV), Peabody Picture Vocabulary Test, Kaufman ABC, Wechsler Preschool and Primary Scale of Intelligence (WPPSI)
Educational achievement	Iowa Test of Basic Skills (ITBS), Iowa Test of Educational Development (ITED), Wide Range Achievement Test—Revised (WRAT-R)
Adaptive behavior	Vineland Adaptive Behavior Scales, Conners' Teacher Rating Scale—Revised
Perceptual-motor abilities	Draw-a-Person Test, Bender-Gestalt, Benton Visual Retention Test, Purdue Pegboard Test, Beery Developmental Test of Visual-Motor Integration
Personality	Thematic Apperception Test, Rorschach Test

bottom threshold is lower and does not require extensive acquisition of knowledge. The Kaufman ABC and the Wechsler Preschool and Primary Scale of Intelligence are appropriate for assessing young children.

The WISC-IV is the standard test for assessing the intelligence of school-age children between the ages of 6 and 16 years. (The Wechsler Adult Intelligence Scale—IV [WAIS-IV] is used for children older than 16 years.) The WISC-IV consists of a group of ten core subtests that assess a variety of cognitive functions (e.g., vocabulary, comprehension, block design, matrix reasoning, digit span, symbol search). These are used to generate a full-scale IQ, verbal and performance IQs, and four composite scores known as indices (verbal comprehension, perceptual organization, processing speed, and working memory).

Examining the scores on individual WISC-IV subtests gives clinicians a sense of the child's overall intellectual skills and weaknesses. The test is scaled to have a mean of 100 and a standard deviation of 15. Sixty-seven percent of children have IQs that fall between 85 and 115, whereas 95% have IQs that fall between 70 and 130. Children from middle-class and culturally advantaged backgrounds tend to perform better on these tests. In such instances, the performance scales of the test may give a somewhat better indication of the child's "culture-free intelligence," although this clearly will not be helpful for those children who have performance deficits for some reason (e.g., visual-motor and/or perception difficulties). Interpretation of the WISC-IV must be made within the context of each child's social background and educational opportunities.

Other briefer and simpler tests are also sometimes used to obtain an approximate estimate of intelligence. For example, the Peabody Picture Vocabulary Test is sometimes used to give a global measure of intelligence. The test uses pictures to provide a measure of oral language comprehension, from which verbal intelligence can be inferred. In general, IQ based on the Peabody or other similar tests tends to be an overestimate.

Educational Achievement

Standardized educational achievement tests are often used in the public school systems. The implementation of the No Child Left Behind Act has increased the use of such tests, because it requires that schools receiving federal funding use the theories of standards-based education and give standard tests of basic skills to all students. Two widely used tests are the Iowa Test of Basic Skills (ITBS) and the Iowa Test of Educational Development (ITED); these are representative of the type of standardized tests now used throughout most of the United States. The former is typically used for younger children, whereas versions of the latter are available for assessment of patients up to completion of high school. For the ITBS and the ITED, national, state, and school-specific norms are available, so that the child's achievement can be assessed within his or her specific environmental context. Achievement tests provide scores for specific areas such as reading, language arts, study skills, arithmetic, and social studies. Evaluating the pattern of achievement can provide some index as to whether the child has a learning disorder.

Adaptive Behavior

Various standard questionnaires can be used to assess adaptive behavior. The Vineland Adaptive Behavior Scales were originally developed to evaluate children with mental retardation but are also used to provide a standardized measure of adaptive skills for children with a broader range of problems, including those with normal intelligence. The Conners' Teacher Rating Scale—Revised was developed to assess the child's behavior in the classroom. It is a pencil-and-paper test specifically targeted to assess behavior associated with ADHD, such as impulsivity, physical activity, or impaired attention. It also has subscales to assess social withdrawal and aggressive behavior. A complementary rating scale to be completed by parents is also available.

Perceptual-Motor Skills

Various standardized tests are used to assess perceptual-motor skills. In the assessment of young children, the Draw-a-Person Test is one of the most popular. The complexity and detail of the person drawn give a crude indication of the child's maturity, whereas the drawing skills shown allow assessment of the child's ability to translate his or her thoughts into a visual representation. The Bender-Gestalt and Benton Visual Retention Test assess the ability to copy a design and to recall it later, which are also fundamental aspects of perceptual-motor skills. The Purdue Pegboard Test is a somewhat pure test of manual dexterity, assessing the child's ability to place pegs in appropriate slots. The Beery Developmental Test of Visual-Motor Integration is popular with school systems.

Personality Style and Social Adjustment

Personality style and social adjustment are typically evaluated in children through projective tests. The Thematic Apperception Test uses a series of cards depicting obscure figures in ambiguous situations; the child is asked to describe what is happening and tell a story about it. The Rorschach Test is the famous inkblot test. In this test, the child is shown cards containing inkblots that have ambiguous and suggestive shapes. The child is asked to identify and label what he or she sees (e.g., two men dancing) and to indicate the basis for his or her perception. Although semistandardized scores can be applied, one of the most common applications of these tests is to provide a standardized structured stimulus to the child, using his or her response as an indication of interpersonal experiences, anxieties, fears, and drives.

Physical Examination

A careful physical examination is an important part of the child's evaluation. In addition to the standard physical examination, the clinician should carefully inspect the child for indications of congenital anomalies, such as a high-arched palate, low-set ears, single palmar creases, unusual carrying angle, webbing, abnormalities of the genitalia, and neuroectodermal anomalies. Congenital anomalies tend to occur together, and midline or neuroectodermal anomalies are more likely to be associated with central nervous system anomalies. The observation of such anomalies is an indication for magnetic resonance imaging (MRI) to assess for the presence of structural brain abnormalities, particularly in the midline.

The clinician should be attentive to assessment of neurological soft signs in children as well. A standardized repertoire should be developed for assessing graphesthesia, left-right discrimination, motor coordination, and simple perceptual-motor skills that can be evaluated at the bedside. For example, left-right discrimination can be examined systematically through a graded series of questions such as the following: "Hold up your right hand. Hold up your left foot. Put your right forefinger on your nose. Use your left forefinger to point to your right foot. Point to my right hand. Use your left forefinger to point to my left hand." Tongue twisters such as "Methodist-Episcopal" or "Luke Luck likes lakes" may be used to assess oral-motor coordination, whereas hopping, walking in tandem, and rapid alternating movements are used to evaluate other motor skills. Fine motor skills are evaluated through drawing and writing. After the clinician has assessed many children across a wide range of ages, he or she will gradually develop a sense of what constitutes normal performance on such tests of neurological soft signs for a given child at a given age. Extensive neurological soft signs may serve as an indicator for ordering a more comprehensive laboratory workup including electroencephalography (EEG) or brain scanning.

■ Mental Retardation

Mental retardation is characterized by subnormal intelligence, as measured by IQ, accompanied by deficits in adaptive functioning. IQ is defined as mental age (as assessed by a standard test such as the WISC-IV) divided by chronological age and multiplied by 100. Thus, a child with an IQ of 50 might have a mental age of 5 years and a chronological age of 10 years; in other words, he or she would be performing with the intellectual skills of a 5-year-old. The specific IQ cutoff point used to define mental retardation is 70. IQs between 70 and 85 are considered to indicate *borderline intellectual functioning*. The criteria for diagnosing mental retardation also require that the individual have problems in coping with social and economic demands or abnormalities in interpersonal adjustment.

The DSM-IV-TR criteria for mental retardation require an onset before age 18 years. In general, mental retardation is typically observed and diagnosed long before age 18 and usually is considered to be present from very early in life. For example, a 13-year-old who sustains a head injury in a car accident and subsequently has a marked decrement in IQ is considered to have a dementia induced by trauma rather than mental retardation. In DSM-IV-TR, mental retardation is coded on Axis II.

Mental retardation is divided into four broad categories: mild, moderate, severe, and profound. Children with *mild mental retardation* have IQs from about 50–55 to 69. They represent the majority of cases of mental retardation, constituting approximately 85% of the individuals with IQs below 70. Children with IQs in this range are considered educable, and they usually are able to attend special classes and to work toward the long-term goal of being able to function in the community and to hold some type of job. They usually can learn to read, write, and perform simple arithmetical calculations. Children with *moderate mental retardation* have IQs ranging from about 35–40 to 50–55 and constitute approximately 10% of the mentally retarded population. They are considered trainable, in that they can learn to talk, to recognize their name and other simple words, to perform activities of self-care such as bathing or doing their laundry, and to handle small change. They require management and treatment in special education classes. The ideal long-term goal for these individuals is care in a sheltered environment, such as a group home. Severely and profoundly mentally retarded children constitute the smallest groups. *Severe mental retardation* is defined as an IQ from about 20–25 to 35–40, and *profound mental retardation* is defined as an IQ below 20–25. Individuals with IQs in this range almost invariably require care in institutionalized settings, usually beginning relatively early in life.

Epidemiology, Clinical Findings, and Course

Mental retardation is very common, affecting 1%–2% of the general population. Mental retardation is more common in males, with a male-to-female ratio of approximately 2:1. Mild mental retardation is more common in the lower social classes, but moderate, severe, and profound mental retardation are equally common among all social classes.

The long-term outcome of mental retardation is variable. Some severe and profound forms may be characterized by progressive physical deterioration and ultimately premature death, as early as the teens or early 20s (e.g., Tay-Sachs disease). Individuals with mild and moderate forms of mental retardation have a somewhat reduced life expectancy, but active intervention may enhance their quality of life. Like all children, children with mental retardation may show maturational spurts that could not be predicted at an earlier age. Typically, mentally retarded children progress through normal milestones, such as sitting, standing, talking, and learning numbers and letters, in a pattern similar to that of nonretarded children but at a slower rate. The educable and trainable mentally retarded children are able to learn to read, write, and calculate at some level, as long as appropriately structured educational settings are provided.

Etiology and Pathophysiology

Mental retardation is a syndrome that represents a final common pathway produced by a variety of factors that injure the brain and affect its normal development. Individuals with IQs below 55 often have an identifiable cause for their mental retardation, whereas those individuals with IQs above 55 often do not and probably develop their mental retardation through some complex multifactorial and polygenetic combination. Down syndrome is the most common *chromosomal* cause of mental retardation. Fragile X syndrome is the most common heritable form of mental retardation and is second only to Down syndrome in frequency. The fragile X gene has been discovered; it contains an unstable segment that expands as it is passed through generations and affects children differently depending on whether it is passed through fathers or mothers (imprinting). Inborn errors of metabolism account for a small percentage of cases; examples include Tay-Sachs disease and untreated phenylketonuria.

In addition to these clearly defined genetic causes, a substantial proportion of cases of mental retardation probably also reflect polygenic inheritance, possibly interacting with nongenetic factors such as nutrition and psychosocial nurturance. Many prenatal factors also may affect fetal development and lead to neurodevelopmental anomalies. The high rate of Down syndrome (trisomy 21) in children born to older mothers is a prime example. Other prenatal factors that may affect fetal development include maternal malnutrition or substance abuse; exposure to mutagens such as radiation; maternal illnesses such as diabetes, toxemia, or rubella; and maternal abuse and neglect. Fetal alcohol syndrome is a common nongenetic cause of mental retardation. Perinatal and early postnatal factors also may contribute. Examples include traumatic deliveries that cause brain injury, malnutrition, exposure to toxins, infections such as encephalitis, and head injuries occurring during infancy or early childhood. Psychosocial factors obviously contribute to some of these biological factors, and some psychosocial factors also may contribute independently. For example, poor prenatal and perinatal care are more likely to occur in children born in impoverished environments.

Differential Diagnosis

As in other childhood disorders, the differential diagnosis of mental retardation (particularly mild mental retardation) can be complex because of the frequent comorbidity of childhood disorders. The differential diagnosis includes ADHD, learning disorders, autism, and childhood psychoses or mood disorders, but all of these conditions can occur with mental retardation. Seizure disorders also are very common in children with mental retardation. Children in whom mental retardation is suspected should be thoroughly evaluated with a careful physical and neurological examination, EEG, and MRI, as well as IQ testing.

Clinical Management

Following a thorough evaluation, a comprehensive program should be developed to determine the best situation in which to place and treat the child, taking the needs and abilities of both the child and the parents into account. Decisions may range from care in the home (supplemented by family support and special education), to placement in a foster or group home, to long-term institutionalization. Because most mentally retarded children are mildly retarded, the majority will remain at home, at least initially. Because the parents of some of these children themselves have mental retardation, ongoing evaluation through social service agencies may be helpful and even necessary to ensure that the child's needs are being adequately met.

Whatever their own intellectual resources, the parents of mentally retarded children are confronted with a host of burdens and stresses and will benefit from both supportive counseling and training in behavioral techniques to help manage their child's behavior problems. Comorbid conditions such as seizures require medical management. Intellectual evaluation will help to determine the appropriate educational placement for the child, but this should be subjected to periodic review. It is not clear whether mildly mentally retarded children benefit more from placement in regular school programs (mainstreaming) or from placement in special settings where education is tailored to their specific needs. To a large extent, however, mainstreaming is currently the dominant trend.

■ Learning Disorders

The learning disorders are characterized by an inability to achieve in a specific area of learning (reading, writing, or arithmetic) at a level consistent with the person's overall IQ. Typically, individuals with these disorders have normal intelligence (although it may be borderline or high) but have a specific inability to learn at least one of these academic skills and sometimes several.

The DSM-IV-TR definitions for *reading disorder, mathematics disorder,* and *disorder of written expression* are similar. In each case, the diagnosis is made on the basis of educational testing that indicates that the individual is performing markedly below a level expected on the basis of the person's IQ. For example, a 14-year-old with reading disorder (developmental dyslexia) may have an IQ of 110 and be reading at a third-grade level.

These disorders are relatively common. A specific disability in reading affects 2%–8% of school-age children. The rates for writing and mathematics disabilities are unknown, but they are probably high as well. These disorders are from two to four times more common in boys than in girls.

Specific learning disabilities tend to be familial, but not uniformly or consistently so. They are assumed to represent a neurodevelopmental defect or cerebral injury affecting the particular brain region involved in developing the academic skill. For example, in the case of some developmental reading or writing disorders, the language regions in the brain (i.e., Broca's area, Wernicke's area) are thought to be affected.

If not diagnosed and treated early and aggressively, learning disorders are extremely handicapping. Although children with these disorders typically have normal intelligence, they often come to view themselves as failures and feel rejected by their peers because of their inability to progress academically in a particular area.

The frustration associated with an impairment in academic skills is also associated with a variety of complications, such as truancy, school refusal, conduct disorder, mood disorder, or substance abuse. Rather than being causal, learning disorders may be comorbid with these conditions, as well as with ADHD. In this instance, it is important for the clinician to recognize the multiple disorders and to treat both (or all) of them appropriately.

Educational intervention proceeds on two fronts. Children or teenagers usually need remedial instruction to shore up skill deficits, as well as instruction in developing "attack" skills that will assist them in learning strategies to compensate for the neural deficits that underlie their condition. With steady, sympathetic educational support, most children with these specific learning disabilities are able to develop acceptable skills in reading, writing, and arithmetic.

■ Autistic Disorder and Related Conditions

Autistic disorder is the most important among the *pervasive developmental disorders* (PDDs). The characteristic features of autism include impaired social interactions, impaired ability to communicate, and a restricted repertoire of activities and interests.

Individuals with autism are usually noted to be developing abnormally relatively soon after birth. Within the first 3–6 months of these children's lives, their parents may note that they do not develop a normal pattern of smiling or responding to cuddling. The first clear sign of abnormality is usually in the area of language. As they grow older, they do not progress through developmental milestones such as learning to say words and speak sentences. They seem aloof, withdrawn, and detached. Instead of developing patterns of relating warmly to their parents, they may instead engage in self-stimulating behavior, such as rocking or head banging. By age 2 or 3 years, it is usually clear that there is something severely wrong, and the features of the disorder continue to become more obvious over time as the child fails to develop normal verbal and interpersonal communication. Children with this disorder are referred to as *autistic* because they appear to be withdrawn and self- (*auto-*) absorbed. Most of the defining features of autistic disorder reflect this autistic pattern of thinking, speaking, feeling, and behaving.

The DSM-IV-TR criteria for autistic disorder appear in Table 16–3. The criteria require that at least 6 of 12 items be present. The items cover the three major domains involved in autism (i.e., social interaction, communication, and behavioral repertoire).

Impaired social interaction is a hallmark of the disorder. Autistic children appear to lack the ability to bond with their parents or with others. In severe cases, these children seem totally withdrawn. In milder cases, they have some interaction but lack warmth, sensitivity, and awareness. Interactions, when they occur, tend to have a detached and mechanical quality to them. Displays of love and affection do not occur, and autistic children (or autistic adults) do not appear to respond to such displays from others.

TABLE 16–3. DSM-IV-TR diagnostic criteria for autistic disorder

A. A total of six (or more) items from (1), (2), and (3), with at least two from (1), and one each from (2) and (3):

    (1) qualitative impairment in social interaction, as manifested by at least two of the following:

        (a) marked impairment in the use of multiple nonverbal behaviors such as eye-to-eye gaze, facial expression, body postures, and gestures to regulate social interaction

        (b) failure to develop peer relationships appropriate to developmental level

        (c) a lack of spontaneous seeking to share enjoyment, interests, or achievements with other people (e.g., by a lack of showing, bringing, or pointing out objects of interest)

        (d) lack of social or emotional reciprocity

    (2) qualitative impairments in communication as manifested by at least one of the following:

        (a) delay in, or total lack of, the development of spoken language (not accompanied by an attempt to compensate through alternative modes of communication such as gesture or mime)

        (b) in individuals with adequate speech, marked impairment in the ability to initiate or sustain a conversation with others

        (c) stereotyped and repetitive use of language or idiosyncratic language

        (d) lack of varied, spontaneous make-believe play or social imitative play appropriate to developmental level

    (3) restricted repetitive and stereotyped patterns of behavior, interests, and activities, as manifested by at least one of the following:

        (a) encompassing preoccupation with one or more stereotyped and restricted patterns of interest that is abnormal either in intensity or focus

        (b) apparently inflexible adherence to specific, nonfunctional routines or rituals

        (c) stereotyped and repetitive motor mannerisms (e.g., hand or finger flapping or twisting, or complex whole-body movements)

        (d) persistent preoccupation with parts of objects

B. Delays or abnormal functioning in at least one of the following areas, with onset prior to age 3 years: (1) social interaction, (2) language as used in social communication, or (3) symbolic or imaginative play.

C. The disturbance is not better accounted for by Rett's Disorder or Childhood Disintegrative Disorder.

The failure to develop spoken language is usually the first thing that leads parents to realize the gravity of the problem and eventually to seek medical attention. The verbal impairments range from the complete absence of verbal speech to mildly deviant speech and language patterns. Even in patients who develop good facility in verbal expression, the speech has an empty, repetitive quality to it, and intonations may be singsong and monotonous. Autistic children and adults seem to lack the capacity to engage in conversation with others, sometimes talking spontaneously without an audience and at other times replying irrelevantly or inappropriately.

Finally, the behavioral repertoire is impaired. There is an intense and rigid commitment to maintaining specific routines, and autistic children tend to become quite distressed if routines are interrupted. They may have to sit in a particular chair, dress in a particular way, or eat particular foods.

Most autistic individuals (70%) show some evidence of mental retardation, but others have normal intelligence, and some have very specific talents or abilities, particularly in the areas of music and mathematics. IQ testing tends to show considerable scatter, and patients with autism tend to perform better on performance scales than on verbal scales.

Children who present with symptoms suggestive of autism should receive comprehensive psychiatric and physical examinations, with an emphasis on neurological components. Children should be screened for other disorders that might explain their symptoms, such as phenylketonuria or Down syndrome. Because these children present with profound social withdrawal, hearing and vision should be checked to rule out sensory defects as a cause. Many children with autism have a comorbid seizure disorder (25%) or eventually develop one. For that reason, an EEG should also be obtained. IQ testing will help assess the child's intellectual strengths and weaknesses.

Epidemiology, Clinical Findings, and Course

Autism has a prevalence of about 10–15 cases per 10,000 individuals. There is some evidence that the prevalence of autism and other forms of pervasive developmental disorders has increased over the past two decades. This is thought to be related primarily to better recognition. Other causes have been advanced, such as environmental toxins or vaccines, but there is no empirical evidence to support these claims. Autism is more common in boys than in girls, with a ratio of 3:1 or 4:1. The onset of autism occurs in early childhood, and problems are typically noted during the first or second year of life.

Autism is chronic and lifelong. Some children show some improvement as they mature, although others may worsen. Very few individuals with autism (2%–3%) are able to progress normally through school or to live independently. Follow-up studies show that most autistic persons have some improvement in social interaction over time, but even the most functional never achieve complete normality. Nearly all of the defining features of the disorder, including social aloofness, language abnormalities, and rigid and ritualistic behavior, tend to persist into adulthood. Good prognostic features include higher IQ and better language and social skills.

Etiology and Pathophysiology

Autism is a neurodevelopmental disorder that manifests shortly after birth. Twin studies have shown that genetic factors play a major role, with heritability explaining about 90% of the risk. Family studies also support a genetic role. The siblings of autistic children have an increased rate of both autistic disorder (2% vs. the population rate of 0.1%) and mental retardation and speech and language disorders. The illness does not appear to follow any classic Mendelian patterns of transmission, however, and multiple different loci and candidate genes have been identified. Recent work also suggests that some cases of autism may be a consequence of copy number variants—spontaneous mutations occurring during meiosis that are not inherited.

Imaging studies have been used in an attempt to identify the nature of the neurodevelopmental abnormality. In autism, unlike in most mental illnesses, children have been found to have large brain size relative to body size, with some evidence for gyral malformation (polymicrogyria). The large cerebral size has been interpreted as reflecting a failure to achieve normal pruning, the process by which neurons are systematically eliminated or "pruned" back. Abnormalities in the cerebellum (particularly the vermis), the temporal lobes, and the hippocampal complex, as well as cerebral asymmetries, also have been reported. Functional imaging studies suggest the presence of an overall impairment in connectivity in brain networks used for attention, consciousness, and self-awareness. Neuropathological studies have reported small, densely packed (and presumably immature) cells in limbic structures in the cerebellum. Physically, autistic children have a variety of soft neurological signs and primitive reflexes, an excess of nonright-handedness, and an apparent failure to achieve normal cerebral dominance of language functions in the left hemisphere. All of these observations are consistent with a pathophysiology that affects multiple brain regions and a failure to achieve normal cerebral asymmetry.

Differential Diagnosis

The major differential diagnoses include childhood psychosis, mental retardation, and congenital deafness, blindness, or language disorders. The most important distinctions are between autism and mental retardation or language disorders such as selective mutism and expressive language disorder. These distinctions can be quite difficult, and the differential turns largely on the quality of the social interactions (in the context of the individual's particular intellectual abilities). Mentally retarded children also typically have pervasive intellectual impairments, whereas autistic children tend to have a much more uneven profile of functional intellectual abilities on the WISC-IV and may be normal to superior in some areas. The major distinction between autism and childhood-onset schizophrenia is the presence or absence of overt psychotic symptoms (delusions and hallucinations), which typically do not occur in autism but are difficult to assess in the noncommunicative child.

Clinical Management

Once the diagnosis is made, the disorder should be described and explained to the parents, making it clear that their child has a neurodevelopmental disease and not a psychological disturbance that they caused through poor parenting. Guidelines for behavioral management should be provided, so that the parents can help reduce the rigid and stereotyped behaviors and improve language and social skills. Children with autism usually require special education or specialized day care programs that also emphasize improvement in social and language skills. Medications are often used as adjuncts to these supportive and behavioral approaches. Children who have seizures require anticonvulsants. Among other medications, both conventional antipsychotics (e.g., haloperidol) and second-generation antipsychotics have been found to decrease aggressive and stereotypical patterns of behavior. The second-generation antipsychotics risperidone and aripiprazole have received U.S. Food and Drug Administration (FDA) approval for the treatment of irritability in children and adolescents with autism. Other medications that have been found to be helpful in some cases include clomipramine, naltrexone, fluoxetine, and carbamazepine.

Autism Spectrum Disorders

Since the early 1990s, the concept of autism has been expanded to include milder conditions now known as autism spectrum disorders (ASDs). These include Asperger's disorder, Rett's disorder, child disintegrative disorder, and a residual category (pervasive developmental disorder not otherwise specified). These conditions are now grouped under the general heading of ASDs in research and clinical studies, particularly those examining genetic etiologies. Taken together, ASDs are considered to affect as many as 1 in 110 to 150 children.

Asperger's disorder is closely related to autism and is considered by some to be simply a milder version of autistic disorder. (It is also referred to as *high-functioning autism.*) Children with Asperger's disorder have a similar early onset of impairment in social interaction and abnormal behavior such as stereotypies and rituals, but they have normal language functions and usually have normal intelligence as well.

Asperger's disorder is relatively new, in that its first description in a standardized nomenclature occurred in DSM-IV in 1994. Although the disorder was initially considered rare, it now appears that it is more common than was previously thought. ASDs are now diagnosed approximately 3–4 times more often than autism. Whether ASDs represent a different disorder or a milder version of autistic disorder remains a matter of debate.

Little is known about the epidemiology, etiology, or pathophysiology of Asperger's disorder. Children with the disorder perform better in school and have a better long-term outcome than do children with autistic disorder. Some complete college and graduate school and have normal careers.

Management strategies for Asperger's disorder are similar to those for autistic disorder, but higher expectations can be set.

Less is known about the other ASDs. *Rett's disorder* involves normal development through the first 5 months, followed by an arrest of developmental functions with deceleration of head growth: loss of previously acquired purposeful hand skills, loss of social engagement, incoordination, and impaired language development. This condition occurs almost exclusively in girls and has been proposed to be caused by an X-linked dominant mutation that is lethal in hemizygous males. *Child disintegrative disorder* involves the loss of adaptive, communicative, and social functioning skills following apparently normal development for the first 2 years after birth. The syndrome is similar to autistic disorder but is more likely to be accompanied by moderate to profound mental retardation. Finally, the category *pervasive developmental disorder not otherwise specified* is used for those children who do not meet the criteria for a more specific disorder (e.g., a child with some but not all features of autistic disorder).

■ Attention-Deficit/Hyperactivity Disorder and Other Disruptive Behavior Disorders

The attention-deficit and disruptive behavior disorders are the staples of child psychiatry. Children with these disorders are experienced as difficult to manage and therefore disruptive by those around them, including parents, teachers, and often peers. Sometimes this group of disorders is referred to as involving *acting-out behavior,* meaning that the child expresses his or her problems outwardly rather than holding them within. For that reason, they are also referred to as *externalizing disorders,* in contrast with the internalizing disorders, such as the anxiety disorders, in which the child is considered to turn his or her suffering inward. Although closer contact with many of the children who manifest disruptive behavior makes it clear that they too may suffer a great deal internally and also may experience considerable anxiety, this aspect of the disorder is not immediately obvious to those who must deal with these children on a day-to-day basis.

Attention-Deficit/Hyperactivity Disorder

Children with ADHD are a caricature of the active child. They are physically overactive, distractible, inattentive, impulsive, and difficult to manage. They may have soft neurological signs and indices of slight delay in reaching developmental milestones. ADHD is typically evident early in childhood, with signs of increased activity being noted very early (e.g., "As soon as he could crawl, he got into everything"; "He never seemed to sleep and kicked constantly, even before he was born"). Although the disorder improves with maturation, in some individuals it may persist into adulthood.

ADHD is defined by two broad groups of symptoms: 1) difficulty focusing and maintaining attention and 2) hyperactivity and impulsivity. The DSM-IV-TR criteria for ADHD are shown in Table 16–4. They require that at least 12 of 18 symptoms (6 from the domain of attention and 6 from the domain of hyperactivity-impulsivity) be present for at least 6 months, with onset before age 7. Subtypes can be specified to indicate whether the presentation is predominantly inattentive, predominantly hyperactive-impulsive, or mixed. Because DSM-IV-TR requires that impairment occur in at least two settings, obtaining a school-teacher's input can be important in preventing the overdiagnosis of ADHD.

The actual manifestation of these symptoms will vary depending on the age of the child. Younger children (in the 4- to 6-year age range) are "little terrors." They run from one part of the room to another, hop on furniture, knock objects off tables, explore the contents of visitors' handbags, talk incessantly, run outside without telling their parents where they are going, have difficulty learning to look both ways before crossing the street, lose and break toys, stay up late, wake up early, and generally exhaust their parents. When these children enter school and begin the task of learning, the difficulties in focusing attention become more obvious. They may miss things that the teacher says, be unable to finish assignments, forget their pencils or notebooks, and answer the teacher's questions without holding up a hand and often without even waiting to have the question completed. They may annoy their school-mates by pushing ahead in line, grabbing equipment on the playground, or violating the rules of games without seeming to be aware of them. These children may begin to fall behind their peers in school and to develop a poor concept of themselves. Teachers may complain about their behavior to their parents and request that help be sought.

The following is a relatively typical case history of a patient with ADHD treated in one of our clinics:

> Charlie, a 6-year-old boy, was brought in by his mother after a recent school conference in which it was pointed out that he seemed to be having difficulty in adjusting to first grade.
>
> Charlie's mother described that he had always been a somewhat difficult child. Even as an infant, he was irritable and overactive. He learned to crawl at 7 months and was soon exploring the entire house, leaving a wake of emptied wastepaper baskets and disrupted cupboards behind him. He did not seem to be able to remember or follow through with parental instructions that he should keep his feet off the furniture, not walk on the tops of tables, and not run through the living room carrying melting chocolate popsicles. As he learned to talk, he seemed to talk incessantly and to be continuously in need of attention from his parents.
>
> He began to attend preschool at age 4 years. His teachers at that time complained that he was disruptive and impulsive, seeming to have little consideration for the other children in the school. Charlie's teacher

TABLE 16–4. DSM-IV-TR diagnostic criteria for attention-deficit/ hyperactivity disorder

A. Either (1) or (2):
    (1) six (or more) of the following symptoms of **inattention** have persisted for at least 6 months to a degree that is maladaptive and inconsistent with developmental level:

    Inattention
      (a) often fails to give close attention to details or makes careless mistakes in schoolwork, work, or other activities
      (b) often has difficulty sustaining attention in tasks or play activities
      (c) often does not seem to listen when spoken to directly
      (d) often does not follow through on instructions and fails to finish schoolwork, chores, or duties in the workplace (not due to oppositional behavior or failure to understand instructions)
      (e) often has difficulty organizing tasks and activities
      (f) often avoids, dislikes, or is reluctant to engage in tasks that require sustained mental effort (such as schoolwork or homework)
      (g) often loses things necessary for tasks or activities (e.g., toys, school assignments, pencils, books, or tools)
      (h) is often easily distracted by extraneous stimuli
      (i) is often forgetful in daily activities
    (2) six (or more) of the following symptoms of **hyperactivity-impulsivity** have persisted for at least 6 months to a degree that is maladaptive and inconsistent with developmental level:

    Hyperactivity
      (a) often fidgets with hands or feet or squirms in seat
      (b) often leaves seat in classroom or in other situations in which remaining seated is expected
      (c) often runs about or climbs excessively in situations in which it is inappropriate (in adolescents or adults, may be limited to subjective feelings of restlessness)
      (d) often has difficulty playing or engaging in leisure activities quietly
      (e) is often "on the go" or often acts as if "driven by a motor"
      (f) often talks excessively

TABLE 16–4. DSM-IV-TR diagnostic criteria for attention-deficit/ hyperactivity disorder *(continued)*

Impulsivity
(g) often blurts out answers before questions have been completed
(h) often has difficulty awaiting turn
(i) often interrupts or intrudes on others (e.g., butts into conversations or games)

B. Some hyperactive-impulsive or inattentive symptoms that caused impairment were present before age 7 years.
C. Some impairment from the symptoms is present in two or more settings (e.g., at school [or work] and at home).
D. There must be clear evidence of clinically significant impairment in social, academic, or occupational functioning.
E. The symptoms do not occur exclusively during the course of a Pervasive Developmental Disorder, Schizophrenia, or other Psychotic Disorder and are not better accounted for by another mental disorder (e.g., Mood Disorder, Anxiety Disorder, Dissociative Disorder, or a Personality Disorder).

Code based on type:
Attention-Deficit/Hyperactivity Disorder, Combined Type: if both Criteria A1 and A2 are met for the past 6 months
Attention-Deficit/Hyperactivity Disorder, Predominantly Inattentive Type: if Criterion A1 is met but Criterion A2 is not met for the past 6 months
Attention-Deficit/Hyperactivity Disorder, Predominantly Hyperactive-Impulsive Type: if Criterion A2 is met but Criterion A1 is not met for the past 6 months
Coding note: For individuals (especially adolescents and adults) who currently have symptoms that no longer meet full criteria, "In Partial Remission" should be specified.

complained that it was difficult to even get through a routine class day because of Charlie's behavior. He would not sit in his seat like the other children and would often get up and run around the room. He could not work on an assignment for more than 5 minutes without being distracted. He would also distract his classmates by talking to them when they were supposed to be working quietly. None of the teacher's efforts seemed to be effective in quieting or calming Charlie.

On initial evaluation, Charlie was noted to be quite active. He entered the doctor's office with a firm, aggressive step. He jumped on his chair rather than sitting down, finally squirming himself into a sitting position, which he maintained for only 2 or 3 minutes. He then jumped up and began pulling books off the bookshelves. When told that they belonged to the doctor and should be placed back on the shelf, he threw one or two on the floor and proceeded to the doctor's desk to examine the pens, pencils, and paperweights. Charlie's mother looked embarrassed and exasperated and tried to get him to sit back down.

The psychiatrist decided to prescribe methylphenidate. Within 1 week, Charlie's mother related that the effects were "amazing." Almost immediately, Charlie's behavior improved, and he showed a distinct increase in his ability to focus attention and a decrease in impulsive, overactive behavior. His teacher also noticed a distinct difference. He was able to complete the first grade with only minimal difficulty and was considered to have appropriate progress for his age in basic skills of learning to read and to do very simple arithmetic.

Although ADHD was originally defined as a childhood disorder, increasing numbers of adults also have been given diagnoses of ADHD during the past few years. The rising incidence of adult ADHD has raised concerns about overdiagnosis, risks of substance abuse because the disorder is treated with psychostimulants, and propensity for secondary gain. DSM-IV-TR specifies very explicitly that ADHD cannot be diagnosed in adults without documentation of a childhood diagnosis, and the clinician should exert great care in documenting evidence of a childhood onset. Individuals with adult ADHD may present with difficulties at work caused by inattentiveness as their chief complaint. Alternatively, they may seek treatment because of problems with impulsive behavior that is troublesome.

Epidemiology, Clinical Findings, and Course

Because the definition of ADHD has changed over time, its prevalence is uncertain, but it is definitely common in young and school-age children; estimates range from 3% to 10%. It is far more common in boys than in girls, with a male-to-female ratio of approximately 3:1.

Approximately one-half of the children with this disorder have a good outcome, completing school on schedule with acceptable grades consistent with their family background and family expectations. Longitudinal studies suggest that childhood ADHD persists into young adulthood in as many as 50% of cases.

Some patients with ADHD have a relatively poor outcome. Twenty-five percent subsequently meet criteria for antisocial personality disorder as adults. Children given this diagnosis also have higher rates of substance abuse, more arrests, more suicide attempts, and more car accidents; they complete fewer years of school than children without ADHD. Problems with confidence and self-esteem may be prominent because the disorder invites rejection by both parents and peers. Interestingly, treatment with stimulant drugs has been associated with *decreased* risk for substance abuse. This suggests that treating the disorder not only brings symptomatic relief but also can lead to a better long-term outcome.

Etiology and Pathophysiology

The etiology and pathophysiology of ADHD are uncertain, but genetic, environmental, neurobiological, and social explanations have been proposed. It is well documented that ADHD runs in families, based principally on family studies. Not only does ADHD itself show a familial aggregation, particularly in males, but other psychiatric disorders aggregate with it as well. There is an association with mood disorder, learning disorders, substance abuse, and antisocial personality disorder. There may be a gender threshold effect, in that girls with ADHD have a stronger family history of ADHD than do boys.

Genetic studies have begun to identify the underlying mechanisms for familial transmission. Because dopamine mediates brain reward systems and because the treatments used for ADHD (i.e., psychostimulants) may work through the dopamine system, genes related to dopamine have received special attention. In particular, the dopamine D_4 receptor, which is prominent in limbic regions and associated with novelty-seeking behavior, has been implicated. In one preliminary study, a mutation in the gene for the dopamine transporter was identified in 55% of the patients with ADHD as compared with 8% of the control subjects.

Nongenetic factors also may be important in the development of ADHD. Initial descriptions of ADHD referred to the disorder as *minimal brain dysfunction*. Most nongenetic explanations have stressed the role of perinatal problems such as maternal smoking, alcohol and drug abuse, obstetrical complications during delivery, maternal malnutrition, exposure to toxins, and viral infections. The possible role of such nongenetic factors is consistent with the higher prevalence of ADHD in males as well as the gender threshold effect, because male children are more vulnerable to prenatal and perinatal injury. Children with well-documented perinatal problems, such as fetal alcohol syndrome, tend to have prominent behavior problems that include inattention, hyperactivity, and impulsivity.

Neuroimaging has added to our knowledge of the neural mechanisms of ADHD. Although clinical MRI scans are typically normal, more-focused research studies have indicated various abnormalities in children and adults with ADHD. Quantitative MRI studies indicate that the prefrontal cortex, basal ganglia, and cerebellum either are reduced in size or have abnormalities in asymmetry in ADHD. These findings correlate well with neuropsychological data, which indicate that individuals with ADHD have difficulties in response inhibition, executive functions mediated through the prefrontal cortex, or timing functions mediated through the cerebellum. Functional imaging studies are generally consistent with the structural and anatomical studies, in that they have shown hypoperfusion in prefrontal and basal ganglia regions that may be reversible with psychostimulant treatment.

Neuropsychological studies have examined the cognitive mechanisms that may explain the clinical symptoms of ADHD. It is not surprising that tests of executive functions mediated through the prefrontal cortex are impaired, such as formulating an abstract plan, structuring and organizing the narration of a story, and multitasking. Working memory, another prefrontal function, is impaired in ADHD. Because encoding is a key component in working memory, and because encoding is closely linked to the ability to focus attention, this deficit may explain some symptoms of the disorder.

Psychosocial explanations for ADHD stress the role of parental anxiety and inexperience as well as failure to extinguish undesirable behavior by ignoring it (often difficult to do with hyperactive children). Parents may become uncertain of their parenting skills when faced with a child who seems so difficult to control or shape, thereby conveying uncertainty or anxiety to him or her.

Differential Diagnosis

The differential diagnosis of ADHD includes a wide variety of disorders. In making a differential diagnosis, the clinician must be aware that a child with this disorder may have comorbidity with other disorders common in childhood, such as seizure disorders, other disruptive behavior disorders (e.g., conduct disorder and oppositional defiant disorder), or learning disorders. When any of these disorders is present, it is often difficult to distinguish which is primary and which is secondary. Other disorders that may present with similar symptoms include childhood bipolar disorder, childhood depression, conduct disorder, a normal response to a pathological or abusive home environment (e.g., physical abuse or neglect by the parents), or a neuroendocrine abnormality such as thyroid disorder.

Clinical Management

Most children respond favorably to psychostimulants. Methylphenidate (10–60 mg/day) is usually the first line of treatment, followed by dextroamphetamine (5–40 mg/day). If neither of these succeeds, atomoxetine (Strattera), an α_2 agonist (e.g., clonidine, guanfacine), tricyclic antidepressants (e.g., imipramine), or bupropion may be used. In general, methylphenidate and dextroamphetamine offer short-term effects, lasting 4–6 hours, whereas the effects of the antidepressants tend to last longer. Stimulant drugs are now available in a number of slow- or extended-release formulations.

Stimulant medication should be initiated at a low dosage and titrated gradually according to response and side effects within the recommended dosage range. Stimulants should be given after meals to reduce the likelihood of suppressing appetite. Starting treatment with a morning dose may be useful in assessing the drug's effect, because morning and afternoon school performance then may be compared. The need for medication on weekends or after school must be determined on an individual basis. Weight should be monitored during the initial titration, and weight and height should be measured several times each year. Feedback from schoolteachers can be enormously helpful in gauging the child's therapeutic response.

Common side effects that usually disappear within 2–3 weeks of initiating therapy or in response to a dosage reduction include appetite suppression, weight loss, irritability, abdominal pain, and insomnia. Mild dysphoria and social withdrawal may occur at higher dosages in some patients. In rare cases, children can develop a mild to moderate depression requiring drug discontinuation. A major concern has been the potential for these drugs to cause growth retardation. Recent research shows that the decrease in expected weight gain is small and probably not significant. This effect appears greater with dextroamphetamine than with methylphenidate. The effect on growth can be minimized by using drug holidays; this side effect does not appear to be mediated by effects on growth hormone. Some researchers have even suggested that growth delay is caused by processes inherent to ADHD itself. Other miscellaneous side effects of the stimulants include dizziness, nausea, nightmares, dry mouth, constipation, lethargy, anxiety, hyperacusis, and fearfulness.

Parents will benefit from learning basic techniques of behavioral management, such as the value of positive reinforcement and firm, nonpunitive limit setting. They can also be taught techniques for reducing stimulation, thereby diminishing distractibility and inattentiveness. For example, young hyperactive children do better playing with only one friend rather than in groups. Noisy or complex toys should be avoided, as should toys that encourage impulsivity and aggression. The parent may want to work closely with the child in completing homework tasks and to teach him or her the value of working on tasks in the single, small increments that are best suited to the child's relatively short attention span, mastering one completely before going on to another.

Conduct Disorder

Conduct disorder is characterized by a pattern of behavior that violates the rights of others, such as stealing, lying, or cheating. In terms of both behavior and diagnostic criteria, conduct disorder can be considered to be a forerunner of antisocial personality disorder in adults because it involves similar antisocial behavior. Nevertheless, not all children who manifest conduct disorder develop antisocial personality disorder as adults. With appropriate treatment and rehabilitation, many of these children go on to lead acceptable and normal adult lives.

The DSM-IV-TR criteria require the presence of at least 3 of 15 antisocial behaviors in the past 12 months (with at least 1 criterion present in the past 6 months) (see Table 16–5). The criteria define four major domains of relevant behavior: aggression toward people and animals, destruction of property, deceitfulness or theft, and serious violations of rules. Individuals who manifest this delinquent behavior are further subdivided into two different types. The *childhood-onset type* begins before age 10 years and probably has a more guarded prognosis, whereas the *adolescent-onset type* begins after age 10 years and is more likely to have a better outcome.

Children or adolescents with conduct disorder typically are angry, sullen, and resentful when placed in the context of the adult world, with its pressures to conform, stay in school, and persist in conspicuously dull activities. School performance usually is average to poor. These children or adolescents typically consider their schoolwork irrelevant or uninteresting, do not complete homework, and are often truant. When they are with their peers, their anger and sullenness often disappear, and they seem to be having a good time. Beneath the veneer of anger, toughness, and rebellion, however, they often have profound feelings of self-doubt and worthlessness, although they may be reluctant to discuss these feelings with either adults or their peers. Some children with conduct disorder have been either physically or sexually abused by their parents.

The following is a case history of a child with conduct disorder:

> Heather, a 14-year-old girl, was brought to the child psychiatry clinic by her mother with the complaint that "Heather is getting out of hand. I just can't seem to discipline her anymore." Heather was the youngest of four children and the only girl in the family. She was the product of a normal pregnancy and delivery and had completed her developmental

TABLE 16–5. DSM-IV-TR diagnostic criteria for conduct disorder

A. A repetitive and persistent pattern of behavior in which the basic rights of others or major age-appropriate societal norms or rules are violated, as manifested by the presence of three (or more) of the following criteria in the past 12 months, with at least one criterion present in the past 6 months:

Aggression to people and animals
(1) often bullies, threatens, or intimidates others
(2) often initiates physical fights
(3) has used a weapon that can cause serious physical harm to others (e.g., a bat, brick, broken bottle, knife, gun)
(4) has been physically cruel to people
(5) has been physically cruel to animals
(6) has stolen while confronting a victim (e.g., mugging, purse snatching, extortion, armed robbery)
(7) has forced someone into sexual activity

Destruction of property
(8) has deliberately engaged in fire setting with the intention of causing serious damage
(9) has deliberately destroyed others' property (other than by fire setting)

Deceitfulness or theft
(10) has broken into someone else's house, building, or car
(11) often lies to obtain goods or favors or to avoid obligations (i.e., "cons" others)
(12) has stolen items of nontrivial value without confronting a victim (e.g., shoplifting, but without breaking and entering; forgery)

Serious violations of rules
(13) often stays out at night despite parental prohibitions, beginning before age 13 years
(14) has run away from home overnight at least twice while living in parental or parental surrogate home (or once without returning for a lengthy period)
(15) is often truant from school, beginning before age 13 years

B. The disturbance in behavior causes clinically significant impairment in social, academic, or occupational functioning.

C. If the individual is age 18 years or older, criteria are not met for Antisocial Personality Disorder.

TABLE 16–5. **DSM-IV-TR diagnostic criteria for conduct disorder** *(continued)*

Code based on age at onset:

    Conduct Disorder, Childhood-Onset Type: onset of at least one criterion characteristic of Conduct Disorder prior to age 10 years

    Conduct Disorder, Adolescent-Onset Type: absence of any criteria characteristic of Conduct Disorder prior to age 10 years

    Conduct Disorder, Unspecified Onset: age at onset is not known

Specify severity:

    Mild: few if any conduct problems in excess of those required to make the diagnosis **and** conduct problems cause only minor harm to others

    Moderate: number of conduct problems and effect on others intermediate between "mild" and "severe"

    Severe: many conduct problems in excess of those required to make the diagnosis **or** conduct problems cause considerable harm to others

milestones on schedule. She had been an average student but had taken a particular interest in sports as a child.

Heather's father was a truck driver and was often away from the family, leaving the mother to rear the four children largely by herself. Heather's mother remained at home with the children until Heather was in second grade and then took a job as a clerk in a store.

Heather's parents had separated and divorced 3 years earlier. This appeared to bother Heather much more than her brothers, because she had always been "her father's little girl." Her father had developed a relationship with a woman in another city, had moved away, saw the children infrequently, and was not dependable in child support payments.

Heather's behavior problems began when she entered junior high school. She began to enter puberty in sixth grade, and by seventh grade her body was markedly feminized. Her mother reported that she seemed to react to this by "acting tougher instead of more like a girl." She started to hang out more with boys her own age or slightly older and began to smoke cigarettes secretly (although the evidence could be smelled all over the house and on her clothes). Her grades, previously average, began to drop steadily. She also showed signs of increasingly devious behavior, lying to her mother about where she was going, returning at night well past predefined deadlines, and staying home "sick" without telling her mother. Items that Heather could not afford, such as expensive costume jewelry and cosmetics, began to appear in the house. Whenever Heather's mother confronted her, Heather became angry and ran out of the house, several times staying away overnight.

When interviewed alone, Heather was initially evasive and defensive, looking at the floor and answering questions very briefly. She was an attractive, slightly overweight, dark-haired girl attired in conventional teenage garb with a slightly punk touch (multiple earrings in her ears, leather boots, sleeveless T-shirt showing a nude couple embracing and bearing an obscene logo). Eventually she admitted to most of the conduct abnormalities that her mother had described.

It was concluded that Heather was having difficulties but that she had many strengths as well: a relatively intact childhood, normal intelligence, a history of adequate school performance, and a mother who appeared to genuinely care about her. Heather was seen in individual therapy on a weekly basis for 3–4 months, with a primary emphasis on supportive and relationship approaches. Heather began to talk freely about her difficulties in adjusting to the loss of her father, her experience of entering puberty, and her confusion about whether it was better to relate to her male peers (from whom she desperately desired love and approval) as a "tough girl" or a "sexy girl." With Heather's permission, she was also seen jointly with her mother in family therapy. Heather responded well to therapy, and it was possible to terminate the therapy successfully at the end of the school year.

Epidemiology, Clinical Findings, and Course

Up to 8% of boys and 3% of girls younger than 18 meet criteria for conduct disorder. The rate in females may be increasing. The long-term course and outcome of conduct disorder are variable, but research shows the continuity of misbehavior from childhood to adulthood. An estimated 40% of boys and 25% of girls with conduct disorder will develop adult antisocial personality disorder. To some extent, outcome depends on the child's degree of socialization and aggressiveness. Children who are able to form relationships and to internalize social norms have a better outcome, as do children who are less aggressive. Another factor may be age at onset. Children who develop behavioral problems at a very early age (e.g., 5 years) are more likely to have an enduring pattern of antisocial behavior than are children who develop behavioral problems linked to teenage peer pressure. Mild antisocial behavior is common in adolescents, but most "shape up" as they mature.

Etiology and Pathophysiology

The etiology and pathophysiology of conduct disorder are almost certainly multifactorial. Family studies indicate that children with conduct disorder tend to come from families that have increased prevalence rates of antisocial personality disorder, mood disorder, substance abuse, and learning disorders. Adopted children may have higher rates of conduct disorder, consistent with reports that the adopted offspring of female felons have a high rate of antisocial behavior, such as traffic violations or arrests for robbery, which suggests that there may be at least some genetic component to conduct disorder. Apart from a possible genetic component, no specific neurobiological factors have been identified in children with conduct disorders to any consistent degree, although a slight increase in neurological soft signs and psychomotor seizures has been observed.

Psychosocial factors probably play a major role in the development of conduct disorders. Psychosocial factors that have been shown to have some relation to conduct disorders include parental separation or divorce; parental substance abuse; forms of poor parenting such as rejection, abandonment, abuse, inadequate supervision, and inconsistent or excessively harsh discipline; and association with a delinquent peer group.

Differential Diagnosis

Conduct disorders have considerable comorbidity with other childhood disorders. Among those that often coexist with conduct disorder are learning disorders, ADHD, and mood disorders. The clinician often will encounter these disorders in the differential diagnosis of conduct disorder, because these disorders most commonly must be distinguished from conduct disorder. From 20% to 30% of the children who present with ADHD also meet criteria for conduct disorder. At least 10% of the children with conduct disorder have specific learning disorders. In general, the greater the comorbidity, the more complicated the case, and the worse the outcome.

Clinical Management

The clinical management of conduct disorder varies greatly, depending on the age of the child, the symptoms with which he or she presents, the extent of comorbidity, the availability of family supports, and the child's intellectual and social assets. A relatively mild case, such as was represented by Heather, typically is treated with individual and family therapy. At the opposite extreme are those cases in which the child comes from a highly deviant family and engages in repeated antisocial acts that bring him or her to legal attention; such cases may require removal from the home and placement in a group home or perhaps even in a juvenile detention facility. In some situations, an important part of managing the child with a conduct disorder involves training his or her parents to become more effective as parents. Parental effectiveness training involves instructing parents on how best to communicate with their child, apply appropriate and consistent discipline, monitor the child's whereabouts, and steer the child away from bad peers. Early reports suggest that this approach may offer the best hope for the errant child.

Children and adolescents with conduct disorder who have comorbid disorders such as hyperactivity or seizures will benefit from medication to treat the comorbid disorder. Apart from such indications, however, medications are not typically used to treat conduct disorder. Nevertheless, lithium carbonate, psychostimulants, and second-generation antipsychotics are sometimes used to reduce aggression in children who are out of control. The use of these medications should be closely monitored because of their potential for serious adverse effects.

Oppositional Defiant Disorder

ODD is a relatively new diagnosis that attempts to provide a category for children and adolescents with difficult behavior but not full-blown conduct disorder. As this category has been increasingly used, it has become apparent that many youngsters who would have received diagnoses of good-prognosis or mild conduct disorder in DSM-III are now being placed in this category.

There is clearly a fine line between normal naughtiness and ODD. Most children at times lose their tempers, argue with their parents, refuse to clean their rooms, or fail to obey a curfew. Thus, the proviso is added that these behaviors must be more frequent than those of most children at the same mental age. Clearly, however, there will be great variation in the definition of *more frequent*, depending on who is rendering the judgment. Religiously conservative or authoritarian families are likely to be less tolerant of opposition and defiance than are families with a background of behavioral abnormalities. Thus, to some extent, the appearance of children with this diagnosis in child psychiatry clinics may partially reflect a given family's threshold for accepting defiant behavior, which must be considered in treatment planning. Unlike conduct disorders, which specify that the child must have violated personal rights and social rules (thereby making it more likely that the child's deviant behavior has come to the attention of people outside the immediate family), ODD is defined almost totally on the basis of annoying, difficult, and disruptive behavior.

Because this is a new disorder, very little is known about its epidemiology, etiology, pathophysiology, comorbidity, or treatment. By definition, it cannot coexist with conduct disorder, but it may coexist with ADHD. Common sense dictates that management will emphasize individual and family counseling, with treatment of comorbid hyperactivity (or possibly mood disorder) with medications as needed.

■ Tourette's Disorder

Tourette's disorder is a fascinating syndrome characterized by stereotypical but nonrhythmic "jerky" movements and vocalizations called *tics*. The vocal tics are typically somewhat socially offensive, such as making loud grunting or barking noises or shouting words. The words are sometimes obscenities such as "shit." The person is aware that he or she is producing the vocal tics and is able to exert a mild degree of control over them, but ultimately has to submit to them. Because people with Tourette's disorder are aware that their tics are socially inappropriate, they find them embarrassing. Motor tics occurring in Tourette's disorder are also often odd or offensive behaviors, such as tongue protrusion, sniffing, hopping, squatting, blinking, or nodding. Because most of the general public is unaware of the nature of Tourette's disorder, the behavior is seen as inappropriate or bizarre. The DSM-IV-TR criteria for Tourette's disorder appear in Table 16–6.

Epidemiology, Clinical Findings, and Course

Once considered relatively rare, the disorder affects from 1 to 10 school-children per 10,000 between the ages of 6 and 17. Up to 20% of children, however, experience transient simple tics. Tourette's disorder is more common in males than in females, with a ratio of 3:1. As with ADHD, a gender threshold effect has been observed; that is, female patients with Tourette's disorder appear to have higher genetic loading than male patients with Tourette's disorder, suggesting that there is a lower penetrance for the disorder in females.

Tourette's disorder begins during childhood or early adolescence. Motor tics often begin between the ages of 3 and 8, several years before the appearance of vocal tics. Tic severity tends to peak during the second decade of life. Twenty percent of patients have a remission of motor and vocal tics during their third decade, and most of the remaining patients with Tourette's disorder have a significant decrease in their symptoms as they grow older. Patients with Tourette's disorder typically

TABLE 16–6. DSM-IV-TR diagnostic criteria for Tourette's disorder

A. Both multiple motor and one or more vocal tics have been present at some time during the illness, although not necessarily concurrently. (A *tic* is a sudden, rapid, recurrent, nonrhythmic, stereotyped motor movement or vocalization.)

B. The tics occur many times a day (usually in bouts) nearly every day or intermittently throughout a period of more than 1 year, and during this period there was never a tic-free period of more than 3 consecutive months.

C. The onset is before age 18 years.

D. The disturbance is not due to the direct physiological effects of a substance (e.g., stimulants) or a general medical condition (e.g., Huntington's disease or postviral encephalitis).

experience shame and embarrassment about their disorder, which may lead them to avoid public or social situations or even close interpersonal relationships.

Etiology and Pathophysiology

Several different mechanisms may explain the onset and occurrence of this syndrome. One clue arises from patterns of familial aggregation. Tourette's disorder is both highly familial and comorbid with obsessive-compulsive disorder (OCD). Clinically, tics and compulsions have a superficial resemblance to each other, suggesting that these symptoms may be on a continuum with each other. Two-thirds of the first-degree relatives of patients with Tourette's disorder have tics, and a substantial number also have OCD.

Some children with Tourette's disorder have their onset of symptoms after infection with group A β-hemolytic *Streptococcus*. Streptococcal infections are a well-known cause of Sydenham's chorea, and it now appears that Tourette's disorder is a related condition. This group of syndromes is now referred to as a pediatric autoimmune neuropsychiatric disorder associated with streptococcal infections (PANDAS). Children with PANDAS have choreiform movements, obsessions, compulsions, and tics, as well as emotional lability, anxiety, and other emotional and behavioral symptoms.

The symptoms of Tourette's disorder can be markedly improved through treatment with antipsychotic medication. Because antipsychotics exert a primary effect by blocking dopaminergic pathways in the brain, abnormalities in dopamine transmission are the most commonly hypothesized neurochemical abnormality. Because Tourette's disorder has a prominent motor component, investigators suspect that its primary abnormalities may lie within nigrostriatal projections, but (given the complex feedback loops of the dopamine system, as described in Chapter 3) many other localizations are also possible.

Differential Diagnosis

The evaluation of a patient presenting with Tourette's disorder should include a comprehensive neurological evaluation to rule out other possible causes of the tics. The patient should be examined for the stigmata of Wilson's disease, and a family history should be obtained to evaluate the possibility of Huntington's disease. The patient also should be evaluated for other psychiatric conditions. Comorbidity with ADHD and learning disorders may occur, as may symptoms of mood and anxiety disorders, or OCD.

Clinical Management

The clinical management of Tourette's disorder has emphasized the use of antipsychotics, although treatment is often started with low dosages of α-adrenergic drugs (e.g., clonidine, 0.2–0.3 mg/day; guanfacine, 1.5–4 mg/day). Haloperidol and pimozide are the best-studied antipsychotics, but due to their many side effects, second-generation antipsychotics (e.g., risperidone, 1–3 mg/day; ziprasidone, 20–40 mg/day) are generally prescribed if adrenergic medications are ineffective. In addition to prescribing medication, it is important to educate the family about the disorder and to assist them in providing psychological support to the patient. Because of the social embarrassment that it produces, Tourette's disorder has a potential for serious long-term social complications, and supportive psychotherapy for the patient or family may help minimize these problems.

■ Separation Anxiety Disorder

Separation anxiety disorder represents a more severe and disabling form of a maturational experience that all children normally have. Most infants and children experience fear at the possibility (or reality) of being separated from their parents. Once infants learn to recognize maternal and paternal faces and shapes, they also learn to cry when the parent leaves the room or hands them to a stranger. (Stranger anxiety first develops at about age 9 months.) No doubt this pattern of behavior reflects some type of primal fear of loss or fear of the unknown. As the child grows older, he or she also experiences natural fears of being left with a babysitter, being sent to preschool, or entering kindergarten. Crying, tenseness, or physical complaints may appear and last for minutes, hours, or days in such situations.

As specified in the DSM-IV-TR criteria, separation anxiety disorder is defined largely by the persistence of such symptoms for a long enough duration to be considered pathological. At least three of eight characteristic symptoms must be present for at least 4 weeks and include three types of distress or worry (distress at being separated from home, worry that some harm will come to the parents, and worry that the child will be lost or somehow separated from them), three types of behaviors (school refusal, sleep refusal, and clinging), and two physiological symptoms (nightmares and physical complaints such as headache or nausea). About 3% of schoolchildren meet criteria for separation anxiety disorder, which tends to be a childhood precursor for adult panic disorder.

Another clinically significant anxiety disorder observed in children is variously referred to as *school phobia, school refusal,* or *school absenteeism.* Although this particular anxiety disorder is classified in DSM-IV-TR among the adult disorders as a type of social phobia, it is an important and common childhood anxiety disorder. In some cases, it may be related to separation anxiety disorder. Children with this problem develop a fear of going to school. It may begin with attendance at preschool or kindergarten, but more typically it develops during grade school or junior high school. Typically, a child who has previously been going to school (albeit with some anxiety) begins to develop methods for staying home. He or she may have repeated episodes of "illness" such as headache or nausea. Such children may be truant, leaving home with the appearance of going to school and then returning home without their parents' knowledge or going to some other environment that they experience as safe. They may simply refuse to go to school and give only some vague explanation such as "I don't like it." These various reasons explain why the problem is variously referred to as a phobia, absenteeism, or refusal. There is some controversy among child psychiatrists as to whether school refusal should be considered strictly a subset of separation anxiety disorder or should be defined more broadly to include all children who do not attend school, for whatever reason (e.g., truancy secondary to conduct disorder, avoidance of school as a complication of mood disorder, school avoidance secondary to a psychosis).

Once discovered, school avoidance should be thoroughly evaluated and treated as quickly as possible to prevent personal, social, and academic complications. The clinician should attempt to determine why the child does not want to go to school. These reasons may be expressed overtly (e.g., "The kids make fun of me because I'm stupid"; "I'm afraid that Jimmy Taylor will beat me up"), but often considerable investigation is needed. The child's intellectual and school performance should be evaluated to determine whether the child has some problem with academic skills that may make him or her feel inferior and avoidant. Teachers and parents should be consulted about the child's relationships with his or her peers, and a specific effort should be made to determine whether a problem with teasing or bullying exists.

Treatment of school avoidance depends on the cause that has been identified. Often the child will need encouragement and support from several directions: at home, at school, and from the clinician. If specific problems with academic skills are identified, remedial training should be initiated. Similar training may be appropriate for problems with athletic or social skills. Whatever the cause, however, it is important to impress on both the child and the family that the child must attend school regularly and that absenteeism or refusal will not be tolerated.

■ Other "Adult" Disorders Frequently Seen in Children

Several common "adult" disorders may have their first onset during childhood or adolescence. Because these are syndromally similar across all ages, they are classified among the adult disorders. Common examples are schizophrenia, major depression, and bipolar disorder. In general, children with these disorders meet the criteria that have been defined for adults. There may be subtle differences in presentation and management, however.

Schizophrenia often presents initially during adolescence, but in rare instances the onset is during childhood. Schizophrenia in adolescents often begins insidiously, with apathy, a change in personal hygiene, and withdrawal. Schizophrenia may be particularly difficult to distinguish from depression, and it is usually preferable to make an initial diagnosis of depression if there is any doubt; after an unsuccessful trial of several different antidepressants, the diagnosis of schizophrenia is more certain, particularly when the clinical picture is consistent with the adult presentation. The major challenge in assessing childhood schizophrenia involves determining the difference between normal childhood fantasies and frank delusions and hallucinations. In addition, the symptoms of disorganization of speech and behavior must be distinguished from abnormalities of speech and behavior that are simply due to developmental slowness or mental retardation. Children with a definite diagnosis of schizophrenia usually are given antipsychotic medications, but the dosage is typically lower than that in adults.

Mood disorders in adolescents are extremely common and are also more common in children than was thought several decades ago. Up to 5% of children and 8% of adolescents meet diagnostic criteria for major depression. In both age groups, the patient with major depression may present initially with physical complaints rather than the psychological complaint of depression. In young children, the complaints may be abdominal pain, nightmares, or trouble sleeping. In teenagers, complaints of fatigue, insomnia or hypersomnia, headache, or tension are common. Depression also may present initially as a disruptive behavior disorder. A combination of medication and psychotherapy might provide the best chance of recovery. Fluoxetine and escitalopram are approved by the FDA for the treatment of pediatric depression and should be used as first-line agents.

In 2003, the FDA also issued a black box warning about the risk of increased suicidal behavior in children, adolescents, and young adults (<25 years) taking antidepressants and advised "close supervision" of such patients. This warning was based on an analysis of pooled results of treatment studies that showed there might be an increased risk for suicidal behavior with short-term antidepressant use in these patients, although no suicides were reported. Unfortunately, this warning had the unintended result of reducing prescriptions for antidepressants, without any increase in doctor visits. There is some evidence that the warning has actually led to an increase in suicidal behaviors, because many cases of depression have gone untreated.

Bipolar disorder presenting with mania is also becoming increasingly recognized in children and adolescents. This has created some controversy, because many of its symptoms overlap with ADHD. Examples include impulsivity, distractibility, and disruptive behavior. The essential element that distinguishes the syndromes is the distinct quality of the mood. In mania, the child will be overly happy, giddy, or even euphoric. Sometimes the child will just be irritable. Bipolar disorder in children is generally treated with the same medications used in adults.

Key points to remember about disorders of children and adolescents

1. In assessing children and adolescents, the clinician should be imaginative and meet each patient on his or her own terms.
   - Problem-solving and motor skills can be evaluated by playing games.
   - Dolls and toys should be used with young children to create pretend situations that will provide insight about personal and social interactions.

2. Normal maturational levels are highly variable in children and adolescents.

3. Children and adolescents often do not have a level of cognitive development suitable for the insight-oriented and introspective approaches used with adults.

4. Establishing rapport with adolescents is difficult but may be crucial to creating a therapeutic alliance.
   - The therapist should find out what the patient is interested in and relate to him or her through these interests.

5. The clinician must not preach or judge.

6. The basic maturational task of adolescents is to disengage themselves from their parents, become independent, and define their own identities; reliance on peers is an important crutch for adolescents in this transitional period.

7. The therapist should remain neutral and try not to criticize either parents or peers.

8. The adolescent's first reaction may be to see the therapist as a parent. The therapist should try to use this to therapeutic advantage, or at least try to prevent it from being a therapeutic handicap.

9. It is best to strike a balance between being perceived as a good parent and being perceived as a good peer, but this balance cannot and should not (usually) be achieved by attacking the real parent or real peer.

10. Because the parents and peers of adolescents may vary in quality, the therapist needs to be flexible, insightful, and creative in dealing with the patient's perceptions of him or her.

11. The clinician must be aware of the pervasiveness of comorbidity in childhood and adolescent disorders.

■ Self-Assessment Questions

1. Describe some techniques that are useful in assessing children and establishing rapport with them.

2. List and describe the various types of nonphysician clinicians who may be helpful in assessing and managing children and adolescents.

3. List the IQ levels that are used to define borderline intelligence and mild, moderate, severe, and profound mental retardation.

4. Discuss the distinction between autism, mental retardation, and learning disorders.

5. List three well-recognized causes of mental retardation.

6. Define *learning disorder* and list the three skills that are commonly affected.

7. Describe the three major domains that are abnormal in autism and give examples of signs and symptoms within these domains. How common is autism? What are its long-term course and outcome? What methods are used to treat it?

8. List the two broad categories of symptoms used to define ADHD and give several examples of each. Describe the long-term course and outcome of ADHD. Identify two medications commonly used to treat ADHD, and specify the appropriate dosage range.

9. Describe the symptoms of conduct disorder. What are the prevalence and gender ratio for conduct disorder?

10. Describe ODD and discuss its relationship to conduct disorder.

11. Describe the clinical features of Tourette's disorder. Describe two pharmacological strategies for treating Tourette's disorder.

12. Describe separation anxiety disorder and discuss its relation to school refusal (phobia, avoidance). List three factors that may predispose to the development of school avoidance. Describe three approaches to treating school avoidance.

CHAPTER 17

Sleep Disorders

The woods are lovely, dark and deep.
But I have promises to keep,
And miles to go before I sleep…

Robert Frost

SLEEP DISORDERS are among the most common complaints that people report to their physicians. Each year up to one-half of patients seen in clinical practice report difficulty sleeping, and for many the problem is considered serious. Examples of everyday sleep problems that physicians encounter are the overweight attorney whose wife reports that he snores loudly at night and is drowsy during the day; the executive who frequently flies to meetings in Asia and reports that she is chronically tired and unable to sleep well; and the mother who reports that her teenaged son occasionally sleepwalks and has injured himself by tripping over furniture. Because sleep disorders are so frequently encountered in clinical practice, students and residents should learn to assess and diagnose these conditions and understand their clinical management. The DSM-IV-TR sleep disorders are listed in Table 17–1.

DSM-IV-TR divides the sleep disorders into the *dyssomnias* and the *parasomnias*. In dyssomnias, the predominant disturbance is in initiating and maintaining sleep. In parasomnias, the predominant disturbance is an abnormal event occurring during sleep. A category exists for *sleep disorders related to another mental disorder,* such as major

TABLE 17–1. DSM-IV-TR sleep disorders

Dyssomnias
  Primary insomnia
  Primary hypersomnia
  Narcolepsy
  Breathing-related sleep disorder
  Circadian rhythm sleep disorder
  Dyssomnia not otherwise specified

Parasomnias
  Nightmare disorder
  Sleep terror disorder
  Sleepwalking disorder
  Parasomnia not otherwise specified

Sleep disorders related to another mental disorder
  Insomnia related to an Axis I or Axis II disorder
  Hypersomnia related to an Axis I or Axis II disorder

Other sleep disorders
  Sleep disorder due to a general medical condition
  Substance-induced sleep disorder

depression or schizophrenia. A residual category also exists for other sleep disorders that may result from the effects of a general medical condition or the physiological effects of a substance.

Although the diagnostic criteria do not include data from laboratory procedures such as polysomnography (a procedure in which electroencephalographic, electrooculographic, and electromyographic tracings are recorded during sleep), these data are necessary in some patients to thoroughly investigate their disorder. Polysomnography provides data on sleep continuity, sleep architecture, rapid eye movement (REM) physiology, sleep-related breathing impairment, oxygen desaturation, cardiac arrhythmias, and periodic movements. The Multiple Sleep Latency Test (MSLT) often is used to measure excessive sleepiness. With the MSLT, the patient is given an opportunity to fall asleep in a darkened room for five 20-minute periods in 2-hour intervals across the patient's usual period of wakefulness. The average latency to sleep onset, assessed using polysomnography, is a measure of the tendency to fall asleep. An average sleep latency of less than 5 minutes indicates the presence of excessive sleepiness.

■ Normal Sleep and Sleep Architecture

The average healthy adult requires about 7.5 hours of sleep per night, although some persons require more and some less to feel sufficiently rested. Normal sleep is influenced by many factors; for example, young persons tend to sleep more than the elderly, whose total sleep time tends to be decreased. Furthermore, the longer a person has been awake, the more quickly he or she will fall asleep (i.e., sleep latency).

Sleep stages in adults are divided into REM and non-REM (NREM) sleep. These sleep stages alternate in a cycle that lasts between 70 and 120 minutes. Generally, four to six NREM/REM cycles occur nightly. The first REM period lasts 5–10 minutes; during the night, REM periods become longer and closer together and show progressively greater density of REM. (Figure 17–1 depicts a polysomnographic recording during the various sleep stages.)

The normal sleep stages in adults are as follows:

- *Stage 0* is a period of wakefulness with eyes closed that occurs just before sleep onset. Electroencephalographic (EEG) recording mainly shows sinusoidal alpha waves over the occiput, which have a frequency of 8–13 cycles per second and a fairly low amplitude (or voltage). Muscle tone is increased. Alpha activity decreases as drowsiness increases.
- *Stage 1* is called the sleep-onset stage, or drowsiness, because it provides a brief transition from wakefulness to sleep. Alpha activity diminishes to less than 50% of the EEG recording. There is a low-amplitude, mixed-frequency signal, composed mainly of beta and the slower theta (4–7 cycles per second) activity. Stage 1 accounts for about 5% of the total sleep period.
- *Stage 2* is dominated by theta activity and the appearance of sleep spindles and K complexes. *Sleep spindles* are brief bursts of rhythmic (12–14 cycles per second) waves with a duration of 500–1500 msec. *K complexes* are sharp, negative, high-voltage EEG waves, followed by slower, positive activity, with a duration of 500 msec. They are thought to represent a central nervous system (CNS) response to internal stimuli; they also can be elicited during sleep with external stimuli (e.g., a loud noise). Stage 2 usually accounts for about 45%–55% of the total sleep time.

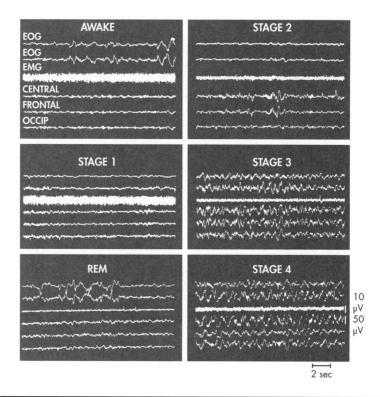

FIGURE 17–1. Polysomnographic recording during the various stages of sleep.

Notice the high electromyogram (EMG) and eye movements during wakefulness, the slow eye movements but absence of rapid eye movements (REMs) during descending Stage 1, and REMs with low EMG during stage REM. Stages 2, 3, and 4 are characterized by the slowing of frequency and an increase in amplitude of the electroencephalogram.

EOG = electrooculogram; OCCIP = occipital.

Source. Reprinted from Bixler EO, Vela-Bueno A: "Normal Sleep: Physiological, Behavioral, and Clinical Correlates." *Psychiatric Annals* 17:437–445, 1987. Used with permission.

- *Stage 3* is characterized by 20%–50% high-voltage delta wave activity having a frequency of 1–2 cycles per second. As in Stage 2, muscle tone is increased, but eye movements are absent.
- *Stage 4* occurs when delta waves comprise more than 50% of the EEG recording. Stages 3 and 4 are often indistinguishable and are collectively referred to as *slow-wave sleep, delta sleep,* or *deep sleep.* These stages together account for about 15%–20% of the total sleep time.

- *REM sleep* is characterized by an EEG recording similar to that seen in Stage 1, along with a burst of rapid conjugate eye movements and reduced muscle tone. REM periods occur in phasic bursts and are accompanied by respiratory and cardiac rate fluctuations as well as penile and clitoral engorgement. This stage constitutes 20%–25% of the total sleep period and is also known as *desynchronized sleep.*

A normal young adult goes from waking into a period of NREM sleep lasting approximately 90 minutes before the first REM period; this portion of NREM sleep is referred to as *REM latency.* The sequence of sleep stages during an early sleep cycle is as follows: NREM Stages 1, 2, 3, 4, 3, and 2; then, a REM period occurs. The number of sleep cycles with REM varies from four to six per night depending on the length of sleep. In young adults, REM sleep constitutes about 25% of the total sleep time but may exceed 50% in newborns.

The sleep cycle (REM time to REM time) is shorter in infants than in adults. REM periods emerge every 50–60 minutes during the sleep of infants and gradually increase to the adult sleep cycle length of 70–100 minutes during adolescence. At birth, REM and NREM periods are equally dispersed throughout the sleep period; as people age, REM periods typically become confined to the final third of the sleep period. Figure 17–2 depicts typical sleep architecture and shows the effects of age on the different sleep stages.

The American Academy of Sleep Medicine recently published guidelines to revise the terminology, recording method, and scoring rules for sleep-related phenomena. In this scheme, Stages 1–4 are referred to as N1, N2, and N3, with N3 reflecting slow-wave sleep (Stages 3 and 4); REM sleep is referred to as stage R. The purpose of the guidelines is to introduce greater reliability in the evaluation of sleep stages, a source of criticism for the current scheme introduced in 1967. The new scoring method is being actively researched but is not yet in wide use.

Serotonin-containing nuclei and pathways play an important role in regulating NREM sleep. Noradrenergic systems are principally involved in the control of REM sleep. The serotonin-containing neurons are mainly located in the group of nuclei in the lower midbrain and upper pons, referred to as the *raphe nuclei.* Activation of these neurons regulates NREM sleep. This knowledge is based on animal models in which destruction of the raphe nuclei induced total insomnia and on models in which animals were injected with parachlorophenylalanine, which inhibits serotonin synthesis.

Noradrenergic neurons are found throughout the brain stem. They achieve their highest concentration in the locus coeruleus in the pons,

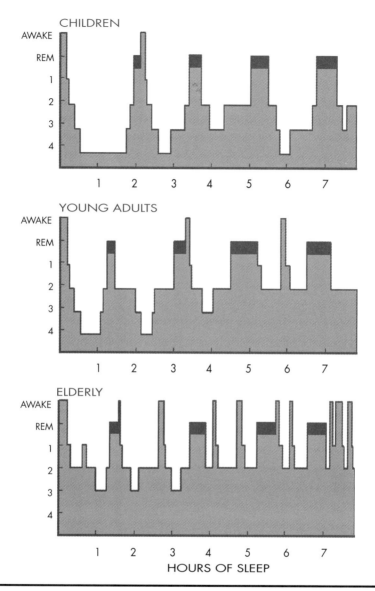

FIGURE 17–2.　The effects of age on the various stages of sleep.

Rapid eye movement (REM) sleep (*shaded area*) occurs cyclically throughout the night at intervals of approximately 90 minutes in all age groups. REM sleep shows little variation in the different age groups, whereas Stage 4 sleep decreases with age. In addition, the elderly have frequent awakenings and a marked increase in total wake time.

Source.　Reprinted from Bixler EO, Vela-Bueno A: "Normal Sleep: Physiological, Behavioral, and Clinical Correlates." *Psychiatric Annals* 17:437–445, 1987. Used with permission.

which is thought to regulate REM sleep; this inference is primarily based on animal research in which lesions of neurons in the locus coeruleus abolished REM sleep and led to hyperactive behavior. REM suppression is brought about by injecting animals with α-methylparatyrosine, a substance that inhibits the synthesis of norepinephrine.

Acetylcholine also plays a major role in sleep, and the reciprocal interaction between serotonergic and noradrenergic systems on the one hand and cholinergic systems on the other may underlie the basic oscillation of the NREM/REM cycle.

■ Dyssomnias

The essential feature of the dyssomnias is a disturbance in the amount, quality, or timing of sleep. These disorders include the *insomnias,* which are disorders of initiating or maintaining sleep or of not feeling rested after sleep; *hypersomnias,* or disorders of excessive daytime sleepiness or sleep attacks; *breathing-related sleep disorder;* and *circadian rhythm sleep disorder,* in which there is a mismatch between the person's sleep-wake pattern and the pattern that is normal for his or her environment. The category *dyssomnia not otherwise specified* is used when a dyssomnia is present but cannot be better classified.

Primary Insomnia

Primary insomnia is characterized by difficulty initiating or maintaining sleep, or having nonrestorative or nonrestful sleep, that lasts for at least 1 month and is not due to another mental disorder, a general medical condition, or the effects of a substance. The subjective report of poor or nonrefreshing sleep may or may not be associated with any objective sleep disturbance and may not accurately reflect the magnitude of the objective sleep disturbances when present. The objective evidence is often relatively minor because subjective estimates of sleep latency and total sleep time tend to exaggerate the degree of any disturbance present. Many people with primary insomnia are anxious worriers who are overaroused and hyperalert.

Insomnia is relatively common in the general population and is even more common among psychiatric patients; however, only a small proportion of persons with insomnia consult a physician. Sleep difficulty occurs more frequently among the elderly, in women, among individuals with limited education and lower socioeconomic status, and in persons with chronic (or multiple) medical problems.

The duration of insomnia is the most helpful factor in evaluating the patient's problem. Transient insomnia (no more than a few nights) typically occurs in persons who usually sleep normally. This form of insomnia occurs at times of acute psychological stress, such as following the death of a loved one. Other situations associated with transient insomnia include a hospital admission, a public speaking engagement, or (for students) a scheduled examination. In these situations, the insomnia is rarely brought to medical attention because it is not regarded as pathological and tends to correct itself.

The estimated one-third to one-half of patients with chronic insomnia with an underlying psychiatric disorder thought responsible for the sleep disturbance do not have primary insomnia. Sleep disorders associated with specific mental disorders are discussed later in the chapter.

The patient with primary insomnia should receive a thorough medical and psychiatric assessment (see Table 17–2). The medical history should include a careful review of drug and medication use. Patients should be asked to maintain a sleep log, in which they record their bedtime, sleep latency (estimated time required to fall asleep), awake time, number of awakenings, daytime naps, and use of drugs or medications. Interviewing the patient's bed partner to learn about the presence of snoring, breathing difficulties, or leg jerks can be helpful.

"Sleep hygiene" measures have been developed for patients with chronic insomnia. These measures include the following:

- Waking up and going to bed at the same time every day, even on weekends
- Avoiding long periods of wakefulness in bed
- Not using the bed as a place to read, watch television, or work
- Leaving the bed and not returning until drowsy if sleep does not begin within a set period (such as 20–30 minutes)
- Avoiding napping
- Exercising at least three or four times a week (but not in the evening if this interferes with sleep)
- Discontinuing or reducing the consumption of alcoholic beverages; beverages containing caffeine; cigarettes; and sedative-hypnotic drugs

Some sleep hygiene measures may be difficult for the patient. For example, asking a patient to quit smoking may be seen as unacceptable, and withdrawal of caffeine could cause temporary headaches and slug-

TABLE 17–2. Sleep history outline

Obtain data from patient, chart, and nursing staff. Review medication history, including illicit drugs, alcohol, and use of hypnotic medication. Obtain information on the following sleep characteristics:

- Usual sleep pattern

- Characteristics of disturbed sleep (for insomnia, difficulty falling asleep, difficulty staying asleep, or early-morning awakenings)

- The clinical course: onset, duration, frequency, severity, and precipitating and relieving factors

- 24-hour sleep-wake cycle (corroborate with staff and chart)

- History of sleep disturbances, including childhood sleep pattern and pattern of sleep when under stress

- Family history of sleep disorders

- Personal history of other sleep disorders

- Sleep pattern at home as described by bed partner

- Consumption of alcoholic beverages; over-the-counter caffeine tablets; coffee, tea, cola, and chocolate; herbals such as kava, which may be stimulating

- Use of prescription and over-the-counter medications

gishness. Nonetheless, many patients motivated to improve their daytime functioning are willing to make a concerted effort to follow these measures.

Sedative-hypnotic medications (i.e., sleeping pills) do not cure insomnia, but for many they can provide dramatic temporary relief. They should be used mainly to treat transient and short-term insomnia, in combination with the sleep hygiene measures just outlined. Long-term benefits are difficult to document, however, and these medications can be habit-forming. Traditionally, the benzodiazepines have been the first choice for reasons of safety and efficacy. Tolerance to their sleep-promoting effects appears to develop less often than it does with barbiturates, barbiturate-like compounds, and antihistamines. Several nonbenzodiazepine alternatives are available, such as zolpidem and eszopiclone. Compared with the benzodiazepines, these agents have less abuse potential, produce little tolerance, and tend not to cause daytime somnolence. Both benzodiazepine and nonbenzodiazepine hypnotics are listed in Table 17–3.

TABLE 17–3. Medications used to treat insomnia

Drug (trade name)	Onset	Half-life, h	Dosage range, mg
Benzodiazepines			
Estazolam (ProSom)	Very fast	10–24	1–2
Flurazepam (Dalmane)	Very fast	50–100	15–30
Quazepam (Doral)	Very fast	15–35	7.5–15
Temazepam (Restoril)	Moderate	8–18	15–30
Triazolam (Halcion)	Very fast	2–3	0.125–0.5
Nonbenzodiazepines			
Eszopiclone (Lunesta)	Very fast	6	1–3
Ramelteon (Rozerem)	Very fast	1–3	8
Zaleplon (Sonata)	Very fast	1	5–20
Zolpidem (Ambien)	Very fast	2–3	5–10

Other drugs frequently used as sleeping aids include chloral hydrate (500–2,000 mg), a nonbarbiturate sedative-hypnotic known more for the fact that it is markedly potentiated by alcohol and forms the basis for "knockout drops" (also known as a Mickey Finn), and the antihistamines diphenhydramine (25–100 mg) and doxylamine (25–100 mg), which are often used as hypnotic agents but are not as potent as the benzodiazepines. The sedating antidepressant trazodone (50–200 mg) is sometimes used as a hypnotic and appears to be effective.

Primary Hypersomnia

Although excessive daytime somnolence is less common than insomnia, it affects about 5% of the adult population, including similar numbers of men and women. According to DSM-IV-TR, the excessive sleepiness lasts at least 1 month, as evidenced by either prolonged sleep episodes or daytime sleep episodes occurring almost daily; the excessive sleepiness causes significant impairment or distress; and the excessive sleepiness is not accounted for by another sleep disorder, a medical condition, or the effects of a substance.

Primary hypersomnia usually involves prolonged nocturnal sleep and continual daytime drowsiness. Nearly one-half of the patients report sleep drunkenness (i.e., excessive grogginess) on awakening, which may last several hours. Patients may report taking one or two naps daily (which can each last more than an hour), unlike the short naps typical of narcoleptic patients.

Polysomnographic studies have shown diminished delta sleep, increased number of awakenings, and reduced REM latency in patients with primary hypersomnia. The MSLT is used to document the short sleep latency. Primary hypersomnia is considered a diagnosis of exclusion, and other more specific disorders should be ruled out, such as narcolepsy.

Treatment of primary hypersomnia involves a combination of sleep hygiene measures, stimulant drugs, and naps for some patients. Stimulants can help maintain wakefulness; both dextroamphetamine and methylphenidate have relatively short half-lives and are taken in multiple divided doses. Modafinil, which is used to treat narcolepsy (see "Narcolepsy" section), can also be used to treat primary hypersomnia. Nonsedating tricyclic antidepressants (e.g., protriptyline) have been reported to be helpful but are rarely used. Because stimulants have substantial abuse potential, their use should be carefully monitored.

The following case example describes a patient with primary hypersomnia:

> Chris, a 24-year-old college student, was being treated for obsessive-compulsive disorder (OCD) consisting mainly of intrusive and unwanted thoughts of harming others. His symptoms were well controlled with paroxetine, a serotonin reuptake inhibitor.
>
> His mother, who usually accompanied him to the clinic, felt that his excessive sleeping and napping were even more of a problem than his OCD. She described how Chris would sleep 12–14 hours nightly and take afternoon naps. Chris admitted that he was frequently late for class and often fell asleep in class. He complained that he was too sleepy to study in the evening. All of these symptoms predated his treatment for OCD.
>
> Chris was referred to a sleep disorders clinic; his polysomnograph was unremarkable. Because there was no evidence of sleep attacks, cataplexy, sleep paralysis, or hypnagogic hallucinations, he received a diagnosis of primary hypersomnia and began treatment with methylphenidate. On this regimen, Chris was able to remain awake and alert during the day without napping. He was more alert in class, and his academic performance improved.

Narcolepsy

Narcolepsy is characterized by excessive sleepiness associated with irresistible sleep attacks that occur either as the only symptoms or in com-

sive sleepiness or sleep attacks. The disorder can have serious psychological consequences, including a general slowing of thought processes, memory impairment, and inattention. Patients often report anxiety, dysphoric mood, or multiple physical complaints. Men and women of all ages and body types can develop sleep apnea, although the typical patient is an overweight middle-aged man.

A thorough medical assessment is necessary and may include a sleep laboratory evaluation with recording of respiration and monitoring of nocturnal oxygen desaturation. Obese patients are counseled to reduce their weight, which in some cases may be sufficient to relieve the apnea. Tricyclic antidepressants (e.g., protriptyline, 10–60 mg nightly) have been used, and reports indicate that buspirone and fluoxetine also may be beneficial. Benzodiazepines should not be used because of their tendency to inhibit alerting responses and to depress respiration at higher dosages.

Continuous positive airway pressure (CPAP) is the most widely used treatment. Room air is blown into the nose through a nasal mask or cushioned cannulae. Some patients do not tolerate CPAP well, but compliance can be enhanced by careful follow-up. Uvulopalatopharyngoplasty is a surgical alternative for patients with redundant oropharyngeal tissue. Tracheostomy is reserved for life-threatening situations in patients whose condition does not respond to CPAP or uvulopalatopharyngoplasty.

Circadian Rhythm Sleep Disorder (Sleep-Wake Schedule Disorder)

Disrupted sleep may result when the sleep-wake cycle is not correctly synchronized with a person's daily schedule. For example, persons with night shift work or who frequently change their work shift (e.g., nurses, factory workers) may develop *circadian rhythm sleep disorder*. Persons who travel frequently and cross time zones also develop disrupted sleep, known as *jet lag*. Persons with these disorders may never feel fully rested. When they want to sleep, they cannot, and when they are expected to be awake and alert, they are sleepy and drowsy.

The best way to avoid these problems is to forgo shift work. Industrial plants have gradually become more aware of these problems, and many have redesigned their schedules, finding that productivity increases and personnel turnover decreases. Some people will always be intolerant to shifting work schedules; these individuals should probably seek other types of employment.

People who travel frequently probably cannot avoid jet lag. Because of the human circadian time-keeping system, it is usually easier for persons to adjust when the cycle is lengthened rather than shortened, traveling west rather than east.

The treatment for jet lag, other than tincture of time, involves the recommendation that usual sleep hours be maintained in the new time zone. Conventional wisdom is that most adults require about 1 day to adjust for each eastward time zone crossed and slightly less after westward travel. Travelers can minimize the loss of sleep by judicious use of hypnotic agents (e.g., zolpidem, 5–10 mg) and by avoiding alcohol and other substances that interfere with sleep. Melatonin, often touted as a cure for jet lag, has not been shown effective in controlled trials.

Dyssomnia Not Otherwise Specified

The category *dyssomnia not otherwise specified* is for insomnias, hypersomnias, or circadian rhythm disturbances that do not meet criteria for any specific dyssomnia. An example is excessive sleepiness attributable to ongoing sleep deprivation. Another example is *restless legs syndrome,* in which uncomfortable sensations lead to an intense urge to move the legs during wakefulness. Restless legs syndrome is considered a sleep disorder because it interferes with sleep and may be associated with periodic limb movements in sleep. The syndrome affects about 5% of the general population. Patients report that symptoms begin in the evening and are relieved by moving the legs or walking. The sensations can delay sleep or waken the person from sleep. Treatment includes the use of dopamine agonists such as pramipexole or ropinirole.

■ Parasomnias

Parasomnias consist of nightmares, sleep terrors, and sleepwalking (or somnambulism). All three disorders are relatively common in children but rarely lead to medical attention unless they are frequent and severe. These disorders generally resolve by late adolescence but can persist into adulthood.

Nightmare Disorder (Dream Anxiety)

Nightmare disorder consists of repeated awakenings with detailed recall of extended and frightening dreams, often involving threats to sur-

Delirium may lead to agitation, combativeness, and wandering during early evening or nighttime hours. Clinically, sleep may be fragmented with frequent awakenings, initial insomnia, or early-morning awakenings. The polysomnographic findings include sleep fragmentation, lower sleep efficiency, decreased Stage 3 and 4 sleep, and a decreased percentage of REM sleep.

Key points to remember about sleep disorders

1. A thorough sleep history is essential for accurate diagnosis and includes the recording of

   - Drug use pattern.

   - Use of caffeine and other stimulant drugs.

   - An interview with the patient's bed partner.

2. For patients with insomnia, the sleep hygiene measures outlined in this chapter are the simplest and most overlooked strategy.

3. Complaints of disturbed sleep should alert the clinician to the possibility of a major psychiatric illness. Major depression and alcohol abuse or dependence are probably the most common causes of disturbed sleep.

4. Prescribing hypnotics for patients with sleep complaints is inappropriate without having first made a diagnosis. For primary insomnia, patients should be told that the sleeping pills are for temporary use only (e.g., days to weeks).

5. Temazepam and estazolam have probably the best therapeutic properties for a benzodiazepine hypnotic: rapid absorption, lack of metabolites, and an intermediate half-life that will allow a full night's sleep. The nonbenzodiazepine hypnotics are excellent alternatives.

6. Some clinicians consider methylphenidate the drug of choice for patients with narcolepsy or primary hypersomnia. It should be titrated up to 60 mg/day. The clinician should keep track of pill use because some patients may be tempted to abuse this medication. Modafinil is an effective alternative to the stimulants.

   - Sodium oxybate is available to treat narcolepsy complicated by cataplexy, although its usefulness is compromised by an awkward administration schedule.

7. If patients have unusual sleep complaints or disorders, a referral should be made to a sleep disorders clinic for a more thorough evaluation, which may include polysomnography and the MSLT.

■ Self-Assessment Questions

1. What are the major categories of sleep disorders?

2. Describe the different dyssomnias. What is the restless legs syndrome?

3. What are sleep hygiene measures?

4. What are the REM and NREM stages? What is their significance?

5. Describe the appropriate use of hypnotic agents. Which are preferred?

6. Distinguish between nightmare disorder and sleep terrors.

7. Does sleepwalking have the same significance in a child that it does in an adult? Describe simple measures that can be taken to reduce the chance of injury in the sleepwalker.

8. How is hypersomnia managed?

9. Do other psychiatric disorders, such as depression, disrupt sleep?

CHAPTER 18

Legal Issues

Lawsuit, *n.* a machine which you go into as a pig and come out as a sausage.

Ambrose Bierce, The Devil's Dictionary

MORE THAN MOST other medical specialists, psychiatrists regularly confront sensitive legal issues. Should this patient be committed to the hospital for treatment against his or her will? Should this patient be forcibly medicated? Can I release information about my patient to someone else without his or her permission?

Because our society values individual freedom and civil liberties, there are rarely easy answers to questions about involuntary hospitalization, the right to treatment (or the right to refuse treatment), confidentiality, and other legal issues. What may seem morally right may not be legally permissible, and conversely, what may be legally permissible may seem morally wrong. The right of a man with schizophrenia to live on the streets, for instance, loses its meaning when he becomes so ill that he lacks the capacity to make important decisions. Thus the psychiatrist often gets caught in the middle between what may be legally right (i.e., not forcing treatment on someone with schizophrenia) and what may be ethically right (i.e., relieving the suffering of the schizophrenic person through involuntary treatment). Because of this interface with the law, psychiatrists should understand the legal issues they are likely to encounter. Although general principles underlie much of the law in the United States, significant variation exists between states and jurisdictions. It is therefore essential that psychiatrists become familiar with relevant laws in the regions where they practice.

Legal issues pertaining to mental illness can be roughly divided into two broad categories: civil and criminal (see Table 18–1). *Civil law* has primarily to do with relationships between citizens, while *criminal law* focuses on the individual's relationship to the state in the maintenance of social order. Civil issues pertinent to the practice of psychiatry include confidentiality, informed consent, and involuntary treatment. Criminal issues that might involve input from mental health practitioners include competence to stand trial (whether the person understands the court process and can assist his lawyer in the present) and criminal responsibility (whether the person accused of a crime was legally insane at the time of the act).

In this chapter, we focus primarily on civil issues encountered by the psychiatrist during the course of his or her day-to-day practice. Forensic psychiatry, a subspecialty within psychiatry, focuses on the interface between psychiatry and the law. Psychiatrists working in this area devote significant time to conducting evaluations of mental capacity, injury, and disability for agencies and courts. Although we offer a general overview of questions asked of psychiatrists by criminal courts, readers interested in these areas are referred to *Clinical Handbook of Psychiatry and the Law.*

■ Civil Issues

Involuntary Treatment

Psychiatrists have a responsibility to provide for the safety of their patients. Legal precedent has extended this duty to include the protection of others who could be physically or emotionally harmed by the actions of a mentally ill person. Thus, when a patient who is thought to be a threat to self or others refuses hospitalization for the treatment of mental illness, the psychiatrist will seek a court order for involuntary hospitalization.

In the past, the court system deferred to the judgment of physicians concerning the detention of patients for treatment, but with increasing emphasis on individual liberties and freedoms articulated during the civil rights movement, the process of *civil commitment* became more a matter for the courts. Because civil commitment involves depriving a person of some of his or her constitutional rights on the basis of a men-

TABLE 18–1. Civil and criminal legal issues involving psychiatrists

Civil	Criminal
Involuntary hospitalization	Competency to stand trial
Confidentiality	Criminal responsibility
Informed consent	
Malpractice	

tal illness, most states now carefully regulate the process in the belief that the courts are more objective in this balancing act than are mental health providers. The appropriateness of this emphasis on civil rights over the right to humane care has been hotly debated. It is sometimes said that the homeless are being allowed to "die with their rights on."

Most commitment laws invoke the concepts of mental illness, dangerousness, and disability. For civil commitment, these laws require the presence of mental illness, although the precise definition of *mental illness* differs from place to place. The law may specify the conditions considered to be mental illness and require that the mental illness be treatable in order to qualify for civil commitment. For example, a diagnosis of a personality disorder may be insufficient for commitment in some jurisdictions while being acceptable in others. The concept of *dangerousness* usually requires that persons present an imminent danger to themselves or others (i.e., within the next 24 hours if not hospitalized). Because psychiatrists are unable to accurately predict dangerousness except in the most obvious of situations, this requirement can be difficult to apply. The third element, *disability*, is a measure of the patient's inability to properly care for him- or herself because of mental illness. Some states use the phrase *gravely disabled* (or similar language) to suggest that a person is unable to take care of his or her personal grooming, to maintain adequate hydration, and to feed him- or herself. A gravely disabled person may not be in imminent danger of harming him- or herself but may still need psychiatric hospitalization and treatment.

Most states allow for patients to be hospitalized on an emergency basis to allow for a more detailed evaluation and short-term psychiatric intervention. This follows the filing of a petition by someone who knows the person and medical certification of the need for emergency commitment. This period may range from 1 to 20 days, depending on the jurisdiction.

Civil commitments occur by court order after a judicial finding of mental illness and potential harm to self or others if released; they provide for continued involuntary hospitalization. There are a variety of legal protections for mentally ill persons facing involuntary commitment. Details vary by jurisdiction, but these protections include a timely court hearing following appropriate notice, ability to be present at all commitment proceedings, representation by an attorney, presentation of evidence by both sides, and privilege against self-incrimination (the right to refrain from saying anything that may make one seem ill). The burden of proof is placed on the petitioner to establish the reason for commitment, and the patient is guaranteed the right to appeal. These requirements contribute to the tension between the individual's legally protected rights and the desire of society to provide necessary mental health treatment.

In general, the case for commitment is made by an attorney representing the state to a magistrate, who makes a decision to commit to inpatient care when the evidence presented is "clear and convincing," a standard generally thought of as the level of proof needed for three of four reasonable people to agree. The judicial decision is intended to favor the best interests of the patient by providing for treatment of the person's mental illness by court order. In all but three states (Iowa, New Hampshire, Kansas), the committed person retains the right to refuse treatment despite being ordered into a hospital. Some facilities and jurisdictions allow for physician reviewers to override patient wishes, while others stipulate that the patient must be found legally incompetent and appointed a guardian before treatment can proceed outside the emergency situation. Psychiatrists find this situation particularly frustrating and ironic; an ill and dangerous person may be involuntarily hospitalized and under their care, yet they are powerless to provide needed treatment.

Much litigation has concerned the right of civilly committed patients to refuse psychotropic medication in nonemergency situations. Antipsychotic medication has been the major focus of this litigation because of the potential risk of serious side effects such as tardive dyskinesia. Although the risks of treatment differ among these drugs (second-generation antipsychotics are associated with lower risk of tardive dyskinesia), some courts have emphasized the potential risk of treatment rather than its potential benefits. In some courts, treatment with antipsychotic medication has been elevated to the status of an "extraordinary" form of medical treatment requiring special scrutiny. In some states, a patient retains the right to refuse medication until the medical treatment team has petitioned the local court to declare the patient incompetent to consent to or refuse medication. In other states, such as Iowa, psychiatrists are allowed to provide mental health treatment (including medication) to patients after a commitment order is issued.

When should the clinician decide to involuntarily hospitalize a patient? In the most typical scenario, a law enforcement officer brings a person thought to be mentally ill to an emergency department because the person was behaving in a bizarre manner or threatened suicide. The psychiatrist is then contacted and asked to assess the individual and to make an appropriate decision about disposition. When the person is deemed mentally ill, dangerous, and/or disabled and refuses hospitalization, the decision is relatively easy to make: the magistrate is contacted, and an order for involuntary hospitalization is requested. From the physician's perspective, it is probably better to err on the side of safety than to allow someone who is potentially dangerous to self or others to leave the emergency department.

Another common scenario occurs when a patient admitted voluntarily requests discharge but is believed to present an ongoing danger to self or others (e.g., a person who has admitted to having suicidal plans). In these situations, a court order should be sought for continued hospitalization.

In addition to involuntary inpatient treatment, most states (41 out of 50) have provisions for involuntary outpatient treatment. Such treatment may be used when the patient is not quite ill enough to merit inpatient care, but presents some risk of harm to self or others because of mental illness and will not voluntarily comply with outpatient treatment. Outpatient commitments can be enormously helpful in improving treatment compliance and reducing the frequency of hospitalization in patients who are otherwise chronically noncompliant. Enforcement is unfortunately limited in most states.

Confidentiality

Maintaining confidentiality is one of the most important ethical and legal obligations that psychiatrists have to their patients. From the time of Hippocrates, physicians have believed that what passes between doctor and patient should remain private and should not be divulged without the patient's consent. Because psychiatrists gather more sensitive information than many medical practitioners, disclosure could be socially embarrassing or harmful and could discourage patients from seeking care. As a practical matter, what this means is that before information is given to a third party, the patient must provide written consent except when disclosure is required by regulation or law.

The U.S. government, recognizing the importance of confidentiality of patient records, devised the Health Insurance Portability and Accountability Act (HIPAA). Under the privacy rule in HIPAA, health care

predict suicide with any acceptable degree of accuracy. Nonetheless, the courts and the public tend to blame psychiatrists for failing to prevent a patient's death. Suicides that occur during hospitalization are probably the ones most likely to result in litigation. This is because suicidal behavior may have been the reason the patient was in the hospital. Potential errors by a psychiatrist include his or her failure to take an adequate history of suicidal behavior, failure to provide adequate protection in the hospital (e.g., one-to-one supervision), or failure to communicate changes in the patient's condition to other doctors and nurses.

Psychiatrists also are sued because of failure to obtain informed consent. Patients may claim that the information provided to them was inadequate, that alternatives were omitted, or that the consent was never obtained. It behooves the clinician to maintain careful records about what happens during an appointment, particularly as it pertains to obtaining consent and providing information. Informed consent should be thought of as an ongoing process, not a slip of paper obtained once.

Psychiatrists are occasionally sued by patients who sustain injuries from psychotropic medications. Situations that have led to claims include failure to disclose relevant information to the patient about adverse effects, failure to obtain an adequate history, and prescription of a drug or drug combination when it is not indicated or when potentially harmful drug interactions might occur. Tardive dyskinesia is an example of an adverse effect that can prompt litigation. Psychiatrists and other prescribers should regularly monitor patients for the presence and severity of side effects such as tardive dyskinesia, and they should educate the patient and family members (or guardian) about the risks of treatment and the continuing need for medication.

Psychiatrists are sometimes sued for abandonment, defined as improperly terminating a doctor–patient relationship despite the continuing need for treatment. Abandonment can give rise to actions for both negligence and breach of contract. Termination may occur because a patient fails to cooperate with treatment, fails to pay bills, threatens or assaults the psychiatrist, or presents a difficult management problem. To avoid litigation, the best course is to notify the patient in writing and provide sufficient time for the patient to find another psychiatrist.

Claims involving ECT are relatively rare but do occur and involve allegations of failure to obtained informed consent, inappropriate or improper treatment, or injury resulting from treatment, such as memory loss. Liability can be minimized by using ECT in accordance with accepted practice standards and monitoring and supervising patients carefully between treatments. The consent process should be fully documented and preferably witnessed.

Although relatively rare in practice, sexual activity with current or former patients has become a well-publicized reason for malpractice litigation. Unlike errors in professional judgment, inappropriate sexual behavior with a patient is a voluntary act by a clinician and is therefore both preventable and excluded under most malpractice insurance policies. A psychiatrist may be expelled from professional associations, have his or her license suspended or revoked, and even face criminal charges for such "boundary violations." The American Psychiatric Association has made it clear that sexual contact with current or previous patients is inappropriate and unethical.

■ Criminal Issues

Psychiatrists rarely encounter situations involving criminal law, whereas these may be "bread and butter" issues for their forensically trained peers. The two most common criminal issues that psychiatrists are asked to comment on are *competency to stand trial* and *criminal responsibility*. To receive a fair trial, a person must be able to understand the nature of the charges against him or her, the possible penalty, and the legal issues and procedures. He or she also must be able to work with the attorney in preparing the defense. The presence of a mental illness, even a psychosis, generally does not render the defendant incompetent to stand trial. Competence to stand trial is assumed unless questioned by someone in the court. Once raised, the court generally hears expert testimony by mental health professionals before deciding the issue.

Competence to stand trial is a legal determination, not a medical one. It is determined by a judge according to national standards established by the U.S. Supreme Court in *Dusky v. United States*. When the court determines that the defendant is incompetent to stand trial, the defendant is typically transferred to a psychiatric hospital for treatment focused on restoring him or her to a competent state. Once competency has been restored, the defendant is returned to court to stand trial. Importantly, competence to stand trial refers to the "here and now" assessment of the person's ability to understand the nature of the proceedings and to assist council, regardless of the presence of mental illness.

Criminal responsibility, or culpability for crime, by contrast has to do with the subject's state of mind at the time of a crime (i.e., "there and then"). Under our current system, a crime is considered to occur only when both bad behavior (*actus rea*) and a blameworthy state of mind (*mens rea*) are present. A person may be so mentally ill as to lack this blameworthy state of mind by virtue of his or her disorder. In such a case, a person is said to lack criminal responsibility and is adjudicated as not guilty by reason of insanity. In practice, a successful insanity defense is rare.

Not all states have an insanity defense, and those that do use different standards for determining criminal responsibility. According to the widely accepted *M'Naghten* standard, modifications of which are used in many states, the person seeking the insanity defense must show that he or she had a mental illness that was so symptomatic that it left him or her unable to know the nature and quality of the act or unable to know that the act was wrong at the time of the alleged offense. The rule is named after a case involving Daniel M'Naghten, who in 1843 shot and killed Edward Drummond, private secretary to British Prime Minister Sir Robert Peel, the intended victim. M'Naghten had suffered delusions for many years and believed that he was being persecuted by the Tory party and their leader (Peel).

Even severely symptomatic patients will only rarely meet the insanity standard. Depending on the jurisdiction, other defenses such as diminished capacity and "guilty but mentally ill" may be used. In diminished capacity, the person is said to be unable to form intent to commit the crime he or she was charged with, but may be found guilty of a lesser charge. In the case of guilty but mentally ill, the person is said to lack the capacity to conform his or her behavior to the requirements of the law at the time of the act despite knowing that the act was wrong. Defendants found "guilty but mentally ill" are usually sentenced to correctional facilities and receive a psychiatric evaluation and appropriate treatment if indicated.

Key points to remember about legal issues

1. In seeking involuntary hospitalization for a patient, there must be evidence of a treatable mental illness, imminent harm to self or others, or grave disability.

   - The psychiatrist should become familiar with the local and state laws.

   - The psychiatrist should know the local judge or magistrate who handles civil commitments.

   - Outpatient commitments are useful in seriously mentally ill patients who are chronically noncompliant with treatment.

Key points to remember about legal issues *(continued)*

2. The psychiatrist should understand applicable state laws on confidentiality and informed consent.

3. Breaching confidentiality under the *Tarasoff* rule may involve contacting the threatened third party.

4. Malpractice lawsuits are common in our litigious society; adequate insurance is essential.

   • The best defense against successful claims of malpractice is to maintain proper documentation.

5. Most psychiatrists do not routinely conduct competency evaluations to determine whether a patient can stand trial. Psychiatrists should get to know their forensic psychiatrist peers.

■ Self-Assessment Questions

1. What is forensic psychiatry?

2. What are the three main categories of legal issues psychiatrists face?

3. What are the major concepts that most civil commitment laws contain?

4. Explain both the right to treatment and the right to refuse treatment. Why is the latter so frustrating to psychiatrists?

5. Explain the *Tarasoff* ruling and the duty to protect. How might the ruling be implemented?

6. Why is confidentiality important? List several situations in which it can (or must) be breached.

7. What are the usual reasons behind malpractice lawsuits filed against psychiatrists?

8. Can a psychotic patient be competent to stand trial?

9. Who was Daniel M'Naghten? Explain the *M'Naghten* standard.

apy works, a substantial empirical base has confirmed the effectiveness of these treatments. For some disorders (e.g., eating disorders) they are first-line treatments, and they have been repeatedly shown to produce good outcomes. For many other disorders (e.g., schizophrenia, mood and anxiety disorders), they have been shown to be an important adjunct to medications by encouraging treatment adherence, educating patients about symptoms and expected outcome, and providing insight or support to deal with the psychological consequences of having a severe illness.

In this chapter, we provide a brief overview of the major classes of psychotherapy that are used by specialists who care for mentally ill patients. Some of these treatments require extensive experience and training on a scale that is outside the range of description of a single chapter. Students who want to explore specific types of psychotherapy in more detail may want to read material cited in the Bibliography. The various psychotherapies include behavior therapy, cognitive-behavioral therapy (CBT), the individual psychotherapies that draw on psychodynamic principles, group therapy, couples and family therapy, and social skills training. The major classes are summarized in Table 19–1.

■ Behavior Therapy

The theoretical underpinnings of behavior therapy derive from British empiricism, Pavlov's studies of conditioning, and subsequent research on stimulus-response relationships conducted by other leading behaviorists such as B. F. Skinner. Behaviorists stress the importance of working with objective, observable phenomena, usually referred to as *behavior,* including physical activities such as eating, drinking, talking, and completing the serial-sequential activities that lead to habit formations and patterns of social interactions. In contrast to psychodynamic psychotherapies, discussed later in this chapter, behavioral techniques do not necessarily help patients to understand their emotions or motivations. Instead of working on thoughts and feelings, the behavior therapist works on *what the patient does.* Indeed, some clinicians who use behavioral approaches argue that changing a patient's behavior may lead to substantial changes in how the patient thinks and feels and that correcting pathological behavior may be more effective than correcting pathological emotions. The motto for this approach is "Change the behavior, and the feelings will follow."

Behavior therapies are particularly helpful for disorders that are associated with abnormal behavioral patterns in need of correction. These

TABLE 19–1. Types of psychotherapy

Behavior therapy

Cognitive-behavioral therapy (CBT)

Individual therapy
  Classical psychoanalysis
  Psychodynamic psychotherapy
  Insight-oriented psychotherapy
  Relationship psychotherapy
  Interpersonal therapy (IPT)
  Supportive psychotherapy

Group therapy

Couples therapy

Family therapy

Social skills training

disorders include alcohol and drug abuse, eating disorders, anxiety disorders, phobias, and obsessive-compulsive behavior. A general knowledge of the principles of behaviorism may be useful in dealing with a broad range of patients, however, including patients with dementias, psychoses, adjustment disorders, childhood disorders, and personality disorders.

The concept of *conditioning* is fundamental to the various behavior therapies. Two types of conditioning have been described: classical (Pavlovian) and operant. Early in the twentieth century, the Russian physiologist Pavlov described the first controlled experiments with conditioning. He demonstrated that by pairing stimuli, such as striking a bell at the same time that dogs were given food, he could eventually produce a conditioned reflex in the animals in the absence of the original triggering stimulus. For example, if the two stimuli (food and the ringing of a bell) were paired frequently enough, the dog would eventually learn to salivate when it heard the bell alone. In this model, the food is regarded as the unconditioned stimulus, the bell as the conditioned stimulus, and salivation in response to the bell the conditioned reflex.

The concept of stimulus pairing can be used both to explain the development of psychopathology and to create behavior therapies through conditioning patients to alter their response patterns.

The study and use of *operant conditioning* involves examining behavior that can control its consequences. For example, a pigeon will increase the frequency of pecking a bar if the pecking behavior is rapidly followed by a food pellet. The food pellet is the reinforcer; the behavior of pecking is increased as a consequence of the reinforcer following the pecking. Behavior may either increase or decrease in frequency, depending on whether the subsequent reinforcers are positive or negative. Praise by a teacher is likely to increase the rate at which a student will raise a hand in response to questions. By contrast, the same student might terminate hand raising in anticipation of critical comments by the teacher. For example, *negative reinforcement* occurs when a child has tantrums following her father's command to "turn off the TV and come to dinner." If the father does not follow through on the command, he has inadvertently negatively reinforced the child's tendency to throw tantrums. In other words, the child is likely to have tantrums more frequently in the future upon hearing a parental command, because such tantrums have been followed by withdrawal of an undesirable command. Operant conditioning is the source of much of the adaptive human learning that occurs during a person's interaction with his or her surrounding environment.

An extensive behavioral literature now suggests that positive reinforcement is more effective in sustaining behavior than negative reinforcement, that failure to provide reinforcements usually will extinguish a behavior, and that variable and unpredictable schedules of reinforcement may be more effective in maintaining behavior than fixed, regular reinforcements. For example, pathological gamblers receive the positive reinforcement of winning only occasionally, but they continue to gamble and are rarely deterred by threats of punishment or even by punishment itself, such as loss of their financial assets or even incarceration. If they won every time they gambled, they would very likely lose interest eventually, and likewise, they would lose interest if they never won at all.

Relaxation Training

Relaxation training is used to teach patients control over their bodies and mental states. Through this procedure, patients learn how to achieve voluntary control over their feelings of tension and relaxation. Relaxation training can be done simply by providing patients with an instructional audio recording that they can listen to in order to practice the techniques on their own. A common form is called *progressive muscle relaxation,* wherein the person is instructed to systematically proceed through each major muscle group, learning to tense and then relax the muscles. Relaxation training can be used alone to help patients who have anxiety or various problems involving pain (e.g., headache, low back pain), or the training can be used in conjunction with systematic desensitization.

Exposure

One of the key principles of behaviorally oriented treatments is that of exposure. Exposure requires that patients place themselves in situations that they usually avoid, in the interest of reducing the adaptive difficulties that are part and parcel of their psychiatric disorders. For example, one of the more harmful aspects of panic disorder is the agoraphobic avoidance that commonly occurs. Panic patients frequently avoid situations in which they fear the onset of panic symptoms, usually based on catastrophic interpretations of what would happen if they panicked. It is this avoidance, more than the somatic experiences themselves, that is responsible for the disability associated with this and other anxiety disorders. Exposure seeks to encourage the patient to place him- or herself directly into situations that evoke feared internal and external circumstances so that new learning and improved adaptive functioning will occur and be maintained. For example, the therapist may ask the agoraphobic patient to imagine what it is like to leave his or her house and visit the shopping mall where he or she typically develops panic attacks, thereby leading the patient to experience the panic attack. This is called *imaginal exposure* because it takes place in one's imagination. (The patient is then encouraged to use relaxation techniques to diminish the sensation of panic and place it under voluntary control.) The patient will gradually become able to enter the feared situation—that is, actually go to the shopping mall—and use relaxation techniques while in the feared setting. This is called *in vivo exposure* because exposure involves a real situation. In complex and difficult situations, the therapist may need to lead the patient gradually to a sense of control by developing a hierarchy of stimuli that increasingly approximate the feared stimulus (e.g., moving from imagination to photographs to photographs plus recorded noises and finally to the actual situation itself).

Flooding

Flooding involves teaching patients to extinguish anxiety produced by a feared stimulus through placing them in continuous contact with the stimulus and helping them learn that the stimulus does not in fact lead to any feared consequences. For example, a patient with a disabling fear of riding on airplanes may be forced to take repeated flights until the fear is extinguished. The patient with a fear of snakes may be requested to go to the zoo and stand in front of the snake cage until his or her anxiety is completely gone. (Handling a snake will provide an even greater flooding experience!)

Behavioral Activation

Many psychiatric disorders are characterized by an inflexible narrowing of the patient's behavioral repertoire. Although exposure is indicated for many such problems, *behavioral activation* is particularly well suited to the treatment of depression. Using a behavioral formulation, depression is conceptualized from a negative reinforcement paradigm in which the depressed patient's withdrawal and isolation is seen to be in the service of avoiding feared punishers. For example, depressed patients frequently expect negative, painful outcomes in their daily lives and begin to avoid such outcomes at the cost of losing important daily routines. Behavioral activation, which is also a component of cognitive therapy, seeks to reengage the patient in those activities, big and small, that lead to a rapid restoration of functioning. In turn, and consistent with behavioral theory, mood improves following restoration of important behavioral sequences in daily life, not the other way around.

Behavior Modification Techniques

Behavior modification techniques tend to use the concept of reinforcement as a way of shaping behavior—in particular, to reduce or eliminate undesirable behavior and to replace it with healthier behaviors or habits. Behavior modification techniques are especially appropriate for disorders characterized by poor impulse control, such as alcohol or other substance abuse, eating disorders, and conduct disorders.

Individual programs must be designed to suit the particular patient by using stimuli that are specific positive and negative reinforcers for that individual. For example, the intermediate goal for a patient with anorexia nervosa is weight gain. Long-term goals are to become less preoccupied with food and body image. Patients with anorexia nervosa typically enjoy exercise. A particular patient with anorexia also may enjoy reading mystery novels and chewing gum. A specific program would be developed for such a patient in which she would be provided with three regular, well-balanced meals per day and told that access to her specific preferred pleasures would be contingent on going to the dining room for meals, eating them, and demonstrating a regular pattern of weight gain. A schedule of reinforcers would be developed to encourage her compliance with eating regularly. For example, she might be restricted to her room initially between meals and given no access to exercise, mystery novels, or chewing gum. After she gains 5 pounds, she will be allowed to leave her room. After she gains an additional 5 pounds, she will be given access to mystery novels. After the gain of another 5 pounds, she will be allowed access to chewing gum. After she reaches her desired target weight (involving a total weight gain of 20 pounds), she will be allowed to exercise regularly. To be permitted to continue exercising, however, she must maintain her target weight for 2 weeks while exercising as much as she desires. If her weight drops, positive reinforcers will gradually be removed until the weight gain is reestablished. In such a program, negative reinforcers, such as tube feeding, also may be built in. As mentioned earlier, however, it is well recognized that these negative reinforcers are much less effective than are the positive reinforcers.

Different mixtures of behavior modification techniques are required for different disorders. For example, a program similar to the one just described, but involving a different schedule of reinforcers and different targets, might be appropriate for the obese patient. Behavior modification programs for patients with substance abuse are more likely to stress teaching the patient the various stimuli that tend to trigger his or her craving, such as diminishing the pent-up irritation of a long day at work by dropping by the bar and socializing with friends. The patient would be taught instead to substitute other positive reinforcers in their place, such as dropping by a health club and releasing his or her hostility by hitting a punching bag, followed by drinking copious amounts of his or her favorite nonalcoholic beverage with a new set of friends developed through contacts with Alcoholics Anonymous (AA).

Combining Therapies

Originally, proponents of behavior therapy were purists, and they tended to denigrate mixing behavior therapy with other types of psychotherapy or with the use of medications. Increasingly, various types of therapy are being combined. Thus, the treatment of panic disorder and agoraphobia may involve the use of a selective serotonin reuptake inhibitor (SSRI) along with exposure therapy. Behavior therapy also may be combined with psychodynamic psychotherapy; for example, a patient with anorexia nervosa may benefit from a behavior modification program and from efforts to help her understand the underlying fears that make her seek a bodily appearance that most people find quite unattractive. A patient with comorbid anxiety and depression may benefit from a program of relaxation training, cognitive therapy, and antidepressant medication.

■ Cognitive-Behavioral Therapy

The theoretical support for CBT derives from a variety of sources, including cognitive psychology, Freudian psychodynamic theory, and some aspects of behaviorism. The theory and techniques of CBT have been developed by many key figures in the field. The best known and most widely used of the CBT models was developed by Aaron Beck, whose model is simply referred to as cognitive therapy. The techniques of CBT are based on the assumption that *cognitive structures* or *schemas* shape the way people react and adapt to a variety of situations that they encounter in their lives. An individual's particular cognitive structures derive from a variety of constitutional and experiential factors (e.g., physical appearance, loss of a parent early in life, previous achievements or failures at school or with friends). Each person has his or her own specific set of cognitive structures that determines how he or she will react to any given stressor in any particular situation. A person develops a psychiatric syndrome, such as anxiety or depression, when these schemas become overactive and predispose him or her to developing a pathological or negative response.

The most widespread use of CBT is for the treatment of depression. In this instance, the individual is typically found to have schemas that lead to negative interpretations. Beck designated the three major cognitive patterns observed in depression as the *cognitive triad:* a negative view of oneself, a negative interpretation of experience, and a negative view of the future. Patients with these cognitive patterns are predisposed to react to situations by interpreting them in the light of these three negative sets. For example, a woman who applies for a highly competitive job and does not receive it, and whose perceptions are shaped by such negative sets, may conclude, "I didn't get it because I'm not really bright, in spite of my good school record, and the employer was able to figure that out" (negative view of self); "Trying to find a decent job is so hopeless that I might as well just give up trying" (negative view of experience); and "I'm always going to be a failure. I'll never succeed at anything" (negative view of the future).

The techniques of CBT focus on teaching patients new ways to change these pathological schemas. CBT tends to be relatively short-term and highly structured. Its goal is to help patients restructure their negative cognitions so that they can perceive reality in a less distorted way and learn to react accordingly.

The actual practice of CBT combines a group of behavioral techniques with a group of cognitive restructuring techniques. The behavioral techniques include a variety of homework assignments and a graded program of activities designed to teach patients that their negative schemas are incorrect and that they are in fact able to achieve small successes and interpret them as such.

For example, the woman described above who failed to obtain the job might be asked to keep a record of her daily activities during the course of a week. Together, the therapist and patient would then review this diary and (in the context of other information about her) develop a set of assignments to be completed during the ensuing week. The diary of activities might indicate a very limited range of social contacts, based on the patient's fear and expectation of rejection. The patient might be assigned to make at least five social contacts during the course of the week by talking to neighbors, phoning friends, and going out on at least one social engagement. These activities also would be recorded in a diary and reviewed the following week with the therapist, including the patient's notes about her responses to the various contacts. She would be helped to see that she tended to initiate each contact with a negative hypothesis or expectation that typically was disconfirmed by her actual experience. In fact, the contacts were largely affirmative. As therapy progressed and her confidence built, the assignments would gradually be made more difficult, until the patient achieved an essentially normal level of behavior and expectation. The diary would serve as a comforting reminder to the patient that based on experience, negative hypotheses are typically disconfirmed. The patient would, of course, have some negative experiences; the therapist then would assist her in understanding that such negative experiences are not a consequence of her own deficiencies and that even negative experiences can be surmounted.

These behavioral techniques are complemented with a variety of cognitive techniques that help the patient identify and correct the dysfunctional schemas that shape the patient's perception of reality. These techniques involve identifying a variety of cognitive distortions that the patient is prone to make and *automatic thoughts* that intrude into the patient's consciousness and produce negative attitudes. Six typical cognitive distortions, identified by Beck, are listed in Table 19–2.

Arbitrary inference involves drawing an erroneous conclusion from an experience. For example, if the patient's hairdresser suggests that she may want to try a new hairstyle, the patient assumes that the hairdresser believes that the patient is becoming older-appearing and unattractive. *Selective abstraction* involves taking a detail out of context and using it to denigrate the entire experience. For example, while playing tennis, the patient may hit the ball out of the court, losing it in a grassy area, and reach the conclusion "That just proves I'm a lousy tennis player." *Overgeneralization* involves making general conclusions about overall experiences and relationships based on a single interaction. For example, after a disagreement with another employee at his or her current (less desirable) job, the patient concludes, "I'm a failure. I can't get along with anybody." *Magnification and minimization* involve altering the significance of specific small events in a way that is structured by negative interpretations. For example, the significance of a success may be minimized (a good grade on an examination is considered trivial because the examination was easy), and the significance of a failure may be maximized (losing a tennis game is seen as indicating that the patient will never succeed at anything). *Personalization* involves interpreting events as reflecting on the patient when they in fact have no specific relation to him or her. For example, a frown from a grouchy traffic policeman is seen as recognition of the patient's overall lack of skill as a driver and general worthlessness. *Dichotomous thinking* represents a tendency to see things in an all-or-none way. For example, an A– student with high expectations receives a B in a course and concludes, "That just proves it. I'm really a terrible student after all."

In addition to these erroneous interpretations, patients are often troubled with a variety of automatic thoughts that spontaneously intrude into their flow of consciousness. The specific automatic thoughts vary from one individual to another but involve negative themes of self-denigration and failure (e.g., "You're so stupid," "You never do anything right," "People wouldn't want to talk to you"). These thoughts intrude spontaneously and produce an accompanying dysphoria. Patients are encouraged to identify these automatic thoughts and to learn ways to counteract them. Such techniques include replacing the automatic thoughts with positive counterthoughts, testing the hypotheses embedded in the thoughts through behavioral techniques as described earlier, and identifying and testing the assumptions behind the thoughts.

The goal of the cognitive component of CBT is to identify and restructure the various negative schemas that shape the patient's per-

TABLE 19-2. Typical cognitive distortions treated through cognitive-behavioral therapy

Distortion	Definition
Arbitrary inference	Drawing an erroneous conclusion from an experience
Selective abstraction	Taking a detail out of context and using it to denigrate the entire experience
Overgeneralization	Making general conclusions about overall experiences and relationships based on a single instance
Magnification and minimization	Altering the significance of specific events in a way that is structured by negative interpretations
Personalization	Interpreting events as reflecting on the patient when they have no relation to him or her
Dichotomous thinking	Seeing things in an all-or-none way

ceptions. The cognitive goal is achieved like the behavioral goals: the patient is encouraged to do homework, to complete assignments that identify the occurrence of dysfunctional cognitions, and to steadily test and correct these cognitions. The therapist also reviews these aspects of the patient's diary and helps formulate an organized program for restructuring the dysfunctional cognitive sets, providing ample empathy and positive reinforcement.

CBT is particularly effective for patients with depression, although its techniques have also been adapted to treat various anxiety disorders through identifying cognitive schemas characterized by fear. It may be used either alone for the treatment of relatively mild disorders or in conjunction with medications for patients with more severe disorders.

■ Individual Psychotherapy

The term *individual psychotherapy* covers a broad range of psychotherapeutic techniques. Both behavior therapy and cognitive therapy usually are done individually (i.e., a single therapist working with a single patient). Countless schools of psychotherapy offer a variety of approaches. The description that follows provides a simplified and selective overview.

The various psychotherapies share some common elements. These include the following, which are characteristic of all psychotherapies:

- Based on an interpersonal relationship
- Use of verbal communication between two (or more) people as a healing element
- Specific expertise on the part of the therapist in using communication and relationships in a healing way
- Based on a rationale or conceptual structure that is used to understand the patient's problems
- Use of a specific procedure in the relationship that is linked to the rationale
- Structured relationship (e.g., contact time, frequency, and duration are prespecified)
- Expectation of improvement

Classical Psychoanalysis and Psychodynamic Psychotherapy

Psychoanalysis was originally developed by Sigmund Freud during the early twentieth century. This technique arose from Freud's experience in attempting to treat patients with hysterical conversion symptoms, such as pains and paralyses. Following the lead of Charcot, his initial efforts involved the use of hypnosis. He observed, however, that this treatment was not always effective and that there was a high recurrence and relapse rate. He began to suspect that these conversion symptoms reflected some sort of painful early psychological experience that had been repressed. Instead of hypnosis, he began to experiment with the technique of having the patient lie down and relax while he placed his hand on the person's forehead to help "release" the repressed thoughts. The patient was instructed to "Talk about whatever comes into your mind." This technique was called *free association.*

This treatment developed at a time when Victorian puritanism and hypocrisy still reigned supreme, and even Freud must have been astonished at the thoughts that flowed from his patients' minds, covering a variety of sexual fantasies and experiences. Based on his many years of experience in applying this approach, initially to conversion symptoms but subsequently to a range of symptoms including anxiety disorders and even psychoses, Freud developed a systematic theory to describe the structure and operations of the human psyche. Basic concepts include stages of psychosexual development (oral, anal, phallic, and genital), the structure of conscious and unconscious thoughts (primary vs. secondary process thinking), the structure of drives and motivations (id, ego, and superego), the symbolism inherent in dreams, theories of infant sexuality, and a host of other concepts that the layperson associates with Freudianism.

Subsequent psychoanalysts elaborated and modified Freud's original work in various ways, such as developing theories of ego psychology and expanding understanding of the mental mechanisms involved in defense, coping, and adaptation. These various ideas and theories are major resources for clinicians trained in either psychoanalysis or psychodynamic psychotherapy. Use of these approaches requires extensive experience and training.

Classical psychoanalysis is now used only in relatively special situations and settings. The form of treatment is best adapted to individuals who are fundamentally healthy (both psychologically and financially) and who have sufficient adaptive resources to go through the intensive process of self-scrutiny required by psychoanalysis. Typical reasons for seeking psychoanalysis include difficulties in relationships and persistent and recurrent anxiety, although neither should be so severe as to be incapacitating.

The core component of classical psychoanalysis is the development of a *transference neurosis*. That is, the patient transfers to the therapist all the thoughts and feelings that he or she experienced during early life; through this transference, he or she is able to make conscious the various unconscious drives and emotions that are troubling him or her and ultimately to modify and heal them as the analyst makes appropriate interpretations during the course of the psychoanalysis.

The patient is typically asked to lie on a couch and to free-associate, saying whatever comes into his or her mind without any type of censorship. The analyst sits behind the patient, remaining a relatively shadowy and neutral figure to encourage the development of transference. (If the analyst becomes too human or "real," then transference cannot develop.) To maintain an appropriate level of intensity, the patient must be seen four to five times per week for 50-minute sessions. The process typically requires 2–3 years. Analysts must go through an extensive period of psychoanalysis themselves to understand their own psychological vulnerabilities and, in particular, the nature of the countertransference that they are likely to develop in relation to their patients.

Psychodynamic psychotherapy uses many of the concepts embodied in psychoanalytic theory, but these concepts are used in ways that make them more suitable for the treatment of larger numbers of patients. Treatment is not necessarily less intensive, in the sense of attempting to focus on and correct problems, but it does not involve the relatively rigidly defined techniques (e.g., use of the couch) that characterize classical psychoanalysis.

Psychodynamic psychotherapy is used to treat patients with a variety of problems, including personality disorders, sexual dysfunctions, somatoform disorders, anxiety disorders, and mild depression. Psychodynamic psychotherapy is typically conducted face to face. Depending on the frequency and duration of therapy, a transference neurosis may or may not occur. The therapist attempts to help the patient in a neutral but empathic way. The patient is encouraged to review early relationships with parents and significant others but also may focus on the here and now. As in classical psychoanalysis, the patient is expected to do most of the talking, while the psychodynamic psychotherapist occasionally interjects clarifications to help the patient understand the underlying dynamics that shape his or her behavior. Psychodynamic psychotherapy typically involves sessions one or two times a week and may involve 2–5 years of treatment.

Insight-Oriented and Relationship Psychotherapy

Insight-oriented psychotherapy and relationship psychotherapy are two other variants of individual psychotherapy that may be somewhat less intensive or long-term.

Insight-oriented psychotherapy draws on many basic psychodynamic concepts but focuses even more on interpersonal relationships and here-and-now situations than does purely psychodynamic psychotherapy. Patients are typically seen once a week for 50 minutes. During the sessions they are encouraged to review and discuss relationships, attitudes toward themselves, and early life experiences. The therapist maintains an involved and supportive attitude and occasionally assists patients with interpretations that will help them achieve insights. This form of psychotherapy does not encourage transference, regression, and abreaction. Instead of re-experiencing and reliving, patients are encouraged to achieve an intellectual understanding of the mainsprings of their behavior that will help them change their behavior as needed.

In *relationship psychotherapy*, the therapist assumes a more active role. The stress is on achieving a corrective emotional experience, with the therapist serving as a loving and trustworthy surrogate parent who assists the patient in confronting unrecognized needs and unresolved drives. The patient is typically seen once per week, and the therapy may last from 6 months to several years, depending on the patient's problems and level of maturity. As in insight-oriented psychotherapy, the content of the sessions focuses primarily on current situations and relationships, with some looking backward to early life experiences. Although the patient may achieve insight, the most important component of this type of psychotherapy is the empathic and caring attitude of the therapist.

Interpersonal Therapy

Interpersonal therapy (IPT) is a specific type of psychotherapy that was developed for the treatment of depression, although it is also potentially useful for the treatment of other conditions, such as personality disorders. Drawing on the ideas of thinkers such as Harry Stack Sullivan, who stressed that mental illnesses may reflect and be expressed in problems in relationships (as opposed to intrapsychic conflict, stressed by psychodynamic approaches), IPT emphasizes working on improving interpersonal relationships during the process of psychotherapy.

During IPT, the emphasis is on the present rather than on the past. During a process of exploration, the therapist helps the patient identify specific problem areas that may be interfering with self-esteem and interpersonal interactions. These usually involve four general domains: grief, interpersonal disputes, role transitions, and interpersonal deficits. After the exploration and identification process, the therapist works systematically with the patient to facilitate the learning of new adaptive behaviors and communication styles.

IPT is usually conducted in weekly sessions, and the overall course of therapy lasts 3 or 4 months. Rigorous empirical testing of its efficacy shows it to be effective for both acute and maintenance treatment of depression. IPT also has been used with some success in treating depressed adolescents and persons with bulimia.

Supportive Psychotherapy

Supportive psychotherapy is used to help patients get through difficult situations. Components of supportive psychotherapy may be incorporated into any of the other types of psychotherapy described in this section, with the exception of classical psychoanalysis.

In conducting supportive psychotherapy, the therapist maintains an attitude of sympathy, interest, and concern. Patients describe and discuss the various problems they are confronting, which could range from marital discord to psychotic experiences such as persecutory delusions. Supportive psychotherapy is appropriate for the full spectrum of psychiatric disorders, ranging from adjustment disorders through the psychoses and even dementia.

As in relationship psychotherapy, the therapist may function much like a healthy and loving parent who provides the patient with encouragement and direction as needed. The goal of supportive therapy is to help the patient cope with difficult situations, experiences, or periods of adjustment. Patients typically describe their problems, and the therapist counters with encouragement and even specific advice. The therapist may suggest specific techniques that patients can use in coping with their problems, such as developing new interests or hobbies, trying new activities that may expand their range of social contacts, achieving emancipation from their parents by moving into independent living circumstances, and developing more organized study habits to improve their school performance. Psychotic patients may be taught to refrain from discussing their delusional ideas, except with the therapist. Alcoholic patients may receive praise and encouragement for refraining from drinking as well as suggestions about ways to increase their self-esteem by achieving mastery and control, such as through improving their skills in a particular sport or developing a new creative hobby. As these examples indicate, the clinician involved in conducting supportive therapy needs to tailor the therapy sessions to the individual needs of each particular patient.

■ Group Therapy

Group therapy provides a highly effective way for clinicians to follow up with and monitor relatively large numbers of patients. It also provides patients with a social environment or even surrogate peer group that will help them learn new and constructive ways to interact with others in a controlled and supportive environment.

Irving Yalom, one of the major leaders of the group therapy movement in the United States, enumerated a variety of factors that summarize the therapeutic mechanisms that occur during the process of group therapy. These include instilling hope, developing socializing skills, using imitative behavior, experiencing catharsis, imparting information, behaving altruistically by attempting to help other members of the group, experiencing a corrective recapitulation of the primary family group, developing a sense of group cohesiveness, diminishing feelings of isolation (universality), and learning through feedback how one's behavior affects others (interpersonal learning).

There are many different kinds of group therapy. The types vary depending on the individuals who compose the group, the problems or disorders that they are confronting, the setting in which the group meets, the type of role that the group leader takes, and the therapeutic goals that have been established.

Group therapy programs have been established in many hospitals for psychiatric inpatients. These groups are typically led by a physician, a nurse, a social worker, or some combination thereof. In very large inpatient hospital settings, several groups may run concurrently and be composed of patients with similar types of problems. For example, one group might consist of patients with severe mood and psychotic disorders, and another group might consist of individuals with eating disorders. Such groups provide patients with a forum to share their problems, diminish their sense of isolation and loneliness, enable them to learn new techniques to cope with their problems either through other patients or through the group leader, and provide support, inspiration, and hope. Such groups also may help patients improve interpersonal and social skills. For example, patients with schizophrenia and other psychoses may improve their skills in relating to others. In many clinical settings, such inpatient groups are supplemented by outpatient or aftercare groups in which patients receive continued follow-up, pursuing goals similar to those described earlier but in the more stressful environment of the real world. These outpatient groups represent an attempt to consolidate and support the learning and skills that have already been developed in the inpatient setting.

Some groups are oriented largely toward providing support. Such groups may or may not have a professional leader. Examples of such support groups include AA meetings, family support groups such as those organized by chapters of the National Alliance on Mental Illness (an organization composed of the family members of patients with serious mental illnesses), support groups for individuals who conceive of themselves as minorities in a particular setting (e.g., women professionals, women medical students, black students), groups composed of military veterans, or groups composed of individuals who have experienced some serious medical illness or difficult surgery (e.g., patients with diabetes, women who have had mastectomies, individuals receiving dialysis). Such groups provide a forum for sharing information, giving encouragement and support, and instilling hope through diminishing feelings of isolation.

Group psychotherapy may also be done as an alternative to individual psychotherapy. Groups are typically led by experienced therapists and are often conducted with a co-therapist. These groups aim to achieve goals similar to those of insight-oriented and interpersonal psychotherapy or cognitive therapy within the context of a group setting. Psychotherapy groups are typically more highly structured than the other types of groups described earlier. The group leaders take an active role in organizing each session, often prescribe exercises within the session, establish ground rules for membership within the group (e.g., no tardiness, regular attendance), resolve conflicts between members of the group, and assume responsibility for providing summaries of each session and access to videos of the sessions. Patients are typically carefully screened before being admitted to a psychotherapy group to ensure that they will be able to participate effectively. Such groups are particularly helpful for individuals with the same type of problems that led them into individual psychotherapy, such as interpersonal and relationship problems, anxiety, mild depression, and personality disorders.

■ Couples Therapy

Couples therapy involves working with two people who see themselves as partners in a committed relationship to help them stabilize and improve their relationship. This therapy once involved seeing a husband and wife. In contemporary society, the partners seeking treatment may be unmarried, gay, or lesbian. Depending on the commitment of the two partners, couples therapy has many variations. Ideally, both partners are willing and cooperative participants who are anxious to initiate change. Sometimes, however, couples therapy is sought because of a crisis: one of the partners may have lost interest in the relationship (and may or may not want to get out), whereas the other is hanging on tight and trying to save the relationship. In the latter instance, one possible outcome might be the eventual decision to end the relationship, and therapy might become divorce mediation and counseling. If children are involved, then what began as couples therapy might turn into family therapy as the couple attempts to work out an equitable arrangement in the context of the larger number of people who will be affected. In some instances, a dysfunctional sexual relationship between the couple will become apparent, and the couple may want referral to a sex therapy clinic for treatment of impotence or anorgasmia.

An individual conducting couples therapy must take care to maintain an atmosphere of fairness, neutrality, and impartiality. Either partner will be particularly sensitive to the possibility that the therapist may take sides and treat him or her unfairly. The therapist's gender may seem quite significant to either partner, even though the therapist may feel quite comfortable with his or her ability to be impartial. Women may believe that only a female therapist is able to understand their point of view and may feel quite defensive if asked to work with a male therapist. Male partners may have similar attitudes or problems.

Couples counseling typically begins with identifying the specific problem. Each partner is asked to identify specific areas in which he or she would like to see change in the other. The therapist attempts to assist the couple in implementing changes in a gradual, graded way, attacking one problem at a time. Typically, in the early sessions, a single, salient problem is the focus of attention. For example, a wife may express feelings of being ignored, whereas a husband may complain of his wife's whining expressions of dependency. Each will identify specific target behaviors in the other that need modification. They then contract with each other to modify these behaviors. Subsequent sessions focus on the steps they have taken to achieve improvement and on continuing work in new areas of concern.

This type of graded behavior change is the minimum component of couples therapy. Often couples also benefit from discussing their hopes for and expectations of each other in the context of personal values, prior family experiences (i.e., role expectations about men and women, based on the behavior of their own parents), changing social norms about the roles of men and women, and needs for both intimacy and independence that occur within the context of a relationship.

■ Family Therapy

Family therapy tends to focus on the larger family unit—at a minimum, one parent and the child (in single-parent families), but more typically both parents and the child (or a parent and stepparent, two separated parents, other parental pairings depending on the family environment in which the child lives), or one or more parents and the child plus siblings. Typically, the child is brought in initially for treatment of a specific problem, such as school difficulties, hyperactivity, delinquency, or aggressive behavior. Often, it rapidly becomes clear that these problems exist in the overall context of the family setting. The family should not necessarily be regarded as dysfunctional, however. Because of changing circumstances or demands (e.g., a recent move), the parents may have difficulty in determining methods for coping with the child's behavior or understanding why it is occurring.

As in couples therapy, it is important for the therapist to be fair and impartial in family therapy. In this instance, however, the therapist is not dealing with two potential equals but rather with a hierarchy in which parents are expected to assume some authority and responsibility for the behavior of their child. The degree of hierarchy in the family will vary depending on the age of the child. For adolescents and teenagers, one important problem may be the challenge that the "child's" growing independence is adding to this hierarchical structure.

As in couples therapy, behavioral approaches are a mainstay of family therapy. The therapist usually begins by focusing on here-and-now problems. Parents and child discuss openly the nature of the problem that has brought about the need for therapy. For example, a 12-year-old boy may be intermittently truant from school, tell lies about his activities, and seek out parties on the weekends, where he has been known to drink beer occasionally. The child may complain of parental pressure and repeated criticism, whereas the parents may express their fears about the child's unreliability and poor school performance. As in couples therapy, graded areas of priority are identified, and contracts are made about changes that both parents and child will implement. Parents are given tactful but explicit suggestions about the value of positive reinforcement instead of criticism as a way of modifying behavior, and the child is led to realize that some hierarchy and structure will remain in his or her life, although to a gradually lessening degree as he or she shows mature and dependable behavior.

Family therapy also may be used to help families in which at least one member has a relatively serious mental illness, such as schizophrenia, bipolar disorder, or recurrent depression. In this type of family therapy, it is important to work firmly within the medical model and to emphasize that the patient has an illness for which neither the patient nor the family can be considered responsible. This approach minimizes guilt, scapegoating, and castigation, and it permits both patient and family members to seek more consoling and constructive methods for coping with the symptoms of the illness. A young schizophrenic patient living at home may need some assistance from his or her family in developing social skills (see the next section, "Social Skills Training," in this chapter), whereas family members may need assistance in learning ways to cope with outbursts of anger or periods of emotional disengagement and withdrawal. Families with high levels of involvement (referred to as high "expressed emotion") may need counseling on ways to be less intensely involved because it has been shown that in some instances, high levels of expressed emotion may be experienced as stressful by the schizophrenic patient and lead to relapse. Thus families may need assistance in finding the right balance between providing needed support and encouragement and setting up excessively high expectations. Education about the symptoms of the illness is also an important component of family therapy for both the patient and the family members.

■ Social Skills Training

Social skills training is a specific type of psychotherapy that focuses primarily on developing abilities in relating to others and in coping with the demands of daily life. It is used primarily for patients with severe mental illnesses, such as schizophrenia, which are often accompanied by marked impairments in social skills.

Social skills training may be done initially on an inpatient basis, but the bulk of the effort is typically done with outpatients because the long-term goal of social skills training is to assist patients in learning to live in the real world. Social skills training is typically done by nurses, social workers, or psychologists. It may be done individually, but it more typically is accompanied by some group work as well, and it may occur in the context of day hospitals or sheltered workshops.

The techniques of social skills training also are primarily behavioral. Specific problems are identified and addressed in a sequentially integrated manner. Severely disabled patients may need assistance initially in grooming and hygiene. They may need encouragement in learning to shave or bathe daily, to keep their clothes laundered, and to eat regular meals. They also may need help in learning how to approach other people and to talk with them appropriately. At higher levels of functioning, they may need assistance in learning how to apply for a job, complete job interviews, and relate to employers and coworkers. Because long-term institutional care is no longer available to most patients with psychotic illnesses, these individuals are literally being forced to learn to live in the community. Many cannot do so without receiving training and assistance in activities of daily living, such as grooming, managing money, and achieving at least a minimal level of social interaction with others. Although the development of such skills may seem elementary or minimal, for some patients it can lead to a substantial improvement in their quality of life.

Key points to remember about psychotherapy

1. Psychotherapy is a key component of comprehensive psychiatric care.

   - Psychotherapy is a first-line treatment for many disorders (e.g., eating disorders).

   - Psychotherapy is an important treatment adjunct for many patients taking psychotropic medication.

   - Combined treatment (psychotherapy plus psychotropic medication) tends to produce the best outcomes.

2. There are many different types of psychotherapy, but most share similar elements including the development of a personal relationship with the therapist, using communication and relationships in a healing way, and conveying a sense of hope and expectation for improvement.

3. With behavioral therapy, the motto is "Change the behavior, and the feelings will follow."

4. CBT aims to change (or restructure) maladaptive cognitive schemas. Through homework and graded exercises, the patient learns to counter negative thoughts and behaviors that tend to promote and maintain psychiatric disorders, such as major depression.

5. Psychodynamic psychotherapies focus on the patient's relationships, attitudes toward himself or herself, and early life experiences. The goal is to help the patient achieve insight into the development and persistence of his or her symptoms and behaviors in order to bring about needed change.

6. Supportive therapy is commonly used to help patients get through difficult times by providing sympathy, encouragement, and even specific advice. This approach is within reach of *all* physicians, not just psychiatrists.

7. Group therapy is an efficient way to deliver care to many patients at once. It provides a surrogate peer group in which patients can learn new ways to interact with others in a controlled environment.

8. Couples and family therapies focus on either a dyad (the couple) or the larger family unit to address specific problems. In either situation, it is essential for the therapist to maintain an atmosphere of fairness, neutrality, and impartiality.

■ Self-Assessment Questions

1. What is the difference between classical conditioning and operant conditioning?

2. What is a positive reinforcer? A negative reinforcer?

3. Describe behavioral activation. How might this be useful with depressed patients?

4. Describe four common techniques for conducting behavior therapy.

5. Describe CBT. What is the cognitive triad? What are automatic thoughts?

6. Describe classical psychoanalysis. How does it differ from psychodynamic psychotherapy? What is transference?

7. Describe two different types of group therapy, and enumerate some situations in which they would be appropriate.

8. Describe the role of the therapist in couples therapy and family therapy.

had powerful calming effects on agitated psychotic patients. Not only were agitated patients calmed, but the new drug seemed to diminish their terrifying hallucinations and troubling delusions. Many antipsychotics have since been developed and marketed, and while they are not curative, improvement can be dramatic. Medication effectiveness is generally sustained over years or even decades.

The antipsychotics can be roughly broken down into two groups. The first group consists of the older, or conventional, antipsychotics. The second group consists of a newer class of drugs, collectively referred to as second-generation antipsychotics (SGAs). They are also known as atypical antipsychotics. The SGAs have rapidly achieved popularity and now account for about 90% of prescriptions for antipsychotic drugs. Both the older antipsychotics and the SGAs ameliorate the symptoms of psychosis, including hallucinations, delusions, bizarre behavior, disordered thinking, and agitation. SGAs tend to have fewer side effects and are better tolerated, but concerns have emerged regarding their potential to induce metabolic side effects, such as impaired glucose tolerance. Although the SGAs were initially seen as more effective than the conventional antipsychotics, this belief is being reappraised in light of recent research. In a large government-funded clinical trial, four SGAs were compared with the conventional antipsychotic perphenazine. There were few differences among the drugs in terms of efficacy or tolerability. The most commonly used antipsychotics are listed in Table 20–1.

Antipsychotic drugs are primarily used to treat schizophrenia and other psychotic disorders, but they are also prescribed to patients with psychotic mood disorders and to patients whose psychoses are medically induced or due to drugs of abuse. Antipsychotics are often used to control aggressive behavior in mentally retarded patients, autistic patients, patients with borderline personality disorder, and patients with delirium or dementia. They also are prescribed to patients with Tourette's disorder to diminish the frequency and severity of vocal and motor tics.

Mechanism of Action

The potency of conventional antipsychotic drugs correlates closely with their affinity for the dopamine 2 (D_2) receptor, blocking the effect of endogenous dopamine at this site. The pharmacological profile of the SGAs differs in that they are weaker D_2 receptor antagonists than conventional antipsychotics, but are potent serotonin type 2A (5-HT_{2A}) receptor antagonists and have significant anticholinergic and antihistaminic activity as

TABLE 20–1. Common antipsychotic agents

Category	Drug (trade name)	Sedation	Orthostatic hypotension	Anticholinergic effects	Extrapyramidal effects	Equivalent dosage, mg	Dosage range, mg/day
Conventional agents							
Phenothiazines							
Aliphatics	Chlorpromazine (Thorazine)	H	H	M	M	100	50–1,200
Piperidines	Thioridazine (Mellaril)	H	H	H	L	95	50–800
Piperazines	Fluphenazine (Prolixin)	L	L	L	VH	2	2–20
	Fluphenazine decanoate	L	L	L	VH	—ᵃ	12.5–50 mg q 2 wk
	Perphenazine (Trilafon)	L	L	L	H	10	12–64
	Trifluoperazine (Stelazine)	L	L	L	H	5	5–40
Thioxanthenes	Thiothixene (Navane)	L	L	L	H	5	5–60
Butyrophenones	Haloperidol (Haldol)	L	L	L	VH	2	2–60
	Haloperidol decanoate	L	L	L	VH	—ᵃ	50–250 mg q 4 wk

TABLE 20–1. Common antipsychotic agents *(continued)*

Category	Drug (trade name)	Sedation	Orthostatic hypotension	Anticholinergic effects	Extrapyramidal effects	Equivalent dosage, mg	Dosage range, mg/day
Second-generation (atypical) agents							
	Aripiprazole (Abilify)	L	VL	L	VL	7.5	10–15
	Asenapine (Saphris)	L	M	L	VL	5	10–20
	Clozapine (Clozaril)	H	H	H	VL	100	200–600
	Iloperidone (Fanapt)	L	M	L	VL	6	12–24
	Olanzapine (Zyprexa)	L	L	M	L	5	15–30
	Quetiapine (Seroquel)	M	L	L	VL	75	300–500
	Paliperidone (Invega)	L	M	L	L	4	3–12
	Risperidone (Risperdal)	L	M	L	L	2	2–6
	Ziprasidone (Geodon)	M	L	VL	L	6	40–160

Note. H = high; L = low; M = moderate; VH = very high; VL = very low.
[a]Long-acting ester; dosage is not directly comparable with that of standard compounds.

well. Central 5-HT$_{2A}$ receptor antagonism is believed to broaden the therapeutic effect of the drug while reducing the incidence of extrapyramidal side effects (EPS) associated with D$_2$ antagonists.

Antipsychotics appear to exert their influence at mesocortical and mesolimbic dopaminergic pathways. Positron emission tomography (PET) studies show that D$_2$ receptor occupancy of 65%–70% correlates with maximal antipsychotic efficacy. These studies also show that antipsychotics block these receptors almost immediately, yet full response to the drugs takes weeks to develop. Although all antipsychotics block these receptors, a patient may respond preferentially to one drug but not to another. These observations suggest that antipsychotic drugs have other effects in the central nervous system (CNS) that may actually be responsible for their therapeutic properties, such as an action on second-messenger systems. Although many drug side effects can be linked to their dopamine-blocking properties (e.g., EPS), these drugs also block noradrenergic, cholinergic, and histaminic receptors to differing degrees, accounting for the unique side effect profile of each agent.

Pharmacokinetics

Absorption of orally administered antipsychotics is variable, and peak plasma levels are generally reached in 1–4 hours. Several antipsychotics are also available in an intramuscular preparation, and administration produces effects within 15 minutes. Injectable antipsychotics have much greater bioavailability than oral medication. Metabolism occurs mostly in the liver, largely by oxidation, so that these highly lipid-soluble agents are converted to water-soluble metabolites and excreted in the urine and feces. Excretion of antipsychotics tends to be slow because of drug accumulation in fatty tissue. Most of the conventional antipsychotics are highly protein bound (85%–90%). Nearly all antipsychotics have a half-life of 24 hours or longer and have active metabolites with longer half-lives. Depot formulations have even longer half-lives and may take 3–6 months to reach steady state.

The majority of conventional antipsychotics are metabolized by the cytochrome P450 (CYP) enzyme subfamilies, including 2D6, 1A2, and 3A4. Because of genetic variation, 5%–10% of whites poorly metabolize medications through the CYP2D6 pathway, as do a significant proportion of African Americans. This can result in higher antipsychotic blood levels than anticipated in some patients.

Plasma concentrations can be measured reliably for many antipsychotic drugs, but studies attempting to correlate plasma level with response have been inconsistent. Haloperidol and clozapine blood levels appear to correlate with clinical response. With haloperidol, response appears to plateau at about 15 ng/mL, and for that reason higher levels are not recommended. Clozapine levels greater than 350 ng/mL appear to be effective for most patients. The other situations in which plasma levels are useful to obtain include the following:

- When patients' symptoms have not responded to standard dosage
- When antipsychotic medications are combined with drugs that can affect their pharmacokinetics (e.g., carbamazepine)
- When patient compliance needs to be assessed

Use in Acute Psychosis

A high-potency conventional antipsychotic such as haloperidol (5–10 mg/ day) or one of the second-generation agents (e.g., risperidone, 4–6 mg/day; olanzapine, 10–20 mg/day; quetiapine, 150–800 mg/day; ziprasidone, 80– 160 mg/day) is recommended as an initial choice for the treatment of acute psychosis. Antipsychotic effects generally start early after the drug is started but are cumulative over the ensuing weeks. An adequate trial should last from 4 to 6 weeks. The trial should be extended for another 4– 6 weeks when the patient shows a partial response to the initial antipsy-chotic. If no response occurs after 4–6 weeks, then another drug should be tried. Clozapine is a second-line choice because of its propensity to cause agranulocytosis and the requirement to monitor the white blood cell count.

Highly agitated patients who are out of control require rapid control of their symptoms and should be given frequent, equally spaced doses of an antipsychotic drug. High-potency antipsychotics (e.g., haloperi-dol) can be given every 30–120 minutes orally or intramuscularly until agitation has subsided. A combination of an antipsychotic and a benzo-diazepine may work even better in calming the patient (e.g., haloperi-dol, 5 mg, plus lorazepam, 2 mg), repeating the doses every 30 minutes until tranquilization is achieved.

Maintenance Treatment

Patients benefiting from short-term treatment with antipsychotic drugs are candidates for long-term maintenance treatment, which has as its goal the sustained control of psychotic symptoms and reduced risk of relapse. The following guidelines regarding relapse prevention were developed at an international conference:

1. Prevention of relapse is more important than risk of side effects because most side effects are reversible, and the consequences of relapse may be irreversible.
2. At least 1–2 years of treatment are recommended following the initial episode because of the high risk of relapse and the possibility of social deterioration from further relapses.
3. At least 5 years of treatment are indicated for multi-episode patients.
4. Chronic, or ongoing, treatment is recommended for patients who pose a danger to themselves or to others.

Research confirms that maintenance treatment with antipsychotics is effective in preventing relapse. When study results are pooled, 30% of those continuing to take medications relapse, compared with 65% of those taking placebo. About 75% of stable patients taken off their medication will relapse within 6–24 months.

Patients with schizoaffective disorder generally receive maintenance treatment with an antipsychotic in combination with a mood stabilizer when the patient has the bipolar type, or an antipsychotic combined with an antidepressant when the patient has the depressed type. Monotherapy with an SGA is a good alternative because these drugs seem to provide both mood stabilization and control of psychotic symptoms. SGAs can also be used for both acute and maintenance treatment of the manic phase of bipolar disorder.

Long-acting antipsychotic preparations are available for patients who are unable to take oral medication on a regular basis or who are noncompliant. There is no universally accepted method for converting a patient from oral to long-acting dosage forms, and dosing with sustained-release formulations must be individualized. A patient can be started on a dosage of 6.25 mg of fluphenazine decanoate intramuscularly every 2 weeks, and the dosage is titrated upward or downward based on the patient's therapeutic response and side effects. For haloperidol, a 400-mg loading dose in the first month, followed by a maintenance dose of 250 mg/month, produces a blood level of 10 ng/mL, and a dose of 150 mg/month produces a blood level between 5 and 6 ng/mL. The SGA risperidone is available in a long-acting injectable preparation (e.g., 25–50 mg every 2 weeks).

Further information about the use of antipsychotics in the treatment of schizophrenia and other psychotic disorders can be found in Chapter 5.

Adverse Effects

Despite their effectiveness in treating psychotic syndromes, antipsychotics have the potential to induce a variety of troublesome side effects. The severity of these effects differs from drug to drug and corresponds with the drug's ability to affect a particular neurotransmitter system (e.g., dopaminergic, noradrenergic, cholinergic, histaminic). Because of their blockade of 5-HT$_{2A}$ receptors, SGAs are less likely to induce EPS than are conventional antipsychotics. Side effect profiles of the antipsychotics are shown in Table 20–1.

Patients receiving long-term treatment with antipsychotic medication should be regularly monitored for the development of *tardive dyskinesia* (TD), a condition that consists of abnormal involuntary movements usually involving the mouth and tongue. Other parts of the body, including the trunk and extremities, may be affected. TD is thought to result when postsynaptic dopamine receptors develop a supersensitivity to dopamine following prolonged receptor blockade from antipsychotics. Second-generation drugs are much less likely to induce TD, although patients taking them should still be monitored.

The movements of TD are generally mild and tolerable, but about 10% of patients with TD develop a more malignant form of the disorder that can be totally disabling. Elderly patients, women, and patients with mood disorders appear more susceptible to developing TD, and it has a reported incidence of 5% per year of exposure to conventional antipsychotics in young persons and 30% after 1 year of treatment in the elderly.

Patients with TD present special problems because the treatment of choice is to stop the offending drug. Many patients will choose to continue taking the drug regardless of the TD because their lives may be intolerable without medication and the TD may be mild. One option is to switch the patient to an SGA, which will help mask the symptoms and will probably not worsen the TD. Vitamin E (i.e., 1,600 IU/day) may help alleviate the abnormal movements to some extent. If patients do not benefit from a 3-month trial, vitamin E should be discontinued.

Antipsychotic medications are also frequently associated with the development of *pseudoparkinsonism*. This side effect usually takes 3 or more weeks to develop. Patients develop symptoms typical of Parkinson's disease, including tremor, rigidity, and hypokinesia. *Akathisia*, the most common form of EPS, may appear in the first few weeks of antipsychotic treatment. This condition causes subjective feelings of anxiety and tension and objective fidgetiness and agitation. Patients may feel compelled to pace, move around in their chairs, or tap their feet. Treatment for both pseudoparkinsonism and akathisia generally consists of reducing the dosage of the antipsychotic drug whenever possible and/ or adding an antiparkinsonian agent to the medication regimen. Akathisia has been treated with β-blockers or amantadine, a drug that potentiates the release of dopamine in the basal ganglia. Benzodiazepines are also helpful in relieving the symptoms of akathisia. Clonidine has been used successfully to treat akathisia, but it may cause sedation and orthostatic hypotension.

Another potential neurological side effect is the *acute dystonic reaction*, which usually occurs during the first 4 days of treatment with antipsychotics. It is more common in younger persons, cocaine users, and in those treated with intramuscular injections of high-potency antipsychotics. A dystonia is a sustained contraction of the muscles of the neck, mouth, tongue, or occasionally other muscle groups that is subjectively distressing and often painful. Acute dystonias typically respond within 20–30 minutes to intramuscular benztropine (i.e., 1–2 mg) or diphenhydramine (i.e., 25–50 mg). There is little need for a standing dose of an antiparkinsonian agent after the dystonia resolves, because dystonic reactions usually do not recur. Patients beginning a course of a conventional antipsychotic can benefit from 2 weeks of prophylactic benztropine (1–4 mg/day) to help head off a dystonic reaction.

Antipsychotics, particularly low-potency compounds (e.g., chlorpromazine), commonly cause anticholinergic side effects including dry mouth, urinary retention, blurry vision, constipation, and exacerbation of narrow-angle glaucoma. These side effects are best treated by reducing the dosage of the drug or switching to a more potent agent (e.g., haloperidol) or to an SGA. Antiparkinsonian drugs commonly used to treat EPS, such as benztropine, can worsen these side effects. If urinary retention continues to be a problem, bethanechol (i.e., 15 mg three times daily) may help the patient empty his or her bladder. Bulk laxatives will help with constipation.

The most common cardiovascular side effect of the antipsychotics is *orthostatic hypotension*, mediated by α-adrenergic blockade. This side effect is caused more frequently by low-potency compounds (e.g., chlorpromazine). Antipsychotics generally do not cause arrhythmogenic effects when used in standard dosages. Chlorpromazine, thioridazine, pimozide, and the second-generation drugs aripiprazole and iloperidone have been associated with QT_c prolongation, which can be of concern for abnormal cardiac conduction or sudden death. Patients with a history of QT_c prolongation, a recent myocardial infarction, or uncompensated heart failure should avoid these drugs.

Agranulocytosis occurs in 0.8% of patients taking clozapine during the first year of treatment and peaks in incidence at 3 months of treatment. The best preventive measure is to be alert to the appearance of malaise, fever, and sore throat early in the course of therapy. Patients prescribed clozapine must have a baseline white blood cell count of no less than 3,500/mm^3 and an absolute neutrophil count of no less than

2,000 mm^3. Weekly complete blood counts and absolute neutrophil counts must be taken for the first 6 months, every 14 days for another 6 months, and monthly thereafter.

Hyperprolactinemia, often considered an unavoidable consequence of treatment with conventional antipsychotics, can induce amenorrhea, galactorrhea, gynecomastia, and impotence. SGAs are less likely to cause hyperprolactinemia, particularly quetiapine and aripiprazole. If it is not possible to reduce the dosage or change antipsychotics, the addition of bromocriptine (e.g., 2.5–7.5 mg twice daily) may be helpful.

The SGAs have been linked to abnormalities in several *metabolic parameters,* including glucose regulation, lipids, and weight gain. Clozapine and olanzapine appear to be the most likely of the drugs to cause weight gain, followed by risperidone and quetiapine; aripiprazole and ziprasidone are relatively weight neutral. Weight gain associated with long-term antipsychotic treatment can be significant and is a risk factor for diabetes and cardiovascular disease. Weight gain is also a frequent cause for treatment noncompliance. When these medications are prescribed, the American Diabetes Association recommends measuring baseline body mass index (BMI), waist circumference, blood pressure, and fasting glucose and lipid panels. BMI should be followed monthly for 3 months and then measured quarterly. Blood pressure, fasting glucose, and lipid panels should be followed up at 3 months and then yearly.

Other miscellaneous side effects of the antipsychotics include nonspecific skin rashes, retinitis pigmentosa (especially with dosages of thioridazine, >800 mg/day), fever (with clozapine), pigmentary changes in the skin (i.e., blue, gray, or tan), weight gain, cholestatic jaundice (with chlorpromazine), reduced libido, and inhibition of ejaculation (with thioridazine). Low-potency conventional antipsychotics are associated with a risk for seizures, especially at higher dosages (e.g., >1,000 mg/ day of chlorpromazine). The drugs are not contraindicated in epilepsy patients as long as they receive adequate treatment with anticonvulsants. All antipsychotics except clozapine are listed as Category C drugs by the U.S. Food and Drug Administration (FDA), meaning that pregnancy risk cannot be ruled out. Clozapine is listed as Category B, meaning that there is no evidence of pregnancy risk in humans.

All conventional antipsychotics have the potential to cause *neuroleptic malignant syndrome* (NMS), a rare idiosyncratic reaction that does not appear to be dose related. SGAs appear to be less likely to induce NMS. Considered a medical emergency, the syndrome is characterized by rigidity, high fever, delirium, and marked autonomic instability. Serum levels of creatinine phosphokinase and of liver enzymes are generally elevated. There is no standard approach to the treatment of NMS. Both the muscle relaxant dantrolene and the dopamine agonist bromocriptine have been used to treat NMS. Stopping the offending antipsychotic drug and providing supportive care may be as effective. ECT can be used in severe cases not responding to medical management. Once the patient has recovered, antipsychotics can be cautiously reintroduced after a 2-week wait. Selecting an agent from a different antipsychotic class (e.g., chlorpromazine rather than haloperidol, if haloperidol caused the NMS) or switching to an SGA is advisable.

Rational use of antipsychotics

1. A high-potency conventional antipsychotic or one of the SGAs should be given as first-line treatment.

   - SGAs are effective and well tolerated and have less potential to induce EPS.

2. Second-line drug choices include the other conventional antipsychotics.

3. A drug trial should last 4–6 weeks.

   - The trial should be extended when there is a partial response that has not plateaued and shortened when no response occurs or side effects are intolerable or unmanageable.

   - Aripiprazole or ziprasidone may be the better choice in patients at risk for weight gain.

   - Quetiapine or aripiprazole may be favored when low EPS and low prolactin levels are desired.

4. All antipsychotics should be started at a low dosage and gradually increased to fall within a therapeutic range.

   - Evidence suggests that blood levels can help guide dosage adjustments for haloperidol and clozapine.

5. There is little reason to prescribe more than one antipsychotic agent. Using two or more such drugs increases adverse effects and adds little clinical benefit.

6. Because of its risk of agranulocytosis and need for monitoring of the white blood cell count, clozapine should be reserved for patients with treatment-refractory illness.

7. Many patients will benefit from chronic antipsychotic administration.

   - Patients should be carefully monitored for evidence of metabolic abnormalities, including weight gain, glucose dyscontrol, and lipid abnormalities.

■ Antidepressants

Not long after chlorpromazine appeared in the late 1950s, the antidepressant imipramine was synthesized in an attempt by researchers to find additional compounds for the treatment of schizophrenia. It soon became apparent that imipramine had little effect on hallucinations and delusions; instead, it alleviated depression in patients who were both psychotic and depressed. This finding led to the development of the tricyclic antidepressants (TCAs). Modifications of the three-ring chemical structure followed as additional TCAs were produced, including amitriptyline and desipramine.

At about the same time that TCAs were synthesized, the antidepressant properties of monoamine oxidase inhibitors (MAOIs) were discovered. Iproniazid, an antibiotic used to treat tuberculosis, was found to relieve depression in tuberculosis patients. Later work showed that the drug also was effective in relieving depression. No longer used as an antidepressant, iproniazid has been succeeded by more effective MAOIs, including phenelzine and tranylcypromine.

A second and third generation of antidepressants have since been developed, some of which differ structurally from both the TCAs and the MAOIs. In the early 1980s, tetracyclic compounds (also referred to as *heterocyclics*) with a somewhat similar structure and comparable properties were marketed, including maprotiline and amoxapine. Another group of antidepressants, collectively known as the *selective serotonin reuptake inhibitors* (SSRIs), was developed in the late 1980s and early 1990s. Other antidepressants also were introduced but do not fit within any particular grouping, including bupropion, mirtazapine, venlafaxine, and duloxetine. The antidepressants are all thought to work by altering levels of neurotransmitters in the CNS. With minor exceptions, all are equally effective, differing primarily in their adverse effects and potency. A comparison of commonly prescribed antidepressants is presented in Table 20–2.

The primary indication for antidepressants is the acute and maintenance treatment of major depression. The effectiveness of antidepressants is unquestioned, and approximately 65%–70% of patients receiving an antidepressant will respond within 4–6 weeks. In contrast, the placebo response rate in depression ranges from 25% to 40%. Depressed patients with melancholic symptoms (e.g., diurnal variation, psychomotor agitation or retardation, terminal insomnia, pervasive anhedonia) may respond better to antidepressants than do other patients. Secondary depressions (i.e., depressions that follow or complicate other

TABLE 20–2. Commonly used antidepressants

Category	Drug (trade name)	Sedation	Anti-cholinergic effects	Orthostatic hypotension	Sexual dysfunction	GI effects	Activation/ Insomnia	Half-life, h	Target dosage, mg	Dosage range, mg/day
Selective serotonin reuptake inhibitors										
	Citalopram (Celexa)	VL	None	None	VH	H	VL	35	20	10–60
	Escitalopram (Lexapro)	VL	None	None	VH	H	VL	25	10	10–30
	Fluoxetine (Prozac)	None	None	None	VH	H	VH	24–72	20	20–80
	Fluvoxamine (Luvox)	M	None	None	VH	H	L	15	200	100–300
	Paroxetine (Paxil)	L	L	None	VH	H	L	20	20	20–50
	Sertraline (Zoloft)	VL	None	None	VH	VH	M	25	100	50–200

TABLE 20–2. Commonly used antidepressants *(continued)*

Category	Drug (trade name)	Sedation	Anti-cholinergic effects	Orthostatic hypotension	Sexual dysfunction	GI effects	Activation/ Insomnia	Half-life, h	Target dosage, mg	Dosage range, mg/day
Other antidepressants										
	Bupropion (Wellbutrin)	None	None	None	None	M	H	12	300	150–450
	Desvenlafaxine (Pristiq)	L	None	VL	H	VH	M	10	50	50–400
	Duloxetine (Cymbalta)	VL	L	None	VL	H	L	8–17	60	40–60
	Mirtazapine (Remeron)	H	None	None	None	VL	None	20–40	30	15–45
	Nefazodone (Serzone)	H	None	L	None	M	VL	2–4	300	100–600
	Trazodone (Desyrel)	VH	VL	VH	None	M	Yes	6–11	400	300–800
	Venlafaxine (Effexor)	L	None	VL	H	VH	M	3–5	225	75–350

TABLE 20–2. Commonly used antidepressants *(continued)*

Category	Drug (trade name)	Sedation	Anti-cholinergic effects	Orthostatic hypotension	Sexual dysfunction	GI effects	Activation/ Insomnia	Half-life, h	Target dosage, mg	Dosage range, mg/day
Tricyclics										
	Amitriptyline (Elavil)	VH	VH	VH	H	VL	None	9–46	150	50–300
	Clomipramine (Anafranil)	VH	VH	VH	VH	VL	None	23–122	150	50–300
	Desipramine (Norpramin)	M	M	M	H	VL	VL	12–28	150	50–300
	Doxepin (Sinequan, Adapin)	VH	VH	VH	H	VL	None	8–25	200	50–300
	Imipramine (Tofranil)	H	VH	VH	H	VL	None	6–28	200	50–300
	Nortriptyline (Pamelor)	M	M	M	H	VL	None	18–56	100	20–150

All of the SSRIs are metabolized by the liver, but only fluoxetine and sertraline have active metabolites. Fluoxetine has the longest half-life at 2–3 days, and its major metabolite, norfluoxetine, has a half-life of 4–16 days. The other SSRIs have half-lives ranging from 15 to 35 hours. The active metabolite of sertraline, norsertraline, has a half-life of 2–4 days. All are well absorbed from the gut and reach peak plasma levels within 4–8 hours.

The SSRIs share a similar side-effect profile, with only subtle differences among them. Side effects are largely dose related and can include mild nausea, loose bowel movements, anxiety or hyperstimulation (which leads to jitteriness, restlessness, muscle tension, and insomnia), headache, insomnia, sedation, and increased sweating. Patients sometimes report other side effects, including weight gain or weight loss, bruxism, vivid dreams, skin rash, and amotivation.

Sexual dysfunction is relatively common in both men and women treated with SSRIs. These drugs can decrease libido and cause ejaculatory delay or failure in men and anorgasmia in women. For this reason, SSRIs are sometimes prescribed to men to treat premature ejaculation. For persistent complaints of sexual dysfunction, management strategies include lowering the dosage, switching to one of the newer non-SSRI antidepressants (e.g., bupropion, duloxetine), or coadministering another medication as an antidote (e.g., bupropion, 75–300 mg/day, or cyproheptadine, 4–8 mg, taken 1–2 hours before sexual activity). Sildenafil and other medications used to treat male erectile dysfunction also appear to be effective in treating SSRI-related sexual dysfunction.

Adverse effects tend to diminish over time, but they persist in some patients. Fluoxetine is the most likely, and escitalopram the least likely, to induce adverse effects. When hyperstimulation is problematic, it can be managed by lowering the dosage, switching to another SSRI, or switching to one of the newer non-SSRI antidepressants. A β-blocker (e.g., propranolol, 10–30 mg three times daily) can be helpful in treating subjective jitteriness and tremor. Benzodiazepines (e.g., lorazepam, 0.5–1 mg twice daily) can be prescribed to counteract this side effect as well. Because complaints of hyperstimulation tend to diminish over time, adjunctive medications may not be needed long-term. Trazodone (e.g., 50–150 mg at bedtime) can be effective in treating insomnia, although men should be warned of its rare propensity to cause priapism (a sustained, painful erection).

When SSRIs are discontinued, many patients develop a *discontinuation syndrome*. The exception is fluoxetine, which self-tapers because of the long half-life of both the parent compound and its major metabolite. Symptoms include nausea, headache, vivid dreams, irritability, and dizziness. These often begin within days of drug discontinuation and continue for 2 weeks or longer. The symptoms can be minimized by tapering the drug slowly over several weeks. The short-term use of a benzodiazepine is often helpful.

Rare cases of a *serotonin syndrome* have been reported with the use of these drugs, particularly among patients who have concurrently taken two or more drugs that boost CNS serotonin levels. Typical symptoms include lethargy, restlessness, mental confusion, flushing, diaphoresis, tremor, and myoclonic jerks. Untreated, the serotonin syndrome can progress to hyperthermia, hypertonicity, rhabdomyolysis, renal failure, and death. Several deaths have been reported in patients taking a combination of an SSRI and MAOI, presumably as a result of this syndrome. Because of the potential lethality of this combination, when a patient is switched from an SSRI to an MAOI, a sufficient time must pass to ensure that the SSRI has been fully eliminated from the body before initiating treatment with an MAOI. With fluoxetine, this means that about 6 weeks must pass.

The SSRIs each inhibit one or more cytochrome P450 isoenzymes to a substantial degree and have the potential to cause clinically important drug interactions. For that reason, care should be taken when prescribing adjunctive or concurrent medication metabolized through this enzyme system. This means that SSRIs may induce a several-fold increase in the levels of coprescribed drugs that are dependent on the inhibited isoenzymes for their clearance. Fluoxetine, fluvoxamine, and paroxetine are the most likely to cause drug interactions, whereas citalopram and escitalopram have less potential to do so. See Table 20–3 for a description of the SSRIs and the isoenzyme systems inhibited and coadministered drugs affected.

Given their widespread use, the SSRIs are undoubtedly being used during pregnancy and breast-feeding. That said, all of the SSRIs are included in FDA risk Category C (pregnancy risk cannot be ruled out), except for paroxetine, which is in Category D (positive evidence of risk). The evidence base is largest with fluoxetine, which appears to be safe. There is some evidence that paroxetine and sertraline are associated with cardiovascular anomalies. The SSRIs are secreted in breast milk and should probably be avoided in women who are breast-feeding.

TABLE 20–3. Selective serotonin reuptake inhibitors (SSRIs) and other newer antidepressants and potentially important drug interactions

Antidepressant	Enzyme system inhibited	Potential drug interactions
Fluoxetine	2D6	Secondary TCAs, haloperidol, type 1C antiarrhythmics
	2C	Phenytoin, diazepam
	3A4	Carbamazepine, alprazolam, terfenadine
Sertraline	2D6	Secondary TCAs, antipsychotics, type 1C antiarrhythmics
	2C	Tolbutamide, diazepam
	3A4	Carbamazepine
Paroxetine	2D6	Secondary TCAs, antipsychotics, type 1C antiarrhythmics, trazodone
Fluvoxamine	1A2	Theophylline, clozapine, haloperidol, amitriptyline, clomipramine, imipramine, duloxetine
	2C	Diazepam
	3A4	Carbamazepine, alprazolam, terfenadine, astemizole
Nefazodone	3A4	Alprazolam, triazolam, terfenadine, astemizole, carbamazepine
Duloxetine	1A2	Fluvoxamine, theophylline, clozapine, haloperidol, amitriptyline, clomipramine, imipramine
	2D6	Secondary TCAs, antipsychotics, type 1C antiarrhythmics, trazodone

Note.   TCAs=tricyclic antidepressants.
Source.   Adapted from Nemeroff et al. 1996.

Other Newer Antidepressants

Bupropion

Bupropion has a unique chemical structure similar to that of psychostimulants, which may account for certain shared properties. Because its primary metabolite, hydroxybupropion, inhibits the reuptake of dopamine and norepinephrine, the drug has been called a dopamine-norepinephrine reuptake inhibitor. Bupropion is used for the treatment of major depression but is also FDA approved for the treatment of smoking cessation under the trade name Zyban. An extended-release form of the drug has been approved as a treatment for seasonal affective disorder. Bupropion also has been used to treat attention-deficit/hyperactivity disorder. It is not effective in treating panic disorder, OCD, social phobia, or other anxiety syndromes.

Bupropion is rapidly absorbed following oral administration, and peak concentrations are achieved within 2 hours, or 3 hours after administration of the sustained-release formulation. Elimination is biphasic, with an initial phase of approximately 1.5 hours and a second phase lasting about 14 hours. The biphasic decline for the sustained-release formulation is less pronounced than that of the immediate-release formulation.

Bupropion is relatively well tolerated, having minimal effects on weight gain, cardiac conduction, or sexual functioning. The most common side effects are headache, nausea, anxiety, tremors, insomnia, and increased sweating. These symptoms generally subside with time. Restlessness and tremor can be treated with propranolol (e.g., 10–30 mg three times daily). The patient may benefit from short-term coadministration of a benzodiazepine tranquilizer.

The main disadvantage of bupropion is that the incidence of seizures increases substantially at dosages greater than 450 mg/day. For this reason, the drug is contraindicated in patients with a seizure disorder or an eating disorder that may be associated with a lower seizure threshold. The main risk of overdose is the development of seizures.

Duloxetine

Duloxetine is a potent inhibitor of both serotonin and norepinephrine and for that reason is designated—along with venlafaxine and desvenlafaxine—as a selective serotonin-norepinephrine reuptake inhibitor (SNRI). The drug is FDA approved to treat major depression and generalized anxiety disorder and also is indicated to treat diabetic neuropathic pain and fibromyalgia. Duloxetine is well absorbed from the gut and is metabolized in the liver mainly through P450 isoenzymes CYP2D6 and CYP1A2. Its major metabolites have minimal pharmacologic activity. The half-life ranges from 8 to 17 hours.

Duloxetine is well tolerated. The most common side effects include insomnia, asthenia, nausea, dry mouth, and constipation. The drug is not associated with weight gain, and rates of sexual dysfunction are low. Duloxetine is metabolized through the CYP isoenzymes, creating a potential for drug interactions (see Table 20–3). Because of reports of hepatotoxicity, the drug should be used with caution in persons with chronic liver disease, or in those with substantial alcohol use. It should not be combined with MAOIs because of the potential for a serotonin syndrome. The drug has been fatal in overdose at doses as low as 1,000 mg.

Mirtazapine

Mirtazapine has a dual mode of action and enhances both serotonergic and noradrenergic neurotransmission but is not a reuptake inhibitor. The drug is also a potent histamine antagonist, a moderate α-adrenergic antagonist, and a moderate antagonist at muscarinic receptors. Mirtazapine is FDA indicated for the treatment of major depression. The drug is well absorbed from the gut and is 85% protein bound. It has a half-life of 20–40 hours. Mirtazapine is well tolerated but may cause somnolence, increased appetite, and weight gain. Because of its long half-life, it needs to be taken only once daily. The drug has little effect on the cardiovascular system and minimally affects sexual functioning. Mirtazapine is unlikely to be associated with cytochrome P450–mediated drug interactions. One potential advantage is its early effect on reducing anxiety symptoms and sleep disturbance.

Somnolence occurs in more than half of the patients receiving mirtazapine, although tolerance develops after the first few weeks of treatment. Rare cases of agranulocytosis have been reported. In these cases, patients recovered after medication discontinuation. Routine laboratory monitoring is not currently recommended because this side effect is rare, but the development of fever, chills, sore throat, or other signs of infection in association with a low white blood cell count warrants close monitoring and discontinuation of the drug. The drug is unlikely to be fatal in overdose. The drug should not be used in combination with an MAOI.

Nefazodone

Nefazodone combines blockade of the 5-HT$_2$ receptor with weak inhibition of neuronal serotonin reuptake and is structurally similar to trazodone. The drug is indicated for the treatment of major depression. Side effects include nausea, somnolence, dry mouth, dizziness, constipation, asthenia, and blurred vision. The drug is generally well tolerated, and these side effects are considered benign. Nefazodone does not appear to alter seizure threshold, does not cause weight gain, and does not impair sexual functioning. The drug has the potential to inhibit the cytochrome P450 3A3/4 isoenzyme, which can lead to drug-drug interactions when other medications metabolized by that isoenzyme are coadministered. Drawbacks include the need for twice-daily dosing and a slow dosage titration. Nefazodone does not appear to be fatal in overdose. In rare cases, potentially irreversible hepatic failure has been associated with the drug. This led the FDA to issue a black box warning in 2002, and later the trade product Serzone was voluntarily withdrawn from the market. Generic formulations remain available.

Trazodone

Trazodone is a weak inhibitor of serotonin but also blocks 5-HT$_2$ receptors. The drug is a triazolopyridine derivative that shares the triazolo ring structure with alprazolam, a benzodiazepine. Trazodone is indicated for the treatment of major depression. The drug is readily absorbed from the gastrointestinal tract, reaches peak plasma levels in 1–2 hours, and has a half-life of 6–11 hours. Trazodone is metabolized by the liver, and 75% of its metabolites are excreted in the urine. Adverse effects are partially mediated by α-adrenergic antagonism and antihistaminic activity. The drug should not be coadministered with MAOIs. Concurrent use with antihypertensives may lead to hypotension.

The most common adverse effects are sedation, orthostatic hypotension, dizziness, headache, nausea, and dry mouth. These effects are mostly benign. Trazodone does not block anticholinergic receptors, so urinary retention and constipation are uncommon. The drug has no significant effect on cardiac conduction, although there are reports of increased ventricular irritability in patients with preexisting cardiac conduction defects or ventricular arrhythmias. It is unlikely to be fatal in overdose. Because trazodone is so sedating, it is widely used to treat insomnia (e.g., 50–150 mg at bedtime).

One concern with trazodone is that in rare cases it has been associated with priapism, which can be irreversible and require surgical intervention. Men prescribed trazodone should be warned of this side effect and be advised to report any change in the frequency or firmness of erections. The drug should be immediately discontinued if these changes occur. Immediate medical treatment should be sought for sustained erections.

Venlafaxine and Desvenlafaxine

Both venlafaxine and its primary active metabolite desvenlafaxine are classified as SNRIs and have minimal effect on other neurotransmitter receptors. Venlafaxine has an indication for the treatment of major depression, but its extended-release formulation is FDA approved for the treatment of generalized anxiety disorder, social anxiety disorder, and panic disorder. The drug is rapidly absorbed from the gut and is 98% bioavailable; its half-life is about 4 hours. Desvenlafaxine is marketed in a sustained-release formulation and is indicated for the treatment of major depression. Like the parent compound, desvenlafaxine is well absorbed orally and has a half-life of about 10 hours. Both venlafaxine and desvenlafaxine are metabolized by the liver and are renally excreted.

The side-effect profile of venlafaxine and desvenlafaxine is similar to that of the SSRIs and includes hyperstimulation, sexual dysfunction, and transient withdrawal symptoms. The drugs do not affect cardiac conduction or lower seizure threshold and generally are not associated with sedation or weight gain. Blood pressure monitoring is recommended with the use of either drug because of dose-dependent increases in mean diastolic blood pressure in some patients, particularly those with hypertension. The drugs are unlikely to inhibit cytochrome P450 isoenzymes, so drug-drug interactions are unlikely. Both drugs are contraindicated in patients taking MAOIs because of the risk of serotonin syndrome. The drugs are generally not fatal in overdose. The main drawback with venlafaxine is that it is generally taken twice daily, although the extended-release formulation can be taken once daily.

Tricyclic and Tetracyclic Antidepressants

TCAs are believed to work by blocking the reuptake of both norepinephrine and serotonin at the presynaptic nerve ending. The tertiary amines (e.g., amitriptyline, imipramine, doxepin) primarily block serotonin reuptake, whereas the secondary amines (e.g., desipramine, nortriptyline, protriptyline) mainly block norepinephrine reuptake. Clomipramine is an exception because it is a relatively selective serotonin reuptake inhibitor. All of these drugs also block muscarinic, histaminic, and α-adrenergic receptors. The degree of blockade corresponds with the side effect profile of the agent as shown in Table 20–2. (The tetracyclics maprotiline and amoxapine are rarely used and are not included in the table.)

TCAs are well absorbed orally; they undergo an enterohepatic cycle, and peak plasma levels develop 2–4 hours after ingestion. They are highly bound to plasma and tissue proteins and are fat soluble. TCAs are metabolized by the liver, and their metabolites are excreted through the kidneys. All TCAs have active metabolites, and there is as much as a tenfold variation in steady-state plasma levels of TCAs among individuals. These differences are primarily caused by individual variations in the way the liver metabolizes the drugs. Their half-lives vary but are generally in the range of 1 day. Steady-state plasma levels are achieved after five half-lives; half-life, in turn, is dependent on metabolism of the drug by hepatic microsomal enzymes. Blood levels tend to be increased by drugs that inhibit the cytochrome P450 system, including chlorpromazine and other antipsychotics, disulfiram, cimetidine, estrogens, methylphenidate, and many of the SSRIs.

The established therapeutic range for imipramine (the total for imipramine plus its metabolite desipramine) is generally thought to be greater than 200 ng/mL. For nortriptyline, the therapeutic range is between 50 and 150 ng/mL. Desipramine plasma levels greater than 125 ng/mL are considered therapeutic. Plasma blood levels can be measured for the other TCAs but are not clinically meaningful. Levels should be obtained 12 hours after the last dose.

There is no reason to routinely obtain plasma levels, particularly when the patient is doing well. Blood levels are helpful in cases of drug overdose but may also be useful when evaluating a patient's failure to respond adequately, significant symptoms of toxicity, or suspected noncompliance; in establishing a therapeutic window; and in setting dosage levels for a patient with significant cardiac or other medical disease (when it is desirable to keep the blood level at the lower range of the therapeutic value).

TCAs commonly cause sedation, orthostatic hypotension, and anticholinergic side effects such as constipation, urinary hesitancy, dry mouth, and visual blurring. Each TCA differs in its propensity to cause these effects. Tertiary amines (e.g., amitriptyline, imipramine, doxepin) tend to cause more pronounced side effects. Tolerance usually develops to anticholinergic side effects and sedation, but TCAs should be used with caution in patients with prostatic enlargement and narrow-angle glaucoma. Elderly patients should have their blood pressure carefully monitored because drug-induced hypotension can lead to falls and resultant fractures.

Antihistaminic effects include sedation and weight gain. α-Adrenergic blockade causes orthostatic hypotension and reflex tachycardia. Miscellaneous side effects of TCAs include tremors, pedal edema, myoclonus, restlessness or hyperstimulation, insomnia, nausea and vomiting, electroencephalographic changes, rashes or allergic reactions, confusion,

TABLE 20–4.   Dietary instructions for patients taking monoamine oxidase inhibitors (MAOIs)

Foods to avoid

Cheese: all cheeses except cottage cheese, farmer cheese, and cream cheese

Meat and fish: caviar; liver; salami and sausage; smoked, dried, pickled, cured, or preserved meats and fish

Vegetables: overripe avocados, fava beans, sauerkraut

Fruits: overripe fruits, canned figs

Other foods: yeast extracts, fermented products, monosodium glutamate

Beverages: red wine, sherry, liquors

Foods to use in moderation

Chocolate

Coffee

Colas

Tea

Soy sauce

Beer, other wine

Medications to avoid

Over-the-counter pain medications except for plain aspirin, acetaminophen, and ibuprofen

Cold or allergy medications

Nasal decongestants and inhalers

Cough medications; plain guaifenesin elixir may be taken, however

Stimulants and diet pills

Sympathomimetic drugs

Meperidine

Selective serotonin reuptake inhibitors (SSRIs), bupropion, desvenlafaxine, mirtazapine, nefazodone, trazodone, venlafaxine

Source.   Adapted from Hyman and Arana 1987; Krishnan 2009.

properties, which act to lower blood pressure when taken sublingually, make it a useful stopgap measure.

All physicians and dentists should be informed when their patients are taking MAOIs, especially when surgery or dental work is indicated, so that drugs that interact adversely with MAOIs can be avoided. It is advisable to wait 2 weeks after discontinuing an MAOI before resuming a normal diet or using a TCA, an SSRI, or another medication that may have an adverse interaction with the MAOI.

Use of Antidepressants

Treatment should begin with one of the SSRIs. Because these drugs are effective, well tolerated, and generally safe in overdose, they have replaced the TCAs as first-line therapy. Most patients will respond to a standard dosage, and frequent dosage adjustments are unnecessary. Patients with a history of cardiac conduction defects should receive one of the SSRIs or another new agent (e.g., bupropion, duloxetine, mirtazapine). Impulsive patients or those with suicidal urges also should receive an SSRI or one of the newer agents because they are unlikely to be fatal in overdose. When a TCA is used, nortriptyline, imipramine, and desipramine are the drugs of choice because meaningful plasma levels can be measured. The TCAs all require close titration, beginning with relatively low dosages. Recommended dosage ranges for the antidepressants are found in Table 20–2.

Patients being treated for their first episode of major depression should be maintained on medication at the same dosage used for acute treatment for at least 4–9 months after achieving remission. When medication is ultimately tapered and discontinued, patients should be carefully monitored to ensure that their remission is stable. Patients with the following characteristics should be considered for chronic maintenance treatment to reduce the risk of relapse:

- Three or more lifetime episodes of major depression
- Double depression (i.e., major depression plus dysthymia)
- Two or more severe episodes of major depression within the past 5 years
- Depressive disorder complicated by comorbid substance use or anxiety disorder
- Age greater than 60 years at onset of major depression

Drug trials generally should last 4–8 weeks. When the patient's symptoms do not respond to an antidepressant after 4 weeks of treatment at the target dosage, the dosage should be increased, or the patient should be switched to another antidepressant, preferably from a different class with a slightly different mechanism of action. When this regimen fails, nonresponders may benefit from the addition of lithium, which will increase the likelihood of response in many patients. Response from lithium augmentation is often evident within a week with relatively low dosages (e.g., 300 mg three times daily). ECT is an option in patients whose depression does not respond to medication.

Other agents have been used to augment the effect of TCAs, including triiodothyronine, tryptophan, methylphenidate, and pindolol, but the effectiveness of these agents in augmenting response has not been adequately studied.

Rational use of antidepressants

1. SSRIs or one of the other newer antidepressants should be used initially, and TCAs and MAOIs should be reserved for nonresponders.

2. Dosages should be adjusted to fall within the recommended range, and each drug trial should last 4–8 weeks.

3. SSRIs generally are given once daily. TCAs can be administered as a single dose, usually at bedtime. MAOIs usually are prescribed twice daily but not at bedtime because they can cause insomnia. Bupropion is administered in two to three divided doses to minimize its risk of causing seizures.

4. Although adverse effects appear within days of starting a drug, therapeutic effects may require 2–4 weeks to become apparent.
   - Improvement should be monitored by following up target symptoms (e.g., mood, sleep, energy, appetite).

5. Patients with heart rhythm disturbances should be given one of the newer antidepressants that do not affect cardiac conduction (e.g., bupropion, mirtazapine, or an SSRI).

6. Antidepressants are usually unnecessary in patients with grief reactions (uncomplicated bereavement) or adjustment disorders with depressed mood, because these disorders are self-limiting.

Rational use of antidepressants *(continued)*

7. When possible, SSRIs should be tapered (except for fluoxetine, which self-tapers) because many patients experience withdrawal symptoms. TCAs also should be tapered slowly because of their tendency to cause withdrawal reactions. No clinically significant withdrawal reaction occurs with MAOIs, but a taper over 5–7 days is sensible.

8. The coadministration of two different antidepressants does not boost efficacy and will only worsen side effects. In rare cases, the combined use of a TCA and an MAOI or a TCA and an SSRI is justified, but these combinations should never be used routinely.

- MAOIs should not be coadministered with SSRIs or with any of the other new antidepressants.

■ Mood Stabilizers

Lithium carbonate, a naturally occurring salt, became available in 1970. Its first use in medicine (in the form of lithium chloride) was as a salt substitute for people with hypertension who needed a low-sodium diet, but its use was abandoned when it was found to make some people sick. In the late 1940s, Australian psychiatrist John Cade found that lithium calmed agitated psychotic patients. Later, it was discovered that lithium was particularly effective in people with mania. The Danish researcher Mogens Schou observed that lithium was effective in relieving the target symptoms of mania and that it also had a prophylactic effect. Lithium has since been joined by valproate, carbamazepine, and lamotrigine for the treatment of bipolar disorder.

In addition to the mood stabilizers, all of the SGAs (except clozapine) have been approved for the treatment of acute mania; two are indicated for maintenance treatment of bipolar disorder (aripiprazole and olanzapine); and four are indicated for the adjunctive treatment of acute mania in combination with lithium or valproate (aripiprazole, olanzapine, quetiapine, and risperidone). Additionally, both quetiapine and a combined form of olanzapine and fluoxetine (Symbyax) are approved to treat the depressed phase of bipolar disorder. The mood stabilizers are listed in Table 20–5. (Further information about the treatment of bipolar disorder is found in Chapter 6.)

TABLE 20–5.   Commonly used mood stabilizers

Drug (trade name)	Therapeutic plasma level	Dosage range, mg/day
Carbamazepine (Tegretol)	6–12 mg/L	400–2,400
Lamotrigine (Lamictal)	N/A	50–200
Lithium carbonate (Eskalith, Lithobid)	0.6–1.2 mEq/L	900–2,400
Valproate (Depakene, Depakote)	50–120 mg/L	500–3,000

Lithium Carbonate

The mechanism of action of lithium is unknown. Lithium has effects on intracellular processes, such as inhibiting the enzyme inositol-1-phosphatase within neurons. The inhibition leads to decreased cellular responses to neurotransmitters that are linked to the phosphatidylinositol second-messenger system.

The onset of action often takes 5–7 days to become apparent. The usual plasma level of lithium for the treatment of acute mania is 0.9–1.4 mEq/L, but some patients do well outside this range. Antipsychotics, which work more quickly, may be preferred when rapid behavioral control is needed, although benzodiazepine-induced sedation may be as effective.

Maintenance dosages may be lower, aiming for a blood level in the range of 0.5–0.7 mEq/L. Lithium has no role in the acute treatment of unipolar major depression but is a first-line treatment for bipolar depression. Lithium is sometimes used to augment the effect of antidepressants in the treatment of major depression.

The most dramatic effect of lithium is in the prophylaxis of manic and depressive episodes in bipolar patients. Lithium appears to work best at reducing the frequency and severity of manic episodes. Although response to lithium tends to remain stable over time, most patients will have breakthrough episodes. Lithium has also been shown to be effective in preventing recurrences of depression in patients with unipolar major depression. It is one of the few drugs demonstrated to reduce suicide attempts and suicides.

Lithium is also used in the treatment of schizoaffective disorder, especially the bipolar subtype. Lithium is sometimes used to treat aggression in patients with dementia, mental retardation, or "acting out" personality disorders (especially the borderline and antisocial types).

Pharmacokinetics of Lithium

Lithium carbonate is administered orally but is available in liquid form as lithium citrate. Lithium is rapidly absorbed from the gut, and peak blood levels are obtained about 2 hours after ingestion. The elimination half-life is about 8–12 hours in manic patients and about 18–36 hours in euthymic patients. (Manic patients are overly active and have a higher glomerular filtration rate and therefore clear lithium from their system more rapidly.) Lithium is not protein bound and does not have metabolites. It is almost entirely excreted through the kidney but may be found in all body fluids (e.g., saliva, semen). Blood plasma levels are checked 12 hours after the last dose is given.

Slow-release preparations are available and are indicated when gastrointestinal toxicity is evident or when twice-daily dosing would enhance compliance. Lithium usually is administered two or three times daily in patients with acute mania. Once-daily dosing with extended-release preparations is recommended in patients receiving the drug prophylactically. Once-daily dosing may offer some protection to the kidneys, although a single large daily dose can cause gastric irritation. Lithium usually is started at 300 mg twice daily in the average patient and is then titrated until a therapeutic blood level is achieved. Dosage may be adjusted every 3–5 days. Levels should be checked monthly for the first 3 months and every 3 months thereafter. Patients receiving chronic lithium administration can be monitored less frequently. Lithium can be safely discontinued without a taper.

Adverse Effects of Lithium

Minor side effects of lithium occur relatively soon after initiating treatment. Thirst or polyuria, tremor, diarrhea, weight gain, and edema are all relatively common side effects but tend to diminish with time. About 5%–15% of the patients undergoing long-term treatment develop clinical signs of hypothyroidism. This side effect is more common in women and tends to occur during the first 6 months of treatment. Hypothyroidism can be managed effectively with thyroid hormone replacement. Baseline thyroid assays should be obtained before starting lithium. Thyroid function should be tested once or twice during the first 6 months of treatment and every 6–12 months thereafter as clinically indicated. Thyroid dysfunction reverses after lithium is discontinued.

Long-term lithium treatment may lead to increased levels of calcium, ionized calcium, and parathyroid hormone. High levels of calcium can cause lethargy, ataxia, and dysphoria, symptoms that may be attributed to depression rather than hypercalcemia.

Commonly reported side effects include gastrointestinal complaints (e.g., nausea, poor appetite, vomiting, diarrhea), asymptomatic serum hepatic transaminase elevation, tremor, sedation, and weight gain. Less frequent side effects include rashes, hematological abnormalities, and hair loss. Hepatic transaminase elevation can occur and is dose related; it generally subsides spontaneously. A rare but fatal hepatotoxic reaction to valproate has been reported. The enteric-coated form of valproate is generally well tolerated and has a low incidence of gastrointestinal side effects; however, it is more expensive than generic formulations.

Neural tube defects have been reported with the use of valproate during the first trimester of pregnancy; therefore, its use in pregnant women is not recommended. Coma and death have occurred from valproate overdoses.

Before valproate treatment is begun, the patient should have a complete blood count and a liver enzyme measurement; the latter should be done periodically during the first 6 months and then about every 6 months thereafter. The drug is started at 250 mg three times daily and can be increased by 250 mg every 3 days. Serum levels can be obtained after 3–4 days. Most patients will need between 1,250 and 2,500 mg/day.

Carbamazepine

Carbamazepine, an anticonvulsant used to treat complex partial and tonic-clonic seizures, has a structure similar to that of the TCAs. It is used as an alternative to lithium and valproate in the treatment of acute mania and may be effective for maintenance treatment of bipolar disorder. The drug has been approved by the FDA for the treatment of acute manic or mixed episodes of bipolar disorder.

The precise mechanism of action of carbamazepine is unknown, but the drug has a wide range of cellular and intracellular effects in the CNS. Of theoretical interest is its dampening effect on kindling, a process in which repeated biochemical or psychological stressors are thought to result in abnormal excitability of limbic neurons.

When carbamazepine is used to treat mania, there is generally a delay of 5–7 days before its effect is apparent. Carbamazepine can safely be combined with antipsychotics, especially when behavioral control is necessary. It may be more effective in patients who cycle rapidly (i.e., more than four episodes per year) and who tend not to respond well to lithium. The usual custom is to aim for typical anticonvulsant blood levels of 8–12 µg/mL, despite the fact that no dose-response curve has been established.

From 10% to 15% of the patients taking carbamazepine develop a skin rash, which is generally transient. Other common side effects include impaired coordination, drowsiness, dizziness, slurred speech, and ataxia. Many of these symptoms can be avoided by increasing the dosage slowly. A transient leukopenia causing as much as a 25% decrease in the white blood cell count occurs in 10% of patients. A smaller reduction in the white blood cell count may persist in some patients as long as they take the drug, but this is not a reason for discontinuation. Aplastic anemia develops in rare cases.

Carbamazepine is typically started at a dosage of 200 mg twice daily and increased to three times daily after 3–5 days. Most patients will need dosages of 600–1,600 mg/day.

Before starting carbamazepine, the patient should have a complete blood count and an electrocardiogram. The patient should be warned about the drug's rare hematological side effects. Any indication of infection, anemia, or thrombocytopenia (e.g., petechiae) should be investigated and a complete blood count should be obtained, but routine blood monitoring is unnecessary. Because carbamazepine is a vasopressin agonist, it can induce hyponatremia; therefore, convulsions or undue drowsiness should be cause for obtaining serum electrolyte measurements. Carbamazepine has been linked with fetal malformations similar to those seen with phenytoin and therefore should be avoided in pregnant women, especially during the first trimester. Breast-feeding by women taking this drug is not recommended.

Lamotrigine

Lamotrigine, also an anticonvulsant, is FDA approved for the maintenance treatment of bipolar I disorder to delay the time to occurrence of mood episodes. It appears to be most effective in delaying the time to occurrence of depressive episodes and may be effective in the treatment of acute depressive episodes as well. Although its mechanism of action is unclear, it affects CNS neurotransmission by blocking sodium channels. This action inhibits the release of presynaptic glutamate, aspartate, and GABA. The drug also is a weak inhibitor of the serotonin-3 receptor.

The target dosage of lamotrigine is 200 mg/day, achieved through a slow titration (i.e., 25 mg/day for 2 weeks, 50 mg/day for 2 weeks, 100 mg/day for 1 week, then 200 mg/day). The oral bioavailability of the drug is 98%, and peak plasma concentrations occur initially at 1–3 hours, with a secondary peak at 4–6 hours. The drug is about 60% protein bound and is widely distributed in the body. Metabolism is through hepatic glucuronidation, and none of the metabolites are active. The half-life ranges from 25 to 35 hours.

Lamotrigine is generally well tolerated, and most side effects are minor. In rare cases, the drug can induce the potentially life-threatening Stevens-Johnson syndrome and toxic epidermal necrolysis. Patients should be instructed to discontinue the drug at the first sign of a rash. Rashes are more common in children. Lamotrigine should probably not be combined with valproate because the combination can substantially increase the risk of serious rash, including Stevens-Johnson syndrome. The drug is listed as Category C in terms of pregnancy risk, which indicates that risk cannot be ruled out.

Rational use of mood stabilizers

1. Lithium, valproate, or carbamazepine should be used initially for the treatment of acute mania.

    *   Monotherapy with SGAs, which are effective and well tolerated, is an excellent alternative.

    *   The combination of lithium and valproate or the combination of a mood stabilizer with one of the SGAs may be effective when monotherapy fails.

2. A clinical trial of lithium, valproate, or carbamazepine should last 3 weeks; at this point, another drug should be added or substituted if there is minimal or inadequate response.

    *   Drug nonresponders may respond to electroconvulsive therapy.

3. Lithium may be given as a single dose at bedtime when the amount is less than 1,200 mg. Lithium should be given with food to minimize gastric irritation.

4. Renal function and thyroid indices should be regularly monitored in patients treated with lithium. Hepatic function should be regularly monitored in patients treated with valproate.

5. Lamotrigine may be particularly helpful in preventing the development of depressive episodes in bipolar I patients.

■ Anxiolytics

Anxiolytics are the most widely prescribed class of psychotropic drugs. They include the barbiturates, the nonbarbiturate sedative-hypnotics

TABLE 20–6. Benzodiazepines commonly used as anxiolytics

Drug (trade name)	Rate of onset	Half-life, h	Long-acting metabolite	Equivalent dosage, mg	Dosage range, mg/day
Alprazolam (Xanax)	Fast	6–20	No	0.5	1–4
Chlordiazepoxide (Librium)	Fast	20–100	Yes	10.0	15–60
Clonazepam (Klonopin)	Moderate	30–40	No	0.25	1–6
Diazepam (Valium)	Very fast	30–100	Yes	5.0	5–40
Lorazepam (Ativan)	Fast	10–20	No	1.0	0.5–10
Oxazepam (Serax)	Slow	5–20	No	15.0	30–120

(e.g., meprobamate), the benzodiazepines, and buspirone. Currently, only the benzodiazepines and buspirone can be recommended because of their superior safety record. There is still a strong belief in the general population that these medications are overprescribed by psychiatrists and other physicians. Despite their reputation, benzodiazepines are generally prescribed for short periods, are prescribed for rational indications, and are used appropriately by most patients.

Benzodiazepines

Benzodiazepines constitute an important class of drugs with clear superiority over the barbiturates and nonbarbiturate sedative-hypnotics. Benzodiazepines have been marketed in the United States since 1964. These drugs have a high therapeutic index, little toxicity, and relatively few drug-drug interactions. The benzodiazepines are indicated for the treatment of anxiety syndromes, sleep disturbances, musculoskeletal disorders, seizure disorders, and alcohol withdrawal and for inducing anesthesia. Their approved indications reflect subtle differences among them (e.g., side effects, potency) and in marketing strategy. Commonly used benzodiazepines are compared in Table 20–6.

Benzodiazepines are believed to exert their effects by binding to specific benzodiazepine receptors in the brain. The receptors are intimately linked to receptors for GABA, a major inhibitory neurotransmitter. By binding to benzodiazepine receptors, the drugs potentiate the actions of GABA, leading to a direct anxiolytic effect on the limbic system.

Indications for Benzodiazepines

Benzodiazepines are useful for the treatment of generalized anxiety disorder, especially when severe. Many patients benefit when their anxiety is acute and problematic; these drugs generally should be given for short periods (e.g., weeks or months). Patients with mild anxiety may not need medication and can be successfully managed with behavioral interventions (e.g., progressive muscle relaxation).

Benzodiazepines have an antipanic effect. Both alprazolam and clonazepam have FDA indications for the treatment of panic disorder but because of their abuse potential are considered second-line treatments after the SSRIs. Similarly, while benzodiazepines are effective in treating social phobia, the SSRIs should be used initially because they do not have an abuse potential.

Anxiety frequently complicates depression. Benzodiazepines are frequently coadministered with an antidepressant because they are more effective in quickly relieving accompanying anxiety than is the antidepressant. When the antidepressant begins to take effect, the benzodiazepine can be withdrawn gradually.

Benzodiazepines are effective in alleviating situational anxiety. These syndromes, called *adjustment disorders with anxiety* in DSM-IV-TR, are characterized by anxiety symptoms (e.g., tremors, palpitations) that occur in response to a stressful event. Adjustment disorders are generally brief, and for that reason, treatment with benzodiazepines is time limited.

Benzodiazepines have established efficacy in the short-term treatment of primary insomnia unrelated to identifiable medical or psychiatric illness. Their use as hypnotic agents is discussed in Chapter 17, which includes a description of the individual drugs, their dosing, and their adverse effects.

Alcohol withdrawal syndromes are commonly treated with benzodiazepines (most often chlordiazepoxide), because benzodiazepines and alcohol are cross-tolerant. The treatment of these syndromes is described in Chapter 9. Other uses of the benzodiazepines include the treatment of akathisia and catatonia and as an adjunct to the treatment of acute agitation and mania.

Pharmacokinetics of Benzodiazepines

Benzodiazepines are rapidly absorbed from the gut and, with the exception of lorazepam, are poorly absorbed intramuscularly. Lorazepam is available for parenteral use, and its versatility contributes to its widespread use in hospitalized patients. Midazolam is a short-acting agent used to induce anesthesia but is not available orally. Benzodiazepines are metabolized chiefly by hepatic oxidation and have active metabolites. Lorazepam, oxazepam, and temazepam are metabolized by glucuronide conjugation and have no active metabolites; they are relatively short acting and are thus the preferred benzodiazepines for elderly patients.

There are differences between single-dose and steady-state kinetics. Rapid-onset drugs tend to be lipophilic, a property that facilitates rapid crossing of the blood-brain barrier. Drugs with longer elimination half-lives accumulate more slowly and take longer to reach steady state. Washout of these drugs is similarly prolonged. Drugs with shorter half-lives reach steady state more rapidly but also have less total accumulation. Drugs with long half-lives tend to have active metabolites.

Because of the differences in metabolism and half-lives, the best therapeutic results are obtained when the needs of the patient and the situation are taken into account. When prescribing, three parameters largely determine drug selection: 1) half-life, 2) presence of metabolites, and 3) route of elimination. For example, in older adults, the clinician should select a benzodiazepine with a short half-life, few metabolites, and renal excretion in order to minimize drug accumulation and adverse side effects.

Adverse Effects of Benzodiazepines

CNS depression is common with benzodiazepines. Symptoms include drowsiness, somnolence, reduced motor coordination, and memory impairment. These may diminish with continued administration or dosage reduction. However, patients should be cautioned not to drive or use machines, especially when starting these drugs.

All benzodiazepines have the potential for abuse and addiction. Because physiological dependence is more likely to occur with longer drug exposure, minimizing the duration of continuous treatment should reduce this risk. Also, benzodiazepines should be prescribed cautiously in patients with histories of alcohol or drug abuse and in patients with unstable personalities (e.g., borderline and antisocial personality disorders). When signs of dependence appear (e.g., drug-seeking behavior, increasing the dosage to get the same effect), the drug should be tapered and discontinued. Patients should be advised to avoid alcohol when taking benzodiazepines because the combination will cause greater CNS depression than either drug alone.

Discontinuation of benzodiazepine therapy after long-term treatment can lead to tremulousness, sweating, sensitivity to light and sound, insomnia, abdominal distress, and systolic hypertension. Serious withdrawal syndromes and seizures are relatively uncommon but are more likely with abrupt discontinuation. Symptom recurrence appears to have a more rapid onset after discontinuation of short-acting benzodiazepines; the effect of drug discontinuation can be minimized by gradually tapering the drug over 1–3 months. Such a slow taper is particularly important for benzodiazepines with short half-lives. When discontinuing short-acting benzodiazepines, it may be helpful to switch the patient to a long-acting drug before initiating a taper (e.g., from alprazolam to clonazepam).

Nearly all benzodiazepines fall into pregnancy risk Category D (positive evidence of risk) or X (contraindicated in pregnancy), mainly on the basis of the occurrence of neonatal toxicity and withdrawal syndromes. For these reasons, their use during pregnancy and breast-feeding should be avoided.

Benzodiazepines can be used safely in medically ill and elderly patients. In general, drugs that do not accumulate (e.g., lorazepam) should be used. Because benzodiazepines can cause respiratory depression, they should not be used in persons with sleep apnea, although small dosages are tolerated even in patients with chronic pulmonary disease. Small dosages are also indicated for the elderly, who are susceptible to the CNS depressant effects of benzodiazepines, which can contribute to memory difficulties and falls.

The least controversial aspect of benzodiazepines is their tremendous index of safety. When they are taken alone, even massive overdoses are rarely fatal.

Buspirone

Buspirone has an FDA indication for the treatment of generalized anxiety disorder. Structurally unlike other anxiolytics, it is a serotonin type 1A (5-HT$_{1A}$) receptor agonist and does not interact with the benzodiazepine receptor. As such, it does not produce sedation, does not interact with alcohol, and does not pose a risk for abuse. Buspirone is ineffective in blocking panic attacks, relieving phobias, or diminishing obsessions or compulsions. Buspirone is well absorbed orally and is metabolized by the liver. Its half-life ranges from 2 to 11 hours. Drowsiness, headache, and dizziness are common side effects.

Buspirone's effect on chronic anxiety is equal to that of diazepam, although its effects are not apparent for 1–2 weeks. The usual dosage range is 20–30 mg/day in divided doses. Alternatives to buspirone for the treatment of generalized anxiety disorder include the SNRIs venlafaxine and duloxetine and the SSRIs.

Rational use of anxiolytics

1. The benzodiazepines should be used for limited periods (e.g., weeks to months) to avoid the problem of dependency, because most conditions they are used to treat are self-limiting.

   - Some patients will benefit from long-term benzodiazepine administration; in these situations, patients should be periodically assessed for continuing need.

2. The benzodiazepines have similar clinical efficacy, so the choice of a specific agent depends on its half-life, the presence of metabolites, and the route of administration.

3. Once- or twice-daily dosing of the benzodiazepines is sufficient for most patients.

   - A dose given at bedtime may eliminate the need for a separate hypnotic.

   - Short-acting agents (e.g., alprazolam) are an exception to this recommendation because their dosing interval is determined by their half-lives.

4. Buspirone is not effective on an as-needed (prn) basis and is useful only for the treatment of generalized anxiety disorder.

5. The SNRIs venlafaxine and duloxetine, or one of the SSRIs, are effective alternatives to the benzodiazepines and buspirone in the treatment of generalized anxiety disorder.

   - Because response to these agents takes several weeks, it is important to educate the patient not to expect quick results.

In treating any EPS, the clinician should begin by reducing the dosage of the antipsychotic drug whenever possible or switching to an SGA with less potential to cause EPS. When these steps fail, anticholinergics, amantadine, or propranolol can be useful adjuncts. Because EPS are unpleasant and reduce the likelihood that the patient will remain compliant with treatment, drugs used to treat these side effects can make a significant difference in the patient's comfort.

■ Electroconvulsive Therapy

ECT is a procedure in which a controlled electric current is passed through the scalp and selected parts of the brain to induce a grand mal seizure. The procedure was introduced in 1938 in Italy by Ugo Cerletti and Lucio Bini to replace less reliable convulsive therapies that used liquid chemicals. ECT is one of the oldest medical treatments still in regular use, a fact that attests to its safety and efficacy. Its mechanism of action is poorly understood, yet it is known to produce multiple effects on the CNS, including neurotransmitter changes, neuroendocrine effects, and alterations in intracellular signaling pathways.

Indications for Electroconvulsive Therapy

ECT is used almost exclusively for the treatment of mood disorders and is generally reserved for patients who fail one or more trials of antidepressant medication, patients who are at high risk for suicide, and patients who are debilitated by their failure to take in adequate food and fluids. Patients at high risk for suicide and in need of rapid treatment are also candidates for ECT because it tends to work more quickly than antidepressant medication. Some patients will choose to have ECT as a first-line treatment rather than take medication. There is growing evidence that the combination of ECT with antidepressant medication produces an even more robust response than either treatment alone.

Patients receive an index course of 6–12 treatments at a rate of two to three per week, although the precise number is individualized based on response. An index series of treatments can be administered in inpatient or outpatient settings, a determination that the physician and patient (and the patient's family) need to make. Generally, if the treatments are given in the outpatient setting, the patient should not be at risk for suicide, should have supportive family members available to help care for the patient at home, and should be medically stable. Some patients will be candidates for maintenance (or prophylactic) ECT to keep them from relapsing. Typically, these patients have failed multiple medication trials yet respond favorably to ECT. With prophylactic ECT, a treatment is given anywhere from once per week to once per month depending on the patient. Because mood disorders tend to be chronic or recurrent, maintenance treatment for some will be indefinite.

As many as 80%–90% of patients receiving ECT as a first-line treatment respond favorably, while those who have failed antidepressants have a 50%–60% response rate. Certain depressive symptoms are associated with a good response to ECT, including psychomotor agitation or retardation; nihilistic, somatic, or paranoid delusions; and acute onset of illness. ECT is not generally recommended for patients with chronic forms of depression or patients with serious personality disorders (e.g., borderline personality disorder).

Mania responds well to ECT, although its use is primarily reserved for patients not responding to medication. Similarly, patients with a schizoaffective disorder may benefit when medication has been ineffective. Schizophrenic patients are sometimes treated with ECT, particularly when a superimposed major depression or a catatonic syndrome is present. As a general rule, patients with schizophrenia of relatively brief duration (i.e., less than 18 months) respond better than those with more chronic forms of the illness, yet sometimes even patients with chronic schizophrenia will respond to ECT. Indications for ECT are summarized in Table 20–8.

TABLE 20–8. Indications for electroconvulsive therapy (ECT)

Medication-refractory depression

Suicidal depression

Depression accompanied by refusal to eat or take fluids

Depression during pregnancy

History of positive response to ECT

Catatonic syndromes

Acute forms of schizophrenia

Mania unresponsive to medication

Psychotic or melancholic depression unresponsive to medication

---

Pre-Electroconvulsive Therapy Workup

Baseline screening should include a physical examination, basic laboratory tests (blood count and electrolytes), and an electrocardiogram. These
will help to rule out physical disorders that may complicate ECT, reveal
occult arrhythmias that may require monitoring during the procedure, or
will uncover electrolyte abnormalities that need correcting prior to ECT
such as hypokalemia. A chest X-ray should be obtained in patients with
pulmonary disease. Spine films are no longer routinely obtained due to
the rarity of fractures with current ECT protocols. Relative contraindications include recent myocardial infarction (i.e., within 1 month), unstable
coronary artery disease, uncompensated congestive heart failure, uncontrolled hypertensive cardiovascular disease, and venous thrombosis.
Space-occupying brain lesions and other causes of increased intracranial
pressure, such as recent intracerebral hemorrhage, unstable aneurysms,
or vascular malformations are the only absolute contraindications to
ECT. Psychotropic medications may be continued, although benzodiazepines should be reduced to the lowest possible dose (or be discontinued
altogether) because they can interfere with the induction of a seizure.

Electroconvulsive Therapy Procedure

ECT sessions are usually scheduled in the morning. The patient's bladder should be emptied, and he or she should not have had food or fluids
for at least 6–8 hours before the procedure. The treatment team usually
consists of a psychiatrist, an anesthesiologist (or nurse anesthetist), and
a specially trained nursing team. The treatment area should have resus-
citative equipment available.

Patients are anesthetized with a short-acting anesthetic (e.g., meth-
ohexital, etomidate), receive oxygen to prevent hypoxia, receive succi-
nylcholine as a muscle relaxant to attenuate convulsions, and receive
atropine or glycopyrrolate to reduce secretions and to prevent bradyarrhythmias. Glycopyrrolate does not cross the blood-brain barrier and
may be associated with less postictal confusion than atropine in the elderly. After the patient is anesthetized, electrodes are placed on the
scalp.

Two different electrode placements are commonly used. Bilateral
placement involves placing the electrode on each side of the head over
the parietal lobes. With unilateral placement, one electrode is placed
over the right temple and the other is placed at the vertex of the skull.
Bilateral placement is associated with a more efficient response while

right unilateral placement is associated with less post-ECT confusion and memory loss.

A brief electrical stimulus is applied after placement of the electrodes. A bidirectional pulse wave is given rather than a continuous sinusoidal waveform commonly used in the past because the pulse wave is associated with less cognitive impairment. Stimulation usually produces a 30- to 90-second tonic-clonic seizure. The seizure is accompanied by a period of bradycardia and a transient drop in blood pressure, followed by tachycardia and a rise in blood pressure. A rise in cerebrospinal fluid pressure parallels the rise in blood pressure. These physiological responses are attenuated by the pre-ECT medications. Minor arrhythmias are frequent but are seldom a problem.

Therapeutic Aspects of Electroconvulsive Therapy

For the treatment to be therapeutic, a seizure must occur. Furthermore, the electrical stimulus must involve sufficient energy. A process called *stimulus dosing* has been developed to deliver the amount of electricity needed to be therapeutic and yet keep the dose to the minimum required to induce a seizure. This will help minimize cognitive impairment. The unit of electrical charge is measured in millicoulombs (mC). Initially, several low doses are given, increasing the charge with each successive stimulation. The dose at which the patient seizes is called the *seizure threshold.* When using bilateral electrode placement, a patient will have a therapeutic response when the dosage is two and one-half times threshold, and about six times threshold when right unilateral placement is used.

Adverse Effects of Electroconvulsive Therapy

Adverse effects during ECT can include brief episodes of hypotension or hypertension, bradyarrhythmias, and tachyarrhythmias; these effects are rarely serious. Fractures were widely reported to occur during ECT-induced seizures in the past but are uncommon now because of the use of muscle relaxants. Other possible adverse effects include prolonged seizures, laryngospasm, and prolonged apnea due to pseudocholinesterase deficiency, a rare genetic disorder. Seizures lasting longer than 2 minutes should be terminated (e.g., with intravenous lorazepam, 1–2 mg). Immediately after treatment, patients experience postictal con-

Bibliography

Introduction

Ackerknecht EH: Short History of Psychiatry. New York, Hafner, 1968
Alexander FG, Selesnick ST: The History of Psychiatry: An Evaluation of Psychiatric Thought and Practice From Prehistoric Times to the Present. New York, Harper & Row, 1966
Andreasen NC: The Broken Brain: The Biological Revolution in Psychiatry. New York, Harper & Row, 1984
Andreasen NC: Brave New Brain: Conquering Mental Illness in the Era of the Genome. New York, Oxford University Press, 2001
Murray CJL, Lopez AD: The Global Burden of Disease. Boston, MA, Harvard University Press, 1996
Zilboorg G: A History of Medical Psychology. New York, WW Norton, 1941

Chapter 1

American Psychiatric Association: Diagnostic and Statistical Manual: Mental Disorders. Washington, DC, American Psychiatric Association, 1952
American Psychiatric Association: Diagnostic and Statistical Manual of Mental Disorders, 2nd Edition. Washington, DC, American Psychiatric Association, 1968
American Psychiatric Association: Diagnostic and Statistical Manual of Mental Disorders, 3rd Edition. Washington, DC, American Psychiatric Association, 1980
American Psychiatric Association: Diagnostic and Statistical Manual of Mental Disorders, 3rd Edition, Revised. Washington, DC, American Psychiatric Association, 1987
American Psychiatric Association: Diagnostic and Statistical Manual of Mental Disorders, 4th Edition. Washington, DC, American Psychiatric Association, 1994
American Psychiatric Association: Diagnostic and Statistical Manual of Mental Disorders, 4th Edition, Text Revision. Washington, DC, American Psychiatric Association, 2000
Feighner JP, Robins E, Guze SB, et al: Diagnostic criteria for use in psychiatric research. Arch Gen Psychiatry 26:57–63, 1972
Kendler KS: Toward a scientific psychiatric nosology: strengths and limitations. Arch Gen Psychiatry 47:969–973, 1990
King LS: Medical Thinking: A Historical Preface. Princeton, NJ, Princeton University Press, 1982

Csernanski JG, Schindler MK, Splinter NR, et al: Abnormalities of thalamic volume and shape in schizophrenia. Am J Psychiatry 161:896–902, 2004

Essock SM, Covell C, Desckersbach T, et al: Effectiveness of switching antipsychotic medications. Am J Psychiatry 163:2090–2095, 2006

Evans JD, Heaton RK, Paulsen JS, et al: Schizoaffective disorder: a form of schizophrenia or affective disorder? J Clin Psychiatry 60:874–882, 1999

Flashman LA, Flaum M, Gupta S, et al: Soft signs and neuropsychological performance in schizophrenia. Am J Psychiatry 153:526–532, 1996

Goldman-Rakic PS: Working memory dysfunction in schizophrenia. J Neuropsychiatry Clin Neurosci 6:348–357, 1994

Green AI, Drake RE, Brunette MF, et al: Schizophrenia and co-occurring substance use disorder. Am J Psychiatry 164:402–408, 2007

Harrison PJ, Weinberger DR: Schizophrenia genes, gene expression, and neuropathology: on the matter of their convergence. Mol Psychiatry 10:40–68, 2005

Hirsch SR, Weinberger DR (eds): Schizophrenia, 2nd Edition. Oxford, UK, Blackwell Science, 2003

Hogarty GE, Flesher S, Ulrich R, et al: Cognitive enhancement therapy for schizophrenia: effect of a 2-year randomized trial on cognition and behavior. Arch Gen Psychiatry 61:866–876, 2004

Holzman PS, Levy DL, Proctor LR: Smooth pursuit eye movements, attention, and schizophrenia. Arch Gen Psychiatry 45:641–647, 1976

Huxley NA, Rendall M, Sederer L: Psychosocial treatments in schizophrenia: a review of the past 20 years. J Nerv Ment Dis 188:187–201, 2000

Kane JM: New-onset schizophrenia: pharmacologic treatment. Focus 6:167–171, 2008

Kasanin J: The acute schizoaffective psychoses. Am J Psychiatry 90:97–126, 1933

Kendler KS: Demography of paranoid psychoses (delusional disorder). Arch Gen Psychiatry 39:890–902, 1982

Langfeldt G: Schizophreniform States. Copenhagen, Denmark, E Munksgaard, 1939

Levinson DF, Mahtani MM, Nancarrow DJ, et al: Genome scan of schizophrenia. Am J Psychiatry 155:741–750, 1998

Lieberman JA: Neurobiology and the natural history of schizophrenia. J Clin Psychiatry 67:e14, 2006

Lieberman JA, Stroup TS, Perkins DO (eds): American Psychiatric Publishing Textbook of Schizophrenia. Washington, DC, American Psychiatric Publishing, 2006

Marder SR: Neurocognition as a treatment target in schizophrenia. Focus 6:180–183, 2008

Marder SR, Wirshing WC, Mintz J, et al: Two-year outcome of social skills training and group psychotherapy for outpatients with schizophrenia. Am J Psychiatry 153:1585–1592, 1996

McElroy SL, Keck PE Jr, Strakowski SM: An overview of the treatment of schizoaffective disorder. J Clin Psychiatry 60 (suppl):16–21, 1999

McGlashan TH: The Chestnut Lodge follow-up study, II: long-term outcome in schizophrenia and the affective disorders. Arch Gen Psychiatry 41:586–601, 1984

McGuire PK, Frith CD: Disordered functional connectivity in schizophrenia. Psychol Med 26:663–667, 1996

McNeil TF, Cantor-Graae E, Weinberger DR: Relationship of obstetric complications and differences in size of brain structures in monozygotic twin pairs discordant for schizophrenia. Am J Psychiatry 157:203–212, 2000

Meltzer HY, Alphs L, Green AI, et al: Clozapine treatment for suicidality in schizophrenia: International Suicide Prevention Trial (InterSePT). Arch Gen Psychiatry 60:82–91, 2003

Montross LP, Zisook S, Kasckow J: Suicide among patients with schizophrenia: a consideration of risk and protective factors. Ann Clin Psychiatry 17:173–182, 2005

Munoz RA, Amado H, Hyatt S: Brief reactive psychosis. J Clin Psychiatry 48:324–327, 1987

Munro A: Psychiatric disorders characterized by delusions: treatment in relation to specific types. Psychiatr Ann 22:232–240, 1992

Murray CJL, Lopez AD: The Global Burden of Disease. Boston, MA, Harvard University Press, 1996

Nicholson R, Lenane M, Singaracharlu S, et al: Premorbid speech and language impairment in childhood-onset schizophrenia associated with risk factors. Am J Psychiatry 157:794–800, 2000

Opjordsmoen S: Long-term course and outcome in delusional disorder. Acta Psychiatr Scand 78:556–586, 1988

Penn DL, Mueser KT: Research update on the psychosocial treatment of schizophrenia. Am J Psychiatry 153:607–617, 1996

Sacks MH: Folie à deux. Compr Psychiatry 29:270–277, 1988

Sedvall G, Terenius L: Schizophrenia: Pathophysiological Mechanisms. Amsterdam, The Netherlands, Elsevier, 2000

Selemon LD, Rajkowska G, Goldman-Rakic S: Abnormally high neuronal density in the schizophrenic cortex. Arch Gen Psychiatry 52:805–818, 1995

Staal W, Hulshoff HE, Schnack HG, et al: Structural brain abnormalities in patients with schizophrenia and their healthy siblings. Am J Psychiatry 157:416–421, 2000

Stroup TS, Lieberman JA, McEvoy JP, et al: Effectiveness of olanzapine, quetiapine, and risperidone in patients with chronic schizophrenia after discontinuing perphenazine: a CATIE study. Am J Psychiatry 164:415–427, 2007

Targum SD: Neuroendocrine dysfunction in schizophreniform disorder: correlation with six-month clinical outcome. Am J Psychiatry 140:309–313, 1983

Tran PV, Tollefson GD, Sanger TM, et al: Olanzapine versus haloperidol in the treatment of schizoaffective disorder: acute and long-term therapy. Br J Psychiatry 174:15–22, 1999

Turetsky BI, Calkins ME, Light GA, et al: Neurophysiological endophenotypes of schizophrenia: the viability of selected candidate measures. Schizophr Bull 33:69–94, 2007

Winokur G: Familial psychopathology and delusional disorder. Compr Psychiatry 26:241–248, 1985

Wright IC, Rabe-Hesketh S, Woodruff P, et al: Meta-analysis of regional brain volumes in schizophrenia. Am J Psychiatry 157:16–25, 2000

Zhang-Wong J, Beiser M, Bean M, et al: Five-year course of schizophreniform disorder. Psychiatry Res 59:109–117, 1995

Swedo SE, Leonard HL, Garvey M: Pediatric autoimmune neuropsychiatric disorders associated with streptococcal infections: clinical descriptions of the first 50 cases. Am J Psychiatry 155:264–271, 1998

Vulink NC, Denys D, Fluitman SB, et al: Quetiapine augments the effect of citalopram in non-refractory obsessive-compulsive disorder: a randomized, double-blind, placebo-controlled study of 76 patients. J Clin Psychiatry 70:1001–1008, 2009

Yates WR: Phenomenology and epidemiology of panic disorder. Ann Clin Psychiatry 21:95–102, 2009

Chapter 8

Allen LA, Escobar JI, Lehrer PM, et al: Psychosocial treatments for multiple unexplained physical symptoms: a review of the literature. Psychosom Med 64:939–950, 2002

American Psychiatric Association: Diagnostic and Statistical Manual of Mental Disorders, 4th Edition, Text Revision. Washington, DC, American Psychiatric Association, 2000

Andreasen NC, Bardach J: Dysmorphophobia: symptom or disease? Am J Psychiatry 134:673–676, 1977

Andreasen PJ, Seidel JA: Behavioral techniques in the treatment of patients with multiple personality disorder. Ann Clin Psychiatry 4:29–32, 1992

Avia MD, Ruiz MA: Recommendations for the treatment of hypochondriac patients. Journal of Contemporary Psychotherapy 35:301–313, 2005

Barsky AJ, Fama JM, Bailey ED, et al: A prospective 4- to 5-year study of DSM-III-R hypochondriasis. Arch Gen Psychiatry 55:737–744, 1998

Blumer D, Heilbronn M: Antidepressant treatment for chronic pain: treatment outcome of 1,000 patients with the pain prone disorders. Psychiatr Ann 14:796–800, 1984

Butler LD: Normative dissociation. Psychiatr Clin North Am 29:45–62, 2006

Coons PM, Bohman ES, Milstein V: Multiple personality disorder: a clinical investigation of 50 cases. J Nerv Ment Dis 176:519–527, 1988

DeWaal MWM, Arnold IA, Eekhof JAH, et al: Somatoform disorders in general practice. Br J Psychiatry 184:470–476, 2004

Eisendrath SJ: Factitious illness: a clarification. Psychosomatics 25:110–117, 1984

Ellason JW, Ross CA: Two year follow-up of inpatients with dissociative identity disorder. Am J Psychiatry 154:832–839, 1997

Foote B, Smolin Y, Kaplan M, et al: Prevalence of dissociative disorders in psychiatric outpatients. Am J Psychiatry 163:623–629, 2006

Grant J, Phillips KA: Recognizing and treating body dysmorphic disorder. Ann Clin Psychiatry 17:205–210, 2005

Guralnik O, Schmeidler J, Simeon D: Feeling unreal: cognitive processes in depersonalization. Am J Psychiatry 157:103–109, 2000

Henningsen P, Jakobsen T, Schiltenwolf M, et al: Somatization revisited: diagnosis and perceived causes of common mental disorders. J Nerv Ment Dis 193:85–92, 2005

Kellner R: Hypochondriasis and somatization. JAMA 258:2718–2722, 1987

Krem MM: Motor conversion disorders reviewed from a neuropsychiatric prospective. J Clin Psychiatry 65:783–790, 2004

Lauer J, Black DW, Keen P: Multiple personality disorder and borderline personality disorder: distinct entities or variations on a common theme? Ann Clin Psychiatry 5:129–134, 1993

Leo RJ: Clinical Manual of Pain Management in Psychiatry. Washington, DC, American Psychiatric Publishing, 2007

Lilienfeld SO, Van Valkenburg C, Larntz K, et al: The relationship of histrionic personality disorder to antisocial personality and somatization disorders. Am J Psychiatry 143:718–722, 1986

Lowenstein RJ: Psychopharmacologic treatments of dissociative identity disorder. Psychiatr Ann 35:666–673, 2005

Noyes R, Reich J, Clancy J, et al: Reduction in hypochondriasis with treatment of panic disorder. Br J Psychiatry 149:631–635, 1986

Noyes R, Kathol RG, Fisher MM, et al: The validity of DSM-III-R hypochondriasis. Arch Gen Psychiatry 50:961–970, 1993

Noyes R, Holt CS, Kathol RG: Somatization: diagnosis and management. Arch Gen Psychiatry 4:790–795, 1995

Noyes R, Langbehn DR, Happel RL, et al: Personality dysfunction among somatizing patients. Psychosomatics 42:320–329, 2001

Perley MJ, Guze SB: Hysteria: the stability and usefulness of clinical criteria. N Engl J Med 266:421–426, 1962

Phillips KA: The Broken Mirror: Understanding and Treating Body Dysmorphic Disorder, Revised and Expanded Edition. New York, Oxford University Press, 2005

Phillips KA, Didie ER, Feusner J, et al: Body dysmorphic disorder: treating an underrecognized disorder. Am J Psychiatry 165:1111–1118, 2008

Piper A: Multiple personality disorder. Br J Psychiatry 164:600–612, 1994

Pope HG Jr, Jonas JM, Jones B: Factitious psychosis: phenomenology, family history, and long-term outcome of nine patients. Am J Psychiatry 139:1480–1483, 1982

Reich P, Gottfried LA: Factitious disorders in a teaching hospital. Ann Intern Med 99:240–247, 1983

Ross CA, Miller SD, Reagor P, et al: Structured interview data on 102 cases of multiple personality disorder from four centers. Am J Psychiatry 147:596–601, 1990

Schenk L, Bear D: Multiple personality and related dissociative phenomena in patients with temporal lobe epilepsy. Am J Psychiatry 138:1311–1315, 1981

Schreiber FR: Sybil. Chicago, IL, Henry Regnery, 1973

Shah KA, Forman MB, Freedman HS: Munchausen's syndrome and cardiac catheterization: a case of a pernicious interaction. JAMA 248:3008–3009, 1982

Sierra M, Berrios GE: Depersonalization: neurobiologic perspectives. Biol Psychiatry 44:898–908, 1998

Simeon D, Gross S, Guralnik O, et al: Feeling unreal: 30 cases of DSM-III-R depersonalization disorder. Am J Psychiatry 154:1107–1113, 1997

Simeon D, Stein DJ, Hollander E: Treatment of depersonalization disorder with clomipramine. Biol Psychiatry 44:302–303, 1998

Jellinek EM: The Disease Concept of Alcoholism. New Haven, CT, College and University Press, 1968

Jones HE, Strain EL, Bigelow GE, et al: Induction with levomethadyl acetate: safety and efficacy. Arch Gen Psychiatry 55:729–736, 1998

Jorenby DE, Leischow SJ, Nides MA, et al: A controlled trial of sustained release bupropion, a nicotine patch, or both for smoking cessation. N Engl J Med 340:685–691, 1999

Kalivas PW, Volkow ND: The neural basis of addiction: a pathology of motivation and choice. Am J Psychiatry 162:1403–1413, 2005

Little KY, Zhang L, Desmond T, et al: Striatal dopamine abnormalities in human cocaine users. Am J Psychiatry 156:238–245, 1999

Malcolm R, Ballenger JC, Sturgis ET, et al: Double-blind controlled trial comparing carbamazepine to oxazepam treatment of alcohol withdrawal. Am J Psychiatry 146:617–621, 1989

McNagney SE, Parker RM: High prevalence of recent cocaine use and the unreliability of patient self-report in an inner city walk-in clinic. JAMA 267: 1106–1108, 1992

Merikangas KR, Stolar M, Stevens DE, et al: Familial transmission of substance use disorders. Arch Gen Psychiatry 55:973–979, 1998

National Consensus Development Panel on Effective Medical Treatment of Opiate Addiction: Effective medical treatment of opiate addiction. JAMA 280:1936–1943, 1998

Nordstrom G, Bergland M: Type I and type II alcoholics (Cloninger & Bohman) have different patterns of long-term adjustment. Addiction 82:761–769, 2006

Nurnberger JI Jr, Weigand R, Bucholz K, et al: A family study of alcohol dependence. Arch Gen Psychiatry 61:1246–1256, 2004

Nutt D: Alcohol and the brain: pharmacologic insights for psychiatrists. Br J Psychiatry 175:114–119, 1999

Peirce JM, Petry NM, Stitzer ML, et al: Effects of lower-cost incentives on stimulant abstinence in methadone maintenance treatment: a National Drug Abuse Treatment Clinical Trials Network study. Arch Gen Psychiatry 63: 201–208, 2006

Perry PJ, Anderson KH, Yates WR: Illicit anabolic steroid use in athletes: a case series analysis. Am J Sports Med 184:422–428, 1990

Perry PJ, Alexander B, Liskow BI, et al: Psychotropic Drug Handbook, 8th Edition. Baltimore, MD, Lippincott Williams & Wilkins, 2006

Pope HG Jr, Yurgelun-Todd D: The residual cognitive effects of heavy marijuana use in college students. JAMA 275:521–527, 1996

Pope HG Jr, Kouri EM, Powell KF, et al: Anabolic-androgenic steroid use among 133 prisoners. Compr Psychiatry 37:322–327, 1996

Schlaepfer TE, Strain EC, Greenberg BD, et al: Site of opioid action in the human brain: mu and kappa agonists' subjective and cerebrospinal blood flow effects. Am J Psychiatry 155:470–473, 1998

Schuckit MA, Smith TL, Anthenelli R, et al: Clinical course of alcoholism in 646 male inpatients. Am J Psychiatry 150:786–792, 1993

Sees KL, Delucchi KL, Masson C, et al: Methadone maintenance vs 180-day psychosocially enriched detoxification for treatment of opioid dependence: a randomized controlled trial. JAMA 283:1303–1310, 2000

Streissguth AP, Clarren SK, Jones KL: Natural history of the fetal alcohol syndrome: a 10 year follow up of 11 patients. Lancet 2:85–91, 1985

Swift RM: Drug therapy for alcohol dependence. N Engl J Med 340:1482–1489, 1999

Toomey R, Lyons MJ, Eisen SA, et al: A twin study of the neuropsychological consequences of stimulant abuse. Arch Gen Psychiatry 60:303–310, 2003

Vaillant GE: A 12-year follow-up of New York narcotic addicts. Arch Gen Psychiatry 15:599–609, 1966

Vaillant GE: The Natural History of Alcoholism: Causes, Patterns, and Paths to Recovery. Cambridge, MA, Harvard University Press, 1983

Van den Bree MBM, Pickworth WB: Risk factors predicting changes in marijuana involvement in teenagers. Arch Gen Psychiatry 62:311–319, 2005

Vereby K, Gold MS: From coca leaves to crack: the effects of dose and routes of administration in abuse liability. Psychiatr Ann 18:513–520, 1988

Volpicelli JR, Alterman AI, Hayashida M, et al: Naltrexone in the treatment of alcohol dependence. Arch Gen Psychiatry 49:876–880, 1992

Warner EA: Cocaine abuse. Ann Intern Med 119:226–235, 1993

Yates WR, Fulton AI, Gabel J, et al: Personality risk factors for cocaine abuse. Am J Public Health 79:891–892, 1989

Chapter 10

American Psychiatric Association: Diagnostic and Statistical Manual: Mental Disorders. Washington, DC, American Psychiatric Association, 1952

American Psychiatric Association: Diagnostic and Statistical Manual of Mental Disorders, 2nd Edition. Washington, DC, American Psychiatric Association, 1968

American Psychiatric Association: Diagnostic and Statistical Manual of Mental Disorders, 3rd Edition. Washington, DC, American Psychiatric Association, 1980

American Psychiatric Association: Diagnostic and Statistical Manual of Mental Disorders, 4th Edition. Washington, DC, American Psychiatric Association, 1994

American Psychiatric Association: Diagnostic and Statistical Manual of Mental Disorders, 4th Edition, Text Revision. Washington, DC, American Psychiatric Association, 2000

Barrett MS, Stanford MS, Felthaus A, et al: The effects of phenytoin on impulsive and premeditated aggression: a controlled study. J Clin Psychopharmacol 17:341–349, 1997

Beck A: Cognitive Therapy of Personality Disorders. New York, Guilford, 1990

Black DW: Bad Boys, Bad Men: Confronting Antisocial Personality Disorder. New York, Oxford University Press, 1999

Black DW, Blum N, Pfohl B, et al: Suicidal behavior in borderline personality disorder: prevalence, risk factors, prediction, and prevention. J Personal Disord 18:226–239, 2004

Blum N, St John D, Pfohl B, et al: Systems Training for Emotional Predictability and Problem Solving (STEPPS) for outpatients with borderline personality disorder: a randomized controlled trial and 1-year follow-up. Am J Psychiatry 165:468–478, 2008

Cadoret RJ, Yates WR, Troughton E, et al: Genetic-environmental interaction in the genesis of aggressivity and conduct disorders. Arch Gen Psychiatry 52:916–924, 1995

Clarkin JF, Levy KN, Lenzenweger MF, et al: Evaluating three treatments for borderline personality disorder: a multiwave study. Am J Psychiatry 164:922–928, 2006

Cleckley H: The Mask of Sanity. St. Louis, MO, Mosby, 1941

Coid JW: Aetiological risk factors for personality disorders. Br J Psychiatry 174:530–538, 1999

Cowdry RW, Gardner D: Pharmacotherapy of borderline personality disorder. Arch Gen Psychiatry 45:111–119, 1988

Donegan NH, Sanislow CA, Blumberg HP, et al: Amygdala hyperreactivity in borderline personality disorder: implications for emotional dysregulation. Biol Psychiatry 54:1284–1293, 2003

Fulton M, Winokur G: A comparative study of paranoid and schizoid personality disorders. Am J Psychiatry 150:1363–1367, 1993

Grant BF, Hasin DS, Stinson FS, et al: Prevalence, correlates, and disability of personality disorders in the United States: results from the National Epidemiologic Survey on Alcohol and Related Conditions. J Clin Psychiatry 65:948–958, 2004

Grant BF, Chou SP, Goldstein RB, et al: Prevalence, correlates, disability, and co-morbidity of borderline personality disorder: results from the Wave 2 National Epidemiologic Survey on Alcohol and Related Conditions. J Clin Psychiatry 69:533–545, 2008

Johnson JG, Cohen P, Brown J, et al: Childhood maltreatment increases risk for personality disorders during young adulthood. Arch Gen Psychiatry 56:600–606, 1999

Kernberg O: Severe Personality Disorders. New Haven, CT, Yale University Press, 1984

Levy KN, Chauhan P, Clarkin JF, et al: Narcissistic pathology: empirical approaches. Psychiatr Ann 39:203–213, 2009

Lieb K, Zanarini MC, Schmahl C, et al: Borderline personality disorder. Lancet 364:453–461, 2004

Linehan MM, Comtois KA, Murray AM, et al: Two-year randomized controlled trial and follow-up of dialectical behavior therapy vs therapy by experts for suicidal behaviors and borderline personality disorder. Arch Gen Psychiatry 63:757–766, 2006

Livesley WJ, Jang LL, Jackson DN, et al: Genetic and environmental contributions to dimensions of personality disorder. Am J Psychiatry 150:1826–1831, 1993

McCrae R, Costa T: Validation of the five-factor model of personality across instruments and observers. J Pers Soc Psychol 52:81–90, 1987

McGlashan TH: Schizotypal personality disorder. Arch Gen Psychiatry 43:329–334, 1986

Nestadt G, Romanoski AJ, Chahal R, et al: An epidemiological study of histrionic personality disorder. Psychol Med 20:413–422, 1990

Pfohl B, Blum N: Obsessive-compulsive personality disorder: a review of available data and recommendations for DSM-IV. J Personal Disord 5:363–375, 1991

Reich J: The morbidity of DSM-III-R dependent personality disorder. J Nerv Ment Dis 84:22–26, 1996

Reich J, Yates W, Nguaguba M: Prevalence of DSM-III personality disorders in the community. Soc Psychiatry Psychiatr Epidemiol 24:12–16, 1989

Ronningstam E, Gundersen J, Lyons M: Changes in pathological narcissism. Am J Psychiatry 152:253–257, 1995

Soeteman DI, Hakkaart-van Roijen L, Verheul R, et al: The economic burden of personality disorders in mental health care. J Clin Psychiatry 69:259–265, 2008

Stinson FS, Dawson DA, Goldstein RB, et al: Prevalence, correlates, and comorbidity of DSM-IV narcissistic personality disorder: results from the Wave 2 National Epidemiologic Survey on Alcohol and Related Conditions. J Clin Psychiatry 69:1033–1045, 2008

Ullrich S, Coid J: Antisocial personality disorder: co-morbid Axis I mental disorders and health service use among a national household population. Personality and Mental Health 3:151–164, 2009

Chapter 11

Balon R, Segraves RT (eds): Clinical Manual of Sexual Disorders. Washington, DC, American Psychiatric Publishing, 2009

Black DW, Goldstein RB, Blum N, et al: Personality characteristics in 60 subjects with psychosexual dysfunction: a non-patient sample. J Personal Disord 9:275–285, 1995

Bodinger L, Hermesh H, Aizenberg D, et al: Sexual function and behavior in social phobia. J Clin Psychiatry 63:874–879, 2002

Briken P, Kafka MP: Pharmacological treatments for paraphilic patients and sexual offenders. Curr Opin Psychiatry 20:609–613, 2007

Brown GR: A review of clinical approaches to gender dysphoria. J Clin Psychiatry 51:57–64, 1990

Brown GR, Wise TN, Costa PT, et al: Personality characteristics and sexual functioning of 188 cross dressing men. J Nerv Ment Dis 184:265–273, 1996

Clayton A, Pradko JF, Croft HA, et al: Prevalence of sexual dysfunction among newer antidepressants. J Clin Psychiatry 63:357–366, 2002

Cohen LJ, McGeoch PG, Watras-Gans S, et al: Personality impairment in male pedophiles. J Clin Psychiatry 63:912–919, 2002

Dunsleith NW, Nelson EB, Brusman-Lovins LA, et al: Psychiatric and legal features of 113 men convicted of sexual offenses. J Clin Psychiatry 65:293–300, 2004

First MB, Frances A: Issues for DSM-V: unintended consequences of small changes: the case of paraphilias. Am J Psychiatry 165:1240–1241, 2008

Gaffney GR, Berlin FS: Is there a gonadal dysfunction in pedophilia? A pilot study. Br J Psychiatry 145:657–660, 1984

Gaffney GR, Lurie SF, Berlin FS: Is there familial transmission of pedophilia? J Nerv Ment Dis 172:546–548, 1984

Grant JE: Clinical characteristics and psychiatric comorbidity in males with exhibitionism. J Clin Psychiatry 66:1367–1371, 2005

Sharp CW, Freeman CPL: The medical complications of anorexia nervosa. Br J Psychiatry 162:452–463, 1993

Yager J, Powers PS (eds): Clinical Manual of Eating Disorders. Washington, DC, American Psychiatric Publishing, 2007

Yates WR, Sieleni B, Reich J, et al: Comorbidity of bulimia nervosa and personality disorder. J Clin Psychiatry 50:57–59, 1989

Chapter 13

American Psychiatric Association: Diagnostic and Statistical Manual of Mental Disorders, 3rd Edition. Washington, DC, American Psychiatric Association, 1980

American Psychiatric Association: Diagnostic and Statistical Manual of Mental Disorders, 4th Edition, Text Revision. Washington, DC, American Psychiatric Association, 2000

Andreasen NC, Hoenk PR: The predictive value of adjustment disorders: a follow-up study. Am J Psychiatry 139:584–590, 1982

Andreasen NC, Wasek P: Adjustment disorders in adolescents and adults. Arch Gen Psychiatry 37:1166–1170, 1980

Derogatis LR, Morrow GR, Fetting J, et al: The prevalence of psychiatric disorders among cancer patients. JAMA 249:751–757, 1983

Despland JN, Monod L, Ferrero F: Clinical relevance of adjustment disorder in DSM-III-R and DSM-IV. Compr Psychiatry 36:454–460, 1995

Fabrega H, Mezzich JE, Mezzich AC: Adjustment disorder as a marginal or transitional illness category in DSM-III. Arch Gen Psychiatry 44:567–572, 1987

Greenberg WM, Rosenfeld DN, Ortega EA: Adjustment disorder as an admission diagnosis. Am J Psychiatry 152:459–461, 1995

Jones R, Yates WR, Williams S, et al: Outcome for adjustment disorder with depressed mood: comparison with other mood disorders J Affect Disord 55:55–61, 1991

Jones R, Yates WR, Zhou HH: Readmission rates for adjustment disorder with depressed mood: comparison with other mood disorders. J Affect Disord 71:199–203, 2002

Kovacs M, Ho V, Pollock MH: Criterion and predictive validity of the diagnosis of adjustment disorder: a prospective study of youths with new-onset insulin dependent diabetes mellitus. Am J Psychiatry 152:523–528, 1995

Looney JG, Gunderson EKE: Transient situational disturbances: course and outcome. Am J Psychiatry 135:660–663, 1978

Oxman TE, Barrett JE, Freeman DH, et al: Frequency and correlates of adjustment disorder related to cardiac surgery in older patients. Psychosomatics 35:557–568, 1994

Pelkonen M, Marttunen M, Henricksson M, et al: Adolescent adjustment disorder: precipitant stressors and distress symptoms in 89 outpatients. Eur Psychiatry 22:288–295, 2007

Popkin MK, Callies AL, Colon EA, et al: Adjustment disorders in medically ill inpatients referred for consultations in a university hospital. Psychosomatics 31:410–414, 1990

Strain JJ, Smith GC, Hammer JS, et al: Adjustment disorder: a multisite study of its utilization and interventions in the consultation-liaison psychiatry setting. Gen Hosp Psychiatry 20:139–149, 1998

Chapter 14

American Psychiatric Association: Diagnostic and Statistical Manual of Mental Disorders, 3rd Edition. Washington, DC, American Psychiatric Association, 1980

American Psychiatric Association: Diagnostic and Statistical Manual of Mental Disorders, 4th Edition, Text Revision. Washington, DC, American Psychiatric Association, 2000

Black DW: A review of compulsive buying disorder. World Psychiatry 6:14–18, 2007

Black DW, Arndt S, Coryell WH, et al: Bupropion in the treatment of pathological gambling: a randomized, placebo-controlled, flexible-dose study. J Clin Psychopharmacol 27:143–150, 2007

Blanco C, Grant J, Petry NM, et al: Prevalence and correlates of shoplifting in the United States: results from the National Epidemiologic Survey on Alcohol and Related Conditions (NESARC). Am J Psychiatry 165:905–913, 2008

Coccaro EF, Lee RJ, Kavoussi RJ: A double-blind, randomized placebo-controlled trial of fluoxetine in patients with intermittent explosive disorder. J Clin Psychiatry 70:653–662, 2009

Goldman MJ: Kleptomania: making sense of the nonsensical. Am J Psychiatry 148:986–996, 1991

Grant JE, Kim SW: Clinical characteristics and psychiatric comorbidity of pyromania. J Clin Psychiatry 68:1717–1722, 2007

Grant JE, Potenza MN, Hollander E, et al: Multicenter investigation of the opioid antagonist nalmefene in the treatment of pathological gambling. Am J Psychiatry 163:303–312, 2006

Grant JE, Kim SW, Odlaug BL: A double-blind, placebo-controlled study of the opiate antagonist naltrexone in the treatment of kleptomania. Biol Psychiatry 65:600–606, 2009

Hollander E, Stein DJ (eds): Clinical Manual of Impulse-Control Disorders. Washington, DC, American Psychiatric Publishing, 2006

Kessler RC, Coccaro EF, Fava M, et al: The prevalence and correlates of DSM-IV intermittent explosive disorder in the National Comorbidity Survey replication. Arch Gen Psychiatry 63:669–678, 2006

Keuthen NJ, O'Sullivan RL, Goodchild P, et al: Retrospective review of treatment outcome for 63 patients with trichotillomania. Am J Psychiatry 155:560–561, 1998

Kolko DJ: Efficacy of cognitive-behavioral treatment and fire safety education for children who set fires: initial and follow-up outcomes. J Child Psychol Psychiatry 42:359–369, 2001

Kuzma J, Black DW: Disorders characterized by poor impulse control. Ann Clin Psychiatry 17:219–226, 2005

Mattes JA: Oxcarbazepine in patients with impulsive aggression: a double-blind, placebo-controlled trial. J Clin Psychopharmacol 25:575–579, 2005

McCloskey MS, Noblett KL, Deffenbacher JL, et al: Cognitive-behavior therapy for intermittent explosive disorder: a pilot randomized clinical trial. J Consult Clin Psychol 76:876–886, 2008

McElroy SL: Recognition and treatment of DSM-IV intermittent explosive disorder. J Clin Psychiatry 60:12–16, 1999

Potenza MN, Kosten TR, Rounsaville BJ: Pathological gambling. JAMA 286: 141–144, 2001

Potenza MN, Steinberg MA, Skudlarski P, et al: Gambling urges in pathological gambling: a functional magnetic resonance imaging study. Arch Gen Psychiatry 60:828–836, 2003

Shaw M, Black DW: Internet addiction: definition, assessment, epidemiology, and clinical management. CNS Drugs 22:353–365, 2008

Shaw M, Forbush K, Schlinder J, et al: The effect of pathological gambling on families, marriages, and children. CNS Spectr 12:615–622, 2007

Stewart LA: Profile of female fire setters: implications for treatment. Br J Psychiatry 163:248–256, 1993

Van Minnen A, Hoogduin KA, Kerjsers GP, et al: Treatment of trichotillomania with behavior therapy or fluoxetine. Arch Gen Psychiatry 60:517–522, 2003

Chapter 15

Alexopoulous GS, Reynolds CF III, Bruce ML, et al: Reducing suicidal ideation and depression in older primary care patients: 24-month outcomes of the PROSPECT study. Am J Psychiatry 166:882–890, 2009

Barraclough B, Bunch J, Nelson B, et al: A hundred cases of suicide: clinical aspects. Br J Psychiatry 125:355–373, 1974

Beck AT, Steer RA, Kovacs M, et al: Hopelessness and eventual suicide. Am J Psychiatry 142:559–563, 1985

Coryell W, Young EA: Clinical predictors of suicide in primary major depressive disorder. J Clin Psychiatry 66:412–417, 2005

Dolan M, Doyle M: Violence risk prediction. Br J Psychiatry 177:303–311, 2000

Ferguson SD, Coccaro EF: History of mild to moderate traumatic brain injury and aggression in physically healthy participants with and without personality disorder. J Person Disord 23:230–239, 2009

Goldstein R, Black DW, Winokur G, et al: The prediction of suicide: sensitivity, specificity, and predictive value of a multivariate model applied to suicide in 1,906 affectively ill patients. Arch Gen Psychiatry 48:418–422, 1991

Gould MS, Fisher F, Parides M, et al: Psychosocial risk factors of child and adolescent completed suicide. Arch Gen Psychiatry 53:1155–1162, 1996

Kaye NS, Soreff SM: The psychiatrist's role, responses, and responsibilities when a patient commits suicide. Am J Psychiatry 148:739–743, 1991

Mann JJ, Ellis SP, Waternaux CM, et al: Classification trees distinguish suicide attempters in major psychiatric disorders: a model of clinical decision making. J Clin Psychiatry 69:23–31, 2008

Marzuk PM, Leon AC, Tardiff K, et al: The effect of access to lethal methods of injury on suicide rates. Arch Gen Psychiatry 49:451–458, 1992

McGirr A, Renaud J, Seguin M, et al: Course of major depressive disorder and suicide outcome: a psychological autopsy study. J Clin Psychiatry 69:966–970, 2008

McNiel DE, Chamberlain JR, Weaver CM, et al: Impact of clinical training on violence risk assessment. Am J Psychiatry 165:195–200, 2008

Miller RJ, Zadolinnyj K, Hafner RJ: Profiles and predictors of assaultiveness for different ward populations. Am J Psychiatry 150:1368–1373, 1993

Murphy GE, Wetzel RD, Robins E, et al: Multiple risk factors predict suicide in alcoholism. Arch Gen Psychiatry 49:459–463, 1992

Patterson WM, Dohn HH, Bird J, et al: Evaluation of suicidal patients: the SAD PERSONS scale. Psychosomatics 24:343–349, 1983

Phillips DP, Carstonson LL: Clustering of teenage suicides after television news stories about suicide. N Engl J Med 55:685–689, 1986

Pulay AJ, Dawson DA, Hasin DS, et al: Violent behavior and DSM-IV psychiatric disorders: results from the National Epidemiologic Survey on Alcohol and Related Conditions. J Clin Psychiatry 69:12–22, 2008

Rich CL, Young D, Fowler RC: San Diego suicide study, I: young versus old subjects. Arch Gen Psychiatry 43:577–582, 1986

Robins E, Murphy GE, Wilkinson RH, et al: Some clinical considerations in the prevention of suicide based on a study of 134 successful suicides. Am J Public Health 49:888–899, 1959

Schneider B, Schnabel A, Wetterling T, et al: How do personality disorders modify suicide risk? J Person Disord 22:233–245, 2008

Stone MH: Violent crimes and their relationship to personality disorders. Personality and Mental Health 1:138–153, 2007

Tardiff K: The Psychiatric Uses of Seclusion and Restraint. Washington, DC, American Psychiatric Press, 1984

Tardiff K, Marzuk PM, Leon AC, et al: Violence by patients admitted to a private psychiatric hospital. Am J Psychiatry 154:88–93, 1997

Chapter 16

American Psychiatric Association: Diagnostic and Statistical Manual of Mental Disorders, 3rd Edition. Washington, DC, American Psychiatric Association, 1980

American Psychiatric Association: Diagnostic and Statistical Manual of Mental Disorders, 4th Edition. Washington, DC, American Psychiatric Association, 1994

American Psychiatric Association: Diagnostic and Statistical Manual of Mental Disorders, 4th Edition, Text Revision. Washington, DC, American Psychiatric Association, 2000

Angold A, Erkanli A, Farmer EMZ, et al: Psychiatric disorder, impairment, and service use in rural African American and white youth. Arch Gen Psychiatry 59:893–901, 2002

Bailey AJ, Bolton P, Butler L, et al: Prevalence of the fragile X anomaly amongst autistic twins and singletons. J Child Psychol Psychiatry 34:673–688, 1993

Barkley RA, Fischer M, Smallish L, et al: Does the treatment of attention-deficit hyperactivity disorder with stimulants contribute to drug use/abuse? A 13-year prospective study. Pediatrics 111:97–109, 2003

Biederman J, Wilens T, Mick E, et al: Pharmacotherapy of attention-deficit hyperactivity disorder reduces risk for substance use disorder. Pediatrics 104: e20, 1999

Biederman J, Monuteaux MC, Spencer T, et al: Stimulant therapy and risk for subsequent substance use disorders in male adults with ADHD: a naturalistic controlled 10 year follow-up study. Am J Psychiatry 165:597–603, 2008

Black DW: Bad Boys, Bad Men: Confronting Antisocial Personality Disorder. New York, Oxford University Press, 1999

Canino G, Shrout PE, Rubio-Stipec M, et al: The DSM-IV rates of child and adolescent disorders in Puerto Rico. Arch Gen Psychiatry 61:85–93, 2004

Cantwell DP, Baker L: Developmental Speech and Language Disorders. New York, Guilford, 1987

Cepeda C: Clinical Manual for the Psychiatric Interview of Children and Adolescents. Washington, DC, American Psychiatric Publishing, 2009

Cohen DJ, Volkmar FR: Handbook of Autism and Pervasive Developmental Disorders, 2nd Edition. New York, Wiley, 1997

Dulcan M (ed): Dulcan's Textbook of Child and Adolescent Psychiatry. Washington, DC, American Psychiatric Publishing, 2009

Findling RL (ed): Clinical Manual of Child and Adolescent Psychopharmacology. Washington, DC, American Psychiatric Publishing, 2008

Findling RL, Aman MG, Eerdekens M, et al: Long-term, open-label study of risperidone in children with severe disruptive behaviors and below-average IQ. Am J Psychiatry 111:677–684, 2004

Geller B, Tillman R, Bolhofner K, et al: Child bipolar I disorder: prospective continuity with adult bipolar I disorder; characteristics of second and third episodes; predictors of 8-year outcome. Arch Gen Psychiatry 65:1125–1133, 2008

Greenspan SI, Wieder S: Infant and Early Childhood Mental Health: A Comprehensive Developmental Approach to Assessment and Intervention. Washington, DC, American Psychiatric Publishing, 2006

Hollander E, Anagnostou E (eds): Clinical Manual for the Treatment of Autism. Washington, DC, American Psychiatric Publishing, 2007

Kanner L: Autistic disturbances of affective contact. Nerv Child 2:217–250, 1943

Klin A, Sparrow SS, Volkmar FR: Asperger Syndrome. New York, Guilford, 2000

Kolevzon A, Mathewson KA, Hollander E: Selective serotonin reuptake inhibitors in autism: a review of efficacy and tolerability. J Clin Psychiatry 67:407–414, 2006

McDougle CJ, Scahill L, Aman MG, et al: Risperidone for the core symptom domains of autism: results from the study by the Autism Network of the Research Units on Pediatric Psychopharmacology. Am J Psychiatry 162:1142–1148, 2005

McGough JJ, Barkley RA: Diagnostic controversies in adult attention deficit hyperactivity disorder. Am J Psychiatry 161:1948–1956, 2004

Morrato EH, Libby AM, Orton HD, et al: Frequency of provider contact after FDA advisory on risk of pediatric suicidality with SSRIs. Am J Psychiatry 165:42–50, 2008

Newcorn JH, Kratochvil CJ, Allen AJ, et al: Atomoxetine and osmotically released methylphenidate for the treatment of attention deficit hyperactivity
disorder: acute comparison and differential response. Am J Psychiatry
165:721–730, 2008

Piven J, Nehme E, Siman J, et al: Magnetic resonance imaging in autism: measurement of the cerebellum, pons, and fourth ventricle. Biol Psychiatry
31:491–504, 1992

Scourfield J, Van den Bree M, Martin N, et al: Conduct problems in children and
adolescents: a twin study. Arch Gen Psychiatry 61:489–496, 2004

Shapiro E, Shapiro AK, Fulop G, et al: Controlled study of haloperidol, pimozide, and placebo for the treatment of Gilles de la Tourette's syndrome.
Arch Gen Psychiatry 46:722–730, 1989

Swedo SE, Leonard HL, Garvey M, et al: Pediatric autoimmune neuropsychiatric disorders associated with streptococcal infections: clinical description of
the first 50 cases. Am J Psychiatry 154:264–271, 1998

Volkmar F, Klin A, Schultz RT, et al: Asperger's disorder. Am J Psychiatry 157:
262–267, 2000

Wassink TH, Hazlett HC, Epping EA, et al: Cerebral cortical gray matter over-
growth and functional variation of the serotonin transporter gene in autism. Arch Gen Psychiatry 64:709–717, 2007

Chapter 17

American Psychiatric Association: Diagnostic and Statistical Manual of Mental
Disorders, 4th Edition, Text Revision. Washington, DC, American Psychiatric Association, 2000

Casola PG, Goldsmith RJ, Daiter J: Assessment and treatment of sleep problems. Psychiatr Ann 36:862–868, 2006

Dashevsky BA, Kramer M: Behavioral treatment of chronic insomnia in psychiatrically ill patients. J Clin Psychiatry 59:693–699, 1998

Driver HS, Shapiro CM: ABC of sleep disorders. Parasomnias. BMJ 306:921–923,
1993

Ford DE, Kamerow DB: Epidemiologic study of sleep disturbances and psychiatric disorders: an opportunity for prevention? JAMA 262:1479–1484, 1989

Goldsmith RJ, Casola PG: An overview of sleep, sleep disorders, and psychiatric medications' effects on sleep. Psychiatr Ann 36:833–840, 2006

Jacobs EA, Reynolds CF, Kupfer DJ, et al: The role of polysomnography in the
differential diagnosis of chronic insomnia. Am J Psychiatry 145:346–349,
1988

Krystal AD, Thakur M, Roth T: Sleep disturbance in psychiatric disorders: effect
of function and quality of life in mood disorders, alcoholism, and schizophrenia. Ann Clin Psychiatry 20:39–46, 2008

Lam SP, Fon SYY, Ho CKW, et al: Parasomnia among psychiatric outpatients: a
clinical, epidemiologic, cross-sectional study. J Clin Psychiatry 69:1374–
1382, 2008

Morin CM, Culbert JP, Schwartz SM: Nonpharmacological interventions for insomnia: a meta-analysis of treatment efficacy. Am J Psychiatry 151:1172–
1180, 1994

Morin CM, Colecchi C, Stone J, et al: Behavioral and pharmacological therapies of late-life insomnia. JAMA 281:991–999, 1999

Moser D, Anderer P, Gruber G, et al: Sleep classification according to the AASM and Rechtschaffen & Kales: effects on sleep scoring parameters. Sleep 32:139–149, 2009

Nofzinger EA, Buysse DJ, Reynolds CF, et al: Sleep disorders related to another mental disorder: a DSM-IV literature review. J Clin Psychiatry 54:244–255, 1993

Nowell PD, Buysse DJ, Reynolds CF, et al: Clinical factors contributing to the differential diagnosis of primary insomnia and insomnia related to mental disorders. Am J Psychiatry 154:1412–1416, 1997

Ohayon MM, Caulet M, Lemoine P: Comorbidity of mental and insomnia disorders in the general population. Compr Psychiatry 39:185–197, 1998

Peterson MJ, Rumble ME, Benca RM: Insomnia and psychiatric disorders. Psychiatr Ann 38:597–605, 2008

Richardson GS: The human circadian system in normal and disordered sleep. J Clin Psychiatry 66 (suppl 9):3–9, 2005

Richardson GS, Zammit G, Wang-Weigand S, et al: Safety and subjective sleep effects of ramelteon administration in adults and older adults with chronic primary insomnia: 1-year, open-label study. J Clin Psychiatry 70:467–476, 2009

Roberts RE, Shema SJ, Kaplan GA, et al: Sleep complaints and depression in an aging cohort: a prospective perspective. Am J Psychiatry 157:81–88, 2000

Rosenberg RP: Sleep maintenance insomnia: strengths and weaknesses of current pharmacologic therapies. Ann Clin Psychiatry 18:49–56, 2006

Shapiro CM, Flanigan MJ: ABC of sleep disorders: function of sleep. BMJ 306:383–385, 1993

Simon GE, VonKorff M: Prevalence, burden, and treatment of insomnia in primary care. Am J Psychiatry 154:1417–1423, 1997

Smith MT, Perlis ML, Park A, et al: Comparative meta-analysis of pharmacotherapy and behavior therapy for persistent insomnia. Am J Psychiatry 159:5–11, 2002

Walsh JK, Fry J, Erwin CW, et al: Efficacy and tolerability of 14-day administration of zaleplon 5 mg and 10 mg for the treatment of primary insomnia. Clinical Drug Investigation 16:347–354, 1998

Winkelman J, Pies R: Current patterns and future directions in the treatment of insomnia. Ann Clin Psychiatry 17:31–40, 2005

Young T, Palta M, Dempsey J, et al: The occurrence of sleep disordered breathing among middle-aged adults. N Engl J Med 328:1230–1235, 1993

Zee PC, Lu BS: Insomnia and circadian rhythm sleep disorders. Psychiatr Ann 38:583–589, 2008

Chapter 18

American Medical Association Board of Trustees: Insanity defense in criminal trials and limitation of psychiatric testimony. JAMA 251:2967–2981, 1984

Appelbaum PS: *Tarasoff* and the clinician: problems in fulfilling the duty to protect. Am J Psychiatry 142:425–429, 1985

Appelbaum PS: Assessment of patients' competence to consent to treatment. N Engl J Med 357:1834–1840, 2007

Appelbaum PS, Gutheil TG: Clinical Handbook of Psychiatry and the Law, 4th edition. Philadelphia, PA, Lippincott Williams & Wilkins, 2007

Appelbaum PS, Zoltek-Jick R: Psychotherapists' duties to third parties: *Ramona* and beyond. Am J Psychiatry 153:457–465, 1996

Buchanan A: Competency to stand trial and the seriousness of the charge. J Am Acad Psychiatry Law 34:458–465, 2006

Dawes SE, Palmer BW, Jeste DV: Adjudicative competence. Curr Opin Psychiatry 21:490–494, 2008

Faust D, Ziskin J: The expert witness in psychology and psychiatry. Science 241:31–35, 1988

Frank B, Gupta S, McGlynn DJ: Psychotropic medications and informed consent: a review. Ann Clin Psychiatry 20:87–95, 2008

Giorgi-Guarnieri D, Janofsky J, Kerem E, et al: AAPL practice guideline for forensic psychiatric evaluation of defendants raising the insanity defense. J Am Acad Psychiatry Law 30 (suppl 2):S3–S40, 2002

Guthiel TG, Gabbard GO: Misuses and misunderstandings of boundary theory in clinical and regulatory settings. Am J Psychiatry 155:409–414, 1998

Lamb HR: Incompetency to stand trial. Arch Gen Psychiatry 44:754–758, 1987

Leang GB, Eth S, Silva JA: The psychotherapist as witness for the prosecution: the criminalization of *Tarasoff*. Am J Psychiatry 149:1011–1015, 1992

McNeil DE, Binder RL, Fulton FM: Management of threats of violence under California's duty-to-protect statute. Am J Psychiatry 155:1097–1101, 1998

Miller RD: Need for treatment criteria for involuntary civil commitment: impact on practice. Am J Psychiatry 149:1380–1384, 1992

Mossman D, Noffsinger SG, Ash P, et al: AAPL practice guideline for the forensic psychiatric evaluation of competence to stand trial. J Am Acad Psychiatry Law 35 (suppl 4): S3–S72, 2007

Simon RI: Concise Guide to Psychiatry and Law for Clinicians, 3rd Edition. Washington, DC, American Psychiatric Publishing, 2001

Simon RI, Gold LH (eds): Textbook of Forensic Psychiatry. Washington, DC, American Psychiatric Publishing, 2004

Simon RI, Sadoff RL: Psychiatric Malpractice: Cases and Comments for Clinicians. Washington, DC, American Psychiatric Press, 1992

Simon RI, Shuman DW: Clinical Manual of Psychiatry and Law. Washington, DC, American Psychiatric Publishing, 2007

Studdert DM, Mello MM, Sage WM, et al: Defensive medicine among high-risk specialist physicians in a volatile malpractice environment. JAMA 293: 2609–2617, 2005

Chapter 19

Baum W: Understanding Behaviorism: Behavior, Culture, and Evolution. Oxford, UK, Blackwell, 2005

Beck AT, Alford BA: Depression: Causes and Treatment, 2nd Edition. Philadelphia, PA, University of Pennsylvania Press, 2008

Clary C, Schweizer E: Treatment of MAOI hypertensive crisis with sublingual nifedipine. J Clin Psychiatry 48:249–250, 1987

Clayton AH, Warnock JK, Kornstein SG, et al: A placebo controlled trial of bupropion SR as an antidote for selective serotonin reuptake inhibitor-induced sexual dysfunction. J Clin Psychiatry 65:62–67, 2004

Clayton AH, Kornstein SG, Rosas G, et al: An integrated analysis of the safety and tolerability of desvenlafaxine compared with placebo in the treatment of major depressive disorder. CNS Spectr 14:183–195, 2009

Correll CV, Leucht S, Kane JM: Lower risk for tardive dyskinesia associated with second-generation antipsychotics: a systematic review of one-year studies. Am J Psychiatry 161:414–425, 2004

Davis JM, Chen N, Glick ID: A meta-analysis of the efficacy of second-generation antipsychotics. Arch Gen Psychiatry 60:553–564, 2003

De Hert M, Schreurs V, Vancampfort D, et al: Metabolic syndrome in people with schizophrenia. World Psychiatry 8:15–22, 2009

Fawcett J, Baskin RL: A meta-analysis of eight randomized, double-blind controlled clinical trials of mirtazapine for the treatment of patients with major depression and symptoms of anxiety. J Clin Psychiatry 59:123–127, 1998

Feighner JP: Mechanism of action of antidepressant medications. J Clin Psychiatry 60 (suppl):4–11, 1999

Geddes J: Efficacy and safety of electroconvulsive therapy in depressive disorders: a systematic review and meta-analysis. Lancet 361:799–808, 2003

Gorman JM: Mirtazapine: clinical overview. J Clin Psychiatry 60 (suppl):9–13, 1999

Hirschfeld RMA: Efficacy of SSRIs and newer antidepressants in severe depression: comparison with TCAs. J Clin Psychiatry 60:326–335, 1999

Hyman SE, Arana GW: Handbook of Psychiatric Drug Therapy. Boston, MA, Little, Brown, 1987

Ichim L, Berk M, Brook S: Lamotrigine compared with lithium in mania: a double-blind randomized controlled trial. Ann Clin Psychiatry 12:5–10, 2000

Igbal MM: Effect of antidepressants during pregnancy and lactation. Ann Clin Psychiatry 11:237–256, 1999

Jones KL, Lacro RV, Johnson KA, et al: Pattern of malformations in the children of women treated with carbamazepine during pregnancy. N Engl J Med 320:1661–1666, 1989

Jones PB, Davies L, Barnes TR, et al: Randomized controlled trial of effect on quality of life of second-generation versus first-generation antipsychotic drugs in schizophrenia. Arch Gen Psychiatry 63:1079–1087, 2006

Kane JM, Fleischhacker WW, Hansen L, et al: Akathisia: an updated review focusing on second-generation antipsychotics. J Clin Psychiatry 70:627–643, 2009

Krishnan KRR: Monoamine oxidase inhibitors, in The American Psychiatric Publishing Textbook of Psychopharmacology, 4th Edition. Edited by Schatzberg AF, Nemeroff CB. Washington, DC, American Psychiatric Publishing, 2009, pp 389–401

Leucht S, Komossa K, Rummel-Kluge C, et al: A meta-analysis of head-to-head comparisons of the second-generation antipsychotics in the treatment of schizophrenia. Am J Psychiatry 166:152–163, 2009

Lieberman JA, Stroup TS, McEvoy JP, et al: Effectiveness of antipsychotic drugs in patients with chronic schizophrenia. N Engl J Med 353:1209–1223, 2005

Lipinsky JF, Zubenko G, Cohen BM, et al: Propranolol in the treatment of neuroleptic induced akathisia. Am J Psychiatry 141:412–415, 1984

Mendelson WB: A review of the evidence for the safety and efficacy of trazodone in the treatment of insomnia. J Clin Psychiatry 66:469–476, 2005

Nemeroff CB, DeVane CL, Pollock BG: Newer antidepressants and the cytochrome P450 system. Am J Psychiatry 153:311–320, 1996

Noyes R, Garvey MJ, Cook BL, et al: Benzodiazepine withdrawal: a review of the evidence. J Clin Psychiatry 49:382–389, 1988

Olajide D, Lader M: A comparison of buspirone, diazepam, and placebo in patients with chronic anxiety states. J Clin Psychopharmacol 75:148–152, 1987

O'Reardon JP, Thase ME, Papacostas GI: Pharmacologic and therapeutic strategies in treatment-resistant depression. CNS Spectr (suppl 4):1–16, 2009

Perry PJ, Alexander B, Liskow BI, et al: Psychotropic Drug Handbook, 8th Edition. Baltimore, MD, Lippincott Williams & Wilkins, 2006

Sackheim HA, Dillingham EM, Prudic J, et al: Effect of concomitant pharmacotherapy on electroconvulsive therapy outcomes. Arch Gen Psychiatry 66:729–737, 2009

Schatzberg AF, Nemeroff CB (eds): The American Psychiatric Publishing Textbook of Psychopharmacology, 4th Edition. Washington, DC, American Psychiatric Publishing, 2009

Stroup TS, Lieberman JA, McEvoy JP, et al: Effectiveness of olanzapine, risperidone, and ziprasidone in patients with chronic schizophrenia following discontinuation of a previous atypical antipsychotic. Am J Psychiatry 163:611–622, 2006

Tyrer P, Murphy S: The place of benzodiazepines in psychiatric practice. Br J Psychiatry 151:719–723, 1987

Vieta E, T'joen C, McQuade RD, et al: Efficacy of adjunctive aripiprazole to either valproate or lithium in bipolar mania patients partially nonresponsive to valproate/lithium monotherapy: a placebo-controlled study. Am J Psychiatry 165:1316–1325, 2008

Weisler RA, Kalali AH, Ketter TA, et al: A multicenter, randomized, double-blind placebo-controlled trial of extended-release carbamazepine capsules as monotherapy for bipolar disorder patients with manic or mixed episodes. J Clin Psychiatry 65:478–484, 2004

Weissman AA, Levy BT, Hartz AJ, et al: Pooled analysis of antidepressant levels in lactating mothers, breast milk, and nursing infants. Am J Psychiatry 161:1066–1078, 2004

Zajecka J, Tracy KA, Mitchell S: Discontinuation syndromes after treatment with serotonin reuptake inhibitors: a literature review. J Clin Psychiatry 58:291–297, 1997

Glossary

A

abreaction Emotional release or discharge after recalling a painful experience that has been repressed because it was not consciously tolerable. A therapeutic effect sometimes occurs through partial or repeated discharge of the painful AFFECT.

acute confusional state 1) A form of delirium in which the most prominent symptoms are disorders of memory and orientation, usually with short-term memory deficit, AMNESIA, and clouding of consciousness (i.e., reduced clarity of awareness of environment with reduced capacity to shift, focus, and sustain ATTENTION to environmental stimuli). See ORGANIC MENTAL DISORDER. 2) An acute stress reaction to new surroundings or new demands; it generally subsides as the person adjusts to the situation.

acute dystonic reaction (ADR) An idiosyncratic drug reaction that involves acute involuntary muscle movements and spasms. Although any muscle group in the body can be involved, the most common symptoms are torticollis, facial grimacing, and body arching. Because of their antidopaminergic properties, traditional antipsychotics often are associated with this reaction and a variety of other motor disorders. Approximately 3%–10% of patients exposed to "traditional" or "typical" antipsychotic drugs will experience an ADR. The movements typically occur at a time when the blood level of medication is dropping.

adaptation Fitting one's behavior to meet the needs of one's environment, which often involves a modification of IMPULSES, emotions, or attitudes.

addiction DEPENDENCE on a chemical substance to the extent that a physiological and/or psychological need is established. This may be

The chief manifestations are difficulty in describing or recognizing one's own emotions, a limited fantasy life, and general constriction in the affective life.

alogia　Literally, speechlessness. Most commonly used to refer to the lack of spontaneity and content in speech and diminished flow of conversation that occur as NEGATIVE SYMPTOMS in schizophrenia.

ambivalence　The coexistence of contradictory emotions, attitudes, ideas, or desires with respect to a particular person, object, or situation. Ordinarily, the ambivalence is not fully conscious and suggests psychopathology only when present in an extreme form.

amines　Organic compounds containing the amino group ($-NH_2$); of special importance in neurochemistry because of their role as neurotransmitters. Dopamine, epinephrine, norepinephrine, and serotonin are amines.

amnesia　Pathological loss of memory; a phenomenon in which an area of experience becomes inaccessible to conscious recall. The loss in memory may be organic, emotional, dissociative, or of mixed origin and may be permanent or limited to a sharply circumscribed time. Two types are distinguished:

> **anterograde**　The inability to form new memories for events following an episode or event that may have produced the amnesia.

> **retrograde**　Loss of memory for events preceding the episode or event presumed to be responsible for the amnesia.

amotivation　One of the NEGATIVE SYMPTOMS of schizophrenia, characterized by lack of interest, passivity, and loss of drive.

amotivational syndrome　A SYNDROME characterized by loss of drive, passivity, lack of concern for one's appearance, no desire to work regularly, and fatigue. Some frequent, long-term marijuana users show signs of amotivational syndrome.

amygdala　In the structure of the brain, part of the basal ganglia located on the roof of the temporal horn of the lateral ventricle at the inferior end of the caudate nucleus. It is a structure in the forebrain that is an important component of the LIMBIC SYSTEM, which is involved in the regulation of emotions.

anal character　A PERSONALITY type that manifests excessive orderliness, miserliness, and obstinacy. Called *obsessive-compulsive character or personality* in other typologies. In PSYCHOANALYSIS, a pattern of behavior in an adult that is believed to originate in the anal phase of infancy, between 1 and 3 years. See also PSYCHOSEXUAL DEVELOPMENT.

anxiety　Apprehension, tension, or uneasiness from anticipation of danger, the source of which is largely unknown or unrecognized. Primarily of intrapsychic origin, in distinction to fear, which is the emotional response to a consciously recognized and usually external threat or danger. May be regarded as pathological when it interferes with social and occupational functioning, achievement of desired goals, or emotional comfort.

attention   The ability to sustain focus on one activity. A disturbance in attention may appear as having difficulty in finishing tasks that have been started, being easily distracted, or having difficulty in concentrating.

atypical depression   In DSM-IV-TR, depressive symptoms that do not meet the criteria for specific depressive disorders.

augmentation strategies   The addition of one or more medications to enhance or magnify the beneficial effects of a medication already used, such as the addition of lithium carbonate, thyroid medication, anticonvulsants, or stimulants to augment a partial response to an antidepressant.

aversion therapy   A BEHAVIOR THERAPY procedure in which stimuli associated with undesirable behavior are paired with a painful or an unpleasant stimulus, resulting in the suppression of the undesirable behavior.

avolition   Lack of initiative or goals; one of the NEGATIVE SYMPTOMS of schizophrenia. The person may wish to do something, but the desire is without power or energy.

B

behavior modification   A technique used in BEHAVIOR THERAPY that focuses on negative habits or behaviors and aims to reduce or eliminate them by the use of reinforcement (e.g., rewarding a desired behavior or punishing an unwanted one).

behavior therapy   A mode of treatment that focuses on substituting healthier ways of behaving for maladaptive patterns used in the past. Most likely to benefit are individuals who want to change habits, those with ANXIETY disorders such as phobias or PANIC ATTACKS, and those with substance abuse or eating disorders. The basic techniques include BEHAVIOR MODIFICATION, operant conditioning, shaping, token economy, systematic desensitization, RELAXATION TRAINING, AVERSION THERAPY, EXPOSURE THERAPY, FLOODING, modeling, social skills training, and PARADOXICAL INTENTION.

benzodiazepine receptors   Receptors located on neurons within the central nervous system (CNS) to which benzodiazepines bind. Benzodiazepine receptors are linked to GABA receptors. Benzodiazepines enhance the affinity of the GABA receptor for GABA, the principal inhibitory neurotransmitter in the CNS, and thereby increase its inhibitory effects, leading to decreased ANXIETY and arousal.

bereavement   Feelings of deprivation, desolation, and grief at the loss of a loved one. The grieving person does not need to seek professional help unless these feelings last for a long time or symptoms such as depression or insomnia become problematic.

beta-blocker   A class of drugs that inhibit the action of β-adrenergic receptors, which modulate cardiac functions, respiratory functions, and the dilation and constriction of blood vessels. β-Blockers are of value in the treatment of hypertension, cardiac arrhythmias, and migraine. In psychiatry, they have been used in the treatment of AGGRESSION and violence, ANXIETY-related TREMORS and lithium-induced TREMORS, antipsychotic-induced AKATHISIA, social phobia, performance anxiety, panic states, and alcohol withdrawal.

binge drinking   A pattern of heavy alcoholic intake that occurs in bouts of a day or more that are set aside for drinking. During periods between bouts, the subject may abstain from alcohol.

binge eating   A period of overeating during which a larger amount of food is ingested than most people would eat during that time. The person feels that he or she cannot stop eating or has no control over what or how much is consumed. During the episode, the person may eat more rapidly than usual, eat until feeling uncomfortably full, eat large amounts of food although not feeling hungry, and eat alone because of embarrassment over how much is being eaten. After a bout of overeating, depression, guilt feelings, and feelings of disgust with oneself are common. When binge eating is accompanied by compensatory behavior such as purging or food restriction to control weight, it is termed *bulimia nervosa.*

biological psychiatry   A school of psychiatric thought that emphasizes physical, chemical, and neurological causes of psychiatric illness and treatment approaches.

blocking   A sudden obstruction or interruption in spontaneous flow of thinking or speaking, perceived as an absence or a deprivation of thought.

borderline intellectual functioning   In DSM-IV-TR, an additional condition that may be a focus of clinical attention, especially when it co-exists with a disorder such as schizophrenia. The intelligence quotient (IQ) is in the 71–84 range.

brain imaging   Any technique that permits the in vivo visualization of the substance of the central nervous system (CNS). The best known of such techniques is computed tomography (CT). Newer methods of brain imaging such as positron emission tomography (PET), single photon emission computed tomography (SPECT), and magnetic resonance imaging (MRI) are based on different physical principles but also yield a series of two-dimensional images (or "slices") of brain regions of interest.

Several other related techniques, such as ultrasound, angiography in its various forms, regional cerebral blood flow (rCBF) measurements, brain electrical activity mapping (BEAM) and its variants, and even the older pneumoencephalogram (PEG), also provide images of some aspect of the CNS. However, these techniques are generally more invasive or limited in the structures visualized, the degree of resolution, or some other parameter, than CT, PET, SPECT, and MRI.

C

cannabinoid receptors Cannabinoids are organic compounds that are present in *Cannabis sativa*. Two subtypes of cannabinoid receptors have been cloned from animal or human sources; however, the therapeutic application of these receptors remains unknown.

Cannabis sativa An India hemp plant from which marijuana is derived. The main psychoactive component of cannabis is delta-9-tetrahydrocannabinol (THC). Marijuana may contain 0.1%–10% THC.

Capgras' syndrome The DELUSION that impostors have replaced others or the self. The SYNDROME typically follows the development of negative feelings toward the other person that the subject cannot accept and attributes, instead, to the impostor. It has been reported in patients with paranoid schizophrenia and other forms of organic brain disease.

catalepsy A generalized condition of diminished responsiveness shown by trancelike states, posturing, or maintenance of physical attitudes for a prolonged period. May occur in organic or psychological disorders, or under hypnosis. See also CATATONIC BEHAVIOR.

cataplexy Sudden loss of postural tone without loss of consciousness, typically triggered by some emotional stimulus such as laughter, anger, or excitement. It is a characteristic of narcolepsy.

catatonia Immobility with muscular rigidity or inflexibility and, at times, excitability.

catatonic behavior Marked motor abnormalities, generally limited to those occurring as part of a psychotic disorder. This term includes catatonic excitement (apparently purposeless AGITATION not influenced by external stimuli), STUPOR (decreased reactivity and fewer spontaneous movements, often with apparent unawareness of the surroundings), NEGATIVISM (apparent motiveless resistance to instructions or attempts to be moved), posturing (the person's assuming and maintaining an inappropriate or a bizarre stance), rigidity (the person's maintaining a stance or posture against all efforts to be moved), and WAXY FLEXIBILITY or CEREA FLEXIBILITAS (the person's limbs can be put into positions that are maintained).

catharsis   The healthful (therapeutic) release of ideas through "talking out" conscious material accompanied by an appropriate emotional reaction. Also, the release into awareness of repressed ("forgotten") material from the UNCONSCIOUS. See also REPRESSION.

cerea flexibilitas   The "WAXY FLEXIBILITY" often present in catatonic schizophrenia in which the patient's arm or leg remains in the position in which it is placed.

cholinergic   Activated or transmitted by acetylcholine (e.g., parasympathetic nerve fibers). Contrast with ADRENERGIC.

circumstantiality   A pattern of speech that is indirect and delayed in reaching its goal because of excessive or irrelevant detail or parenthetical remarks. The speaker does not lose the point, as is characteristic of loosening of associations, and clauses remain logically connected, but to the listener it seems that the end will never be reached.

clanging   A type of thinking in which the sound of a word, rather than its meaning, gives the direction to subsequent associations. Punning and rhyming may substitute for logic, and language may become increasingly a senseless COMPULSION to associate and decreasingly a vehicle for communication. For example, in response to the statement "That will probably remain a mystery," a patient said, "History is one of my strong points."

codependency   A term referring to the effects that people who are dependent on alcohol or other substances have on those around them, including the attempts of those people to manage the chemically dependent person. The term implies that the family's actions tend to perpetuate (enable) the person's DEPENDENCE.

cognition   A general term encompassing all the various modes of knowing and reasoning.

cognitive-behavioral therapy (CBT)   A form of PSYCHOTHERAPY focused on changing thoughts and behaviors that are related to specific target symptoms. Treatment is aimed at symptom reduction and improved functioning. The patient is taught to recognize the negative and unrealistic COGNITIONS that contribute significantly to the development or maintenance of symptoms and to evaluate and modify such thinking patterns. Problematic behaviors are also focused on and changed with the use of behavioral strategies (e.g., response prevention, scheduling pleasant activities).

cognitive development   Beginning in infancy, the acquisition of intelligence, conscious thought, and problem-solving abilities. An orderly sequence in the increase in knowledge derived from sensorimotor activity was empirically shown by Jean Piaget (1896–1980), who described four stages in the cognitive development of the child:

sensorimotor stage   The senses receive a stimulus, and the body reacts to it in a stereotyped way. This occurs from birth to 16–24 months. Object permanence develops during this time.

preoperational thought   Prelogical thought that occurs between ages 2 and 6 years. During this time, symbolic function and language develop and change the child's ability to interact. Egocentric thinking predominates, and the child believes that everything revolves around him or her. MAGICAL THINKING arises, and reality and fantasy are interwoven.

concrete operations   Rational and logical thought process. This stage occurs between ages 7 and 11. Includes the development of the ability to understand another's viewpoint and the concept of conservation.

formal operations   Cognitive stage that includes abstract thinking, conceptual thinking, and deductive reasoning. Formal operational thinking is generally achieved by age 12. See also PSYCHOSEXUAL DEVELOPMENT.

cognitive rehabilitation   Modification of cognitive and role functioning in seriously and persistently mentally ill patients, directed at improving visual and verbal memory and social and emotional perception.

cognitive restructuring   A technique of COGNITIVE THERAPY that enables one to identify negative, irrational beliefs and replace them with truthful, rational statements.

cognitive therapy   A type of PSYCHOTHERAPY, usually focused and problem oriented, directed primarily at identifying and modifying distorted COGNITIONS and behavioral dysfunction. This technique is based on the assumption that certain thought patterns, called *cognitive structures* or *schemas,* shape the way people react to the situations in their lives. Individuals with major depression, ANXIETY disorders, eating disorders, and substance abuse disorders are more likely to benefit.

combat fatigue   An outmoded term for posttraumatic stress disorder (PTSD). Disabling physical and emotional reaction incident to military combat. Paradoxically, the reaction may not necessarily include fatigue.

combination treatment   Refers to the addition of another treatment modality to an existing one to achieve a desired effect, such as the addition of COGNITIVE-BEHAVIORAL THERAPY (CBT) to an antidepressant to treat panic disorder. It also may refer to the use of two or more medications with different mechanisms of action but within the same overall class, such as the use of two different antidepressants to treat refractory depression.

community mental health center (CMHC) A MENTAL HEALTH service delivery system first authorized by the federal Community Mental Health Centers Act of 1963 to provide a comprehensive program of mental health care to Catchment Area residents. The CMHC is typically a community facility or a network of affiliated agencies that serves as a locus for the delivery of the various services included in the concept of COMMUNITY PSYCHIATRY.

community psychiatry That branch of psychiatry concerned with the provision and delivery of a coordinated program of MENTAL HEALTH care to residents of a geographic area. These efforts include working with patients, their families, and agencies within the community. Goals are the prevention of mental illness as well as care and treatment for persons with MENTAL DISORDERS.

comorbidity The simultaneous appearance of two or more illnesses, such as the co-occurrence of schizophrenia and substance abuse or of ALCOHOL DEPENDENCE and depression. The association may reflect a causal relation between one disorder and another or an underlying vulnerability to both disorders; however, the co-occurrence of the illnesses may be unrelated to any common etiology or vulnerability.

compulsion Repetitive ritualistic behavior or thoughts, such as frequent hand washing, arranging objects according to a rigid formula, counting, or repeating words silently. The purpose of these behaviors or thoughts is to prevent or reduce distress or to prevent some dreaded event or situation. The person feels driven to perform such actions in response to an OBSESSION (a recurrent thought, IMPULSE, or image that is intrusive and distressing) or according to rules that must be applied rigidly, even though the behaviors or thoughts are recognized to be excessive or unreasonable.

concrete thinking Thinking characterized by immediate experience rather than abstractions. It may occur as a primary, developmental defect, or it may develop secondary to organic brain disease or schizophrenia.

concussion An impairment of brain function caused by injury to the head. The speed and degree of recovery depend on the severity of the brain injury. Symptoms may include headache, DISORIENTATION, paralysis, and unconsciousness.

conditioning Establishing new behavior as a result of psychological modifications of responses to stimuli.

confabulation Fabrication of stories in response to questions about situations or events that are not recalled.

confidentiality The ethical principle that a physician may not reveal any information disclosed in the course of medical attendance.

conflict A mental struggle that arises from the simultaneous operation of opposing IMPULSES, drives, and external (environmental) or internal demands. Termed *intrapsychic* when the conflict is between forces within the PERSONALITY and *extrapsychic* when it is between the self and the environment.

confusion   Disturbed orientation in respect to time, place, person, or situation.

conscience   The morally self-critical part of one's standards of behavior, performance, and value judgments. Commonly equated with the SUPEREGO.

consultation-liaison psychiatry   An area of special interest in general psychiatry that addresses the psychiatric and psychosocial aspects of medical care, particularly in a general hospital setting. The consultation-liaison psychiatrist works closely with medical-surgical physicians and nonphysician staff to enhance the diagnosis, treatment, and management of patients with primary medical-surgical illness and concurrent psychiatric disorders or symptoms. Consultation may occasionally lead to a recommendation for more specific aftercare referral, but more typically it consists of short-term intervention by a "consultation team" with a biopsychosocial approach to illness.

conversion   A DEFENSE MECHANISM, operating unconsciously (see UNCONSCIOUS), by which intrapsychic conflicts that would otherwise give rise to ANXIETY are instead given symbolic external expression. The repressed ideas or IMPULSES, and the psychological defenses against them, are converted into a variety of somatic symptoms such as paralysis, pain, or loss of sensory function.

coping mechanisms   Ways of adjusting to environmental stress without altering one's goals or purposes. Includes both conscious and UNCONSCIOUS mechanisms.

coprolalia   The involuntary use of profane words seen in patients with Tourette's disorder.

Cotard's syndrome   A NIHILISTIC DELUSION in which one believes that one's body, or parts of it, is disintegrating; that one is bereft of all resources; or that one's family has been exterminated. It has been reported in depressive disorders, schizophrenia, and lesions of the nondominant hemisphere. Named after the French neurologist Jules Cotard (1840–1889).

countertransference   The therapist's emotional reactions to the patient that are based on the therapist's UNCONSCIOUS needs and CONFLICTS, as distinguished from his or her conscious responses to the patient's behavior. Countertransference may interfere with the therapist's ability to understand the patient and may adversely affect the therapeutic technique. However, countertransference also may have positive aspects and may be used by the therapist as a guide to a more empathic and accurate understanding of the patient.

distractibility   Inability to maintain ATTENTION. The person shifts from one area or topic to another with minimal provocation. Distractibility may be a manifestation of an underlying medical disease, a medication side effect, or a MENTAL DISORDER such as an ANXIETY disorder, mania, or schizophrenia.

dynamic psychiatry   The study of psychiatry from the point of view of motivation, emphasizing both psychological meaning and biological instincts as forces relevant to understanding human behavior in health and illness.

dystonia   Irregular muscle tone due to central nervous system disorder, which can result in grotesque movements or distorted positions.

E

echolalia   Parrotlike repetition of overheard words or fragments of speech. It may be part of a developmental disorder, a neurological disorder, or schizophrenia. Echolalia tends to be repetitive and persistent and is often uttered with a mocking, mumbling, or staccato intonation.

echopraxia   Imitative repetition of the movements, gestures, or posture of another. It may be part of a neurological disorder or of schizophrenia.

ego   In psychoanalytic theory (see PSYCHOANALYSIS), one of the three major divisions in the model of the psychic apparatus, the others being the id and the SUPEREGO. The ego represents the sum of certain mental mechanisms, such as perception and memory, and specific DEFENSE MECHANISMS. It serves to mediate between the demands of primitive instinctual drives (the id), of internalized parental and social prohibitions (the SUPEREGO), and of reality. The compromises between these forces achieved by the ego tend to resolve intrapsychic CONFLICT and serve an adaptive and executive function. Psychiatric usage of the term should not be confused with common usage, which connotes self-love or selfishness.

ego-dystonic   Referring to aspects of a person's behavior, thoughts, and attitudes that are viewed by the self as repugnant or inconsistent with the total PERSONALITY. Contrast with EGO-SYNTONIC.

ego-syntonic   Referring to aspects of a person's behavior, thoughts, and attitudes that are viewed by the self as acceptable and consistent with the total PERSONALITY. Contrast with EGO-DYSTONIC.

electroencephalogram (EEG)   A graphic (voltage vs. time) depiction of the brain's electrical potentials (brain waves) recorded by scalp electrodes. It is used for the diagnosis of neurological and neuropsychiatric disorders (especially seizure disorders) and in neurophysiological research. Sometimes used interchangeably with *electrocorticogram* and *depth record*, in which the electrodes are in direct contact with brain tissue.

encephalopathy   An imprecise term referring to any disorder of brain function (metabolic, toxic, neoplastic) but often implying a chronic degenerative process.

entitlement   The right or claim to something. In health law, the term *entitlement programs* refers to legislatively defined rights to health care, such as Medicare and Medicaid programs.

In psychodynamic psychiatry, *entitlement* usually refers to an unreasonable expectation or unfounded claim. An example is a person with narcissistic PERSONALITY DISORDER who feels deserving of preferred status and special treatment in the absence of apparent justification for such treatment.

Epidemiologic Catchment Area (ECA) study   This study was initiated in response to the 1977 report of the President's Commission on Mental Health. The purpose was to collect data on the prevalence and incidence of MENTAL DISORDERS and on the use of, and need for, services by the mentally ill. Research teams at five universities (Yale University, Johns Hopkins University, Washington University, Duke University, and the University of California at Los Angeles), in collaboration with the NATIONAL INSTITUTE OF MENTAL HEALTH (NIMH), conducted the studies with a core of common questions and sample characteristics. All data were collected between 1980 and 1985.

epidemiology   In psychiatry, the study of the incidence, distribution, prevalence, and control of MENTAL DISORDERS in a given population. Common terms in epidemiology are

endemic   Native to or restricted to a particular area.

epidemic   The outbreak of a disorder that affects significant numbers of persons in a given population at any time.

pandemic   Occurring over a very wide area, in many countries, or universally.

epilepsy, temporal lobe   Also called *complex partial seizures*. Usually originating in the temporal lobes, it involves recurrent periodic disturbances of behavior, during which the patient carries out movements that are often repetitive and highly organized but semiautomatic in character.

erotomania   An abnormally strong sexual desire.

euphoria   An exaggerated feeling of physical and emotional well-being, usually of psychological origin. Also seen in ORGANIC MENTAL DISORDERS and in toxic and drug-induced states.

evoked potential   Electrical activity produced by the brain in response to any sensory stimulus; a more specific term than *event-related*

level of prolactin in the blood, which can be caused by a tumor in the pituitary gland or by taking certain medications, such as conventional antipsychotic medications.

globus hystericus   The disturbing sensation of a lump in the throat. See also *hysterical neurosis, conversion type,* under NEUROSIS.

glutamate   An excitatory amino acid used by brain neurons as a primary neurotransmitter that appears to play a role in protecting against the symptoms of PSYCHOSIS.

glutamate receptors   Glutamate is the major excitatory neurotransmitter in the central nervous system, and, as such, the glutamate receptors play a vital role in the mediation of excitatory synaptic transmission.

grandiosity   Exaggerated belief or claims of one's importance or identity, often manifested by DELUSIONS of great wealth, power, or fame.

grief   Normal, appropriate emotional response to an external and a consciously recognized loss; it is usually time-limited and subsides gradually. To be distinguished from depression.

group (psycho)therapy   Application of psychotherapeutic techniques by a therapist who uses the emotional interactions of the group members to help them get relief from distress and possibly modify their behavior. Typically, a group is composed of 4–12 persons who meet regularly with the therapist.

H

halfway house   A specialized residence for patients who do not require full hospitalization but who do need an intermediate degree of domiciliary care before they return to independent community living.

hypertensive crisis   Sudden and sometimes fatal rise in blood pressure; may occur as a result of combining monoamine oxidase inhibitors (MAOIs) with food containing high amounts of tyramine (e.g., certain cheeses, fava beans, red wine) or with other sympathomimetic substances (e.g., cough remedies and nose drops).

hyperventilation   Overbreathing sometimes associated with ANXIETY and marked by reduction of blood carbon dioxide, producing complaints of light-headedness, faintness, tingling of the extremities, palpitations, and respiratory distress.

hypnagogic   Referring to the semiconscious state immediately preceding sleep; may include hallucinations that are of no pathological significance.

hypnopompic   Referring to the state immediately preceding awakening; may include hallucinations that are of no pathological significance.

hypomania   A psychopathological state and abnormality of mood falling somewhere between normal positive mood and mania. It is characterized by unrealistic optimism, pressure of speech and activity, and a decreased need for sleep. Some people show increased creativity during hypomanic states, whereas others show poor JUDGMENT, irritability, and irascibility.

hysteria   A psychiatric SYNDROME first described by the French neurologist Jean-Martin Charcot (1825–1893). The patient with hysteria may show shallow or unmodulated AFFECT, self-absorption, sexual preoccupation or promiscuous sexual behavior, and THOUGHT DISORDER. Hysteria is also referred to as *conversion disorder* because it is a CONVERSION of ANXIETY related to UNCONSCIOUS CONFLICTS into somatic symptoms.

hysterics   Lay term for uncontrollable emotional outbursts.

I

iatrogenic illness   A disorder precipitated, aggravated, or induced by the physician's attitude, examination, comments, or treatment.

ideas of reference   Incorrect interpretations of casual incidents and external events as having direct reference to oneself. May reach sufficient intensity to constitute DELUSIONS.

impulse   A desire or propensity to act in a certain way, typically in order to ease tension or gain pleasure.

inappropriate affect   A display of emotion that is out of harmony with reality or with the verbal or intellectual content that it accompanies. See AFFECT.

incoherence   Lacking in unity or consistency; often applied to speech or thinking that is not understandable because of any of the following: lack of logical connection between words or phrases; excessive use of incomplete sentences; many irrelevancies or abrupt changes in subject matter; idiosyncratic word usage; or distorted grammar.

incompetency   Lack of the capacity to understand the nature of, to assess adequately, or to manage effectively a specified transaction or situation that the ordinary person could reasonably be expected to handle. As used in the law, the term refers primarily to cognitive defects that interfere with JUDGMENT.

insight   Self-understanding; the extent of a person's understanding of the origin, nature, and mechanisms of his or her maladaptive attitudes and behavior. Sometimes used to indicate whether an individual is aware that he or she has a MENTAL DISORDER or that his or her symptoms have a psychiatric cause.

intellectualization   A DEFENSE MECHANISM in which the person engages in excessive abstract thinking to avoid confrontation with CONFLICTS or disturbing feelings.

International Classification of Diseases (**ICD**)   The official list of disease categories issued by the World Health Organization; subscribed to by all member nations, who may assign their own terms to each ICD category. The ICDA (*International Classification of Diseases*, U.S. Public Health Service adaptation) represents the official list of diagnostic terms to be used for each ICD category in the United States.

introjection   A DEFENSE MECHANISM, operating unconsciously (see UN-CONSCIOUS), whereby loved or hated external objects are symbolically absorbed within oneself. The converse of PROJECTION. May serve as a defense against conscious recognition of intolerable hostile IMPULSES. For example, in severe depression, the individual may unconsciously direct unacceptable hatred or AGGRESSION toward herself or himself. Related to the more primitive fantasy of oral incorporation.

introspection   Self-observation or the examination of one's feelings, often as a result of PSYCHOTHERAPY.

introversion   Preoccupation with oneself and accompanying reduction of interest in the outside world. Contrast with EXTRAVERSION. Also used to indicate shyness and decreased sociability.

isolation   An unconscious DEFENSE MECHANISM often used by obsessive-compulsive patients. Isolation separates AFFECT from memory. Thoughts or affects are treated as if they were untouchable, therefore requiring distance. An example is a patient talking about a painful event with a bland expression.

J

judgment   Mental act of comparing choices between a given set of values in order to select a course of action.

K

kindling   A progressively increasing response to successive electrical stimuli. In bipolar disorder, it is important to prevent the onset of mania because with each manic episode, the shorter the period until the next episode. In this regard, it is believed that the manic episode "kindles" the brain by making it more susceptible to a subsequent manic episode.

Kleine-Levin syndrome   Periodic episodes of hypersomnia accompanied by bulimia. The SYNDROME first appears in ADOLESCENCE, usually in boys. It is not classified as either an eating disorder or a sleep disorder. It is considered a neurological syndrome and is believed to reflect a frontal lobe or hypothalamic disturbance.

L

la belle indifférence Literally, "beautiful indifference." Seen in certain patients with CONVERSION disorders who show an inappropriate lack of concern about their disabilities. See *hysterical neurosis, conversion type,* under NEUROSIS.

learning disability A SYNDROME affecting school-age children of normal or above-normal intelligence characterized by specific difficulties in learning to read (dyslexia, word blindness), write (dysgraphia), and calculate (dyscalculia). The disorder is believed to be related to slow developmental progression of perceptual motor skills.

light therapy The use of a balanced-spectrum light box that delivers between 5,000 and 10,000 lux in the treatment of seasonal mood disorder, jet lag, PREMENSTRUAL DYSPHORIC DISORDER, premenstrual syndrome, and some sleep disorders. Also known as *phototherapy.*

limbic system Visceral brain; a group of brain structures—including the AMYGDALA, hippocampus, septum, cingulate gyrus, and subcallosal gyrus—that help regulate emotion, memory, and certain aspects of movement.

lobotomy A type of psychosurgery in which one or more nerve tracts in the cerebrum are severed. This procedure is now rarely used in the United States except for intractable obsessive-compulsive disorder.

M

magical thinking A conviction that thinking equates with doing. Occurs in dreams in children and in patients under a variety of conditions. Characterized by lack of realistic relationship between cause and effect.

managed care A system organized to create a balance among the use of health care resources, control of health costs, and enhancement of the quality of care. Managed care systems seek to provide care in the most cost-effective manner by closely monitoring the intensity and duration of treatment as well as the settings in which it is provided. Managed care systems also organize physicians and other providers into coordinated networks of care to ensure that those who enroll in the system receive all medically necessary care. A wide array of mechanisms is used to control utilization and reduce costs.

nomenclature. In current usage, some clinicians limit the term to its descriptive meaning, NEUROTIC DISORDER, whereas others include the concept of a specific etiological process. Common neuroses are as follows:

anxiety neurosis   Chronic and persistent apprehension manifested by autonomic hyperactivity (e.g., sweating, palpitations, dizziness), musculoskeletal tension, and irritability. Somatic symptoms may be prominent.

depersonalization neurosis   Feelings of unreality and of estrangement from the self, body, or surroundings. Different from the process of DEPERSONALIZATION, which may be a manifestation of ANXIETY or of another MENTAL DISORDER.

depressive neurosis   An outmoded term for excessive reaction of depression due to an internal CONFLICT or to an identifiable event such as loss of a loved one or of a cherished possession.

hysterical neurosis, conversion type   Disorders of the special senses or of the voluntary nervous system, such as blindness, deafness, anesthesia, paresthesia, pain, paralysis, and impaired muscle coordination for which no organic cause is found. A patient with this disorder may show LA BELLE INDIFFÉRENCE to the symptoms, which may actually provide secondary gains by winning the patient sympathy or relief from unpleasant responsibilities. See also CONVERSION.

hysterical neurosis, dissociative type   Alterations in the state of consciousness or in identity, producing symptoms such as AMNESIA.

obsessive-compulsive neurosis   Persistent intrusion of unwanted and uncontrollable EGO-DYSTONIC thoughts, urges, or actions. The thoughts may consist of single words, ruminations, or trains of thought that are seen as nonsensical. The actions may vary from simple movements to complex rituals, such as repeated hand washing. See also COMPULSION.

phobic neurosis   An intense fear of an object or a situation that the person consciously recognizes as harmless. Apprehension may be experienced as faintness, fatigue, palpitations, perspiration, nausea, TREMOR, and even panic.

neurotic disorder   An older term for a MENTAL DISORDER in which the predominant disturbance is a distressing symptom or group of symptoms that one considers unacceptable to one's PERSONALITY. There is no marked loss of REALITY TESTING; behavior does not actively violate gross social norms, although it may be quite disabling. The disturbance is relatively enduring or recurrent without treatment and is not limited to a mild transitory reaction to stress. There is no demonstrable organic etiology. See also NEUROTIC PROCESS.

neurotic process   A specific etiological process involving the following sequence: UNCONSCIOUS CONFLICTS between opposing wishes or between wishes and prohibitions lead to unconscious perception of anticipated danger or dysphoria, which leads to use of DEFENSE MECHANISMS that result in either symptoms, PERSONALITY disturbance, or both. See also NEUROSIS; NEUROTIC DISORDER.

nihilistic delusion   The DELUSION of nonexistence of the self or part of the self, or of some object in external reality.

O

object relations   The emotional bonds between one person and another, as contrasted with interest in and love for the self; usually described in terms of capacity for loving and reacting appropriately to others. Melanie Klein (1882–1960) is generally credited with founding the British object relations school.

obsession   Recurrent and persistent thought, IMPULSE, or image experienced as intrusive and distressing. Recognized as being excessive and unreasonable even though it is the product of one's mind. This thought, impulse, or image cannot be expunged by logic or reasoning.

organic mental disorder   A condition showing behavioral or psychological symptoms that is secondary to or based on detectable disturbances in brain functioning. Recent advances in genetics, neurophysiology, and BRAIN IMAGING have made it possible to identify several biological and physiological factors that contribute to many MENTAL DISORDERS traditionally characterized as "functional" or nonorganic. Consequently, there is general agreement that it is difficult, if not impossible, to make clear distinctions between "organic" and "nonorganic." DSM-IV-TR includes delirium, dementia, and amnestic disorders in a section labeled "Delirium, Dementia, and Amnestic and Other Cognitive Disorders." The remaining disorders in DSM-III-R labeled "organic" (mood, ANXIETY, PERSONALITY, and delusional disorders and organic hallucinosis) are placed in DSM-IV-TR within the diagnostic categories with which they share phenomenology and are identified as substance-induced or due to a general medical condition.

P

panic attack   A period of intense fear or discomfort, with the abrupt development of a variety of physical symptoms and fears of dying, going crazy, or losing control that reach a crescendo within 10 minutes. The symptoms may include shortness of breath or smothering sensations; dizziness, faintness, or feelings of unsteadiness; trembling or shaking; sweating; choking; nausea or abdominal distress; flushes or chills; and chest pain or discomfort.

Panic attacks occur in several ANXIETY disorders. In panic disorder, they are typically unexpected and happen "out of the blue." In disorders such as social phobia, simple phobia, obsessive-compulsive disorder, and body dysmorphic disorder, they are cued and occur when exposed to or in anticipation of a situational trigger. These attacks occur also in posttraumatic stress disorder (PTSD).

paradoxical intention   A technique used in BEHAVIOR THERAPY in which individuals are encouraged to engage in whatever behavior they are trying to stop. For example, a compulsive hand washer might be instructed to wash even more frequently. This helps because it often illustrates the irrationality of the behavior and reduces resistance to change.

paranoia   A condition characterized by the gradual development of an intricate, complex, and elaborate system of thinking based on (and often proceeding logically from) misinterpretation of an actual event; it may meet criteria for a type of delusional disorder. Despite its often chronic course, this condition does not seem to interfere with other aspects of thinking and PERSONALITY. To be distinguished from paranoid schizophrenia.

paranoid   A lay term commonly used to describe an overly suspicious person. The technical use of the term refers to persons with paranoid ideation or to a type of schizophrenia or a class of disorders.

pathognomonic   A symptom or group of symptoms that are specifically diagnostic or typical of a disease.

personality   The characteristic way in which a person thinks, feels, and behaves; the ingrained pattern of behavior that each person evolves, both consciously and unconsciously, as his or her style of life or way of being.

personality disorder   Enduring patterns of perceiving, relating to, and thinking about the environment and oneself that begin by early adulthood and are exhibited in a wide range of important social and personal contexts. These patterns are inflexible and maladaptive, causing either significant functional impairment or subjective distress.

Many types of PERSONALITY or personality disorder have been described. The following are those specified in DSM-IV-TR, which groups them into three clusters:

Cluster A   Paranoid, schizoid, schizotypal

Cluster B   Antisocial, borderline, histrionic, narcissistic

Cluster C   Avoidant, dependent, obsessive-compulsive

antisocial   Called *psychopathic personality* in the older literature; descriptions have tended to emphasize either antisocial behavior or interpersonal and affectional inadequacies. Among the more commonly cited descriptors are superficiality; lack of empathy and remorse, with callous unconcern for the feelings or rights of others; disregard for social norms; poor behavioral controls, with irritability, impulsivity, and low frustration tolerance; and inability to feel guilt or to learn from experience or punishment. Often, there is evidence of conduct disorder (disruptive behavior disorder) in childhood or of overtly irresponsible and antisocial behavior in adulthood, such as inability to sustain consistent work behavior, conflicts with the law, repeated failure to meet financial obligations, and repeated lying or "conning" of others.

avoidant Characterized by social discomfort and reticence, low self-esteem, and hypersensitivity to negative evaluation. Manifestations may include avoiding activities that involve contact with others because of fears of criticism or disapproval; experiencing inhibited development of relationships with others because of fears of being foolish or being shamed; having few friends despite the desire to relate to others; or being unusually reluctant to take personal risks or engage in new activities because they may prove embarrassing.

borderline Characterized by instability of interpersonal relationships, self-image, AFFECTS, and control over IMPULSES. Manifestations may include frantic efforts to avoid real or imagined abandonment; unstable, intense relationships that alternate between extremes of idealization and DEVALUATION; repetitive self-mutilation or suicide threats; and inappropriate, intense, or uncontrolled anger.

dependent Characterized by an excessive need to be taken care of, resulting in submissive and clinging behavior and fears of separation. Manifestations may include excessive need for advice and reassurance about everyday decisions, encouragement of others to assume responsibility for major areas of one's life, inability to express disagreement because of possible anger or lack of support from others, and preoccupation with fears of being left to take care of oneself.

histrionic Characterized by excessive emotional instability and attention seeking. Behavior includes discomfort if not the center of attention; excessive attention to physical attractiveness; rapidly shifting and shallow emotions; speech that is excessively impressionistic and lacking in detail; viewing relationships as being more intimate than they actually are; and seeking immediate gratification.

narcissistic Characterized by a pervasive pattern of GRANDIOSITY in fantasy or behavior and an excessive need for admiration. Manifestations may include having an exaggerated sense of self-importance, having a feeling of being so special that one should associate only with other special people, exploiting others to advance

psychosis   A severe MENTAL DISORDER characterized by gross impairment in REALITY TESTING, typically manifested by DELUSIONS, hallucinations, disorganized speech, or disorganized or CATATONIC BEHAVIOR. Persons with these disorders are termed *psychotic*. Among these illnesses are schizophrenia, delusional disorders, some secondary or symptomatic disorders ("organic psychoses"), and some mood disorders.

psychotherapy   A form of treatment in which a person who wishes to relieve symptoms or resolve problems through verbal interaction seeks help from a qualified MENTAL HEALTH professional and enters into an implicit or explicit contract to interact in a prescribed way with a psychotherapist.

R

rationalization   A DEFENSE MECHANISM, operating unconsciously, in which an individual attempts to justify or make consciously tolerable by plausible means feelings or behavior that otherwise would be intolerable. Not to be confused with conscious evasion or dissimulation. See also PROJECTION.

reaction formation   A DEFENSE MECHANISM, operating unconsciously, in which a person adopts AFFECTS, ideas, and behaviors that are the opposites of IMPULSES harbored either consciously or unconsciously (see UNCONSCIOUS). For example, excessive moral zeal may be a reaction to strong but repressed asocial impulses.

reality testing   The ability to evaluate the external world objectively and to differentiate adequately between it and the internal world. Falsification of reality, as with massive denial or PROJECTION, indicates a severe disturbance of EGO functioning and/or of the perceptual and memory processes on which it is partly based. See also PSYCHOSIS.

relaxation training   Use of relaxation techniques to help individuals control their physical and mental state in the treatment of psychiatric disorders, such as ANXIETY disorders. Although there are many different techniques, most involve the alternate tensing and relaxing of different muscle groups, along with visualization of a pleasant scene or the use of a simple mantra to control distracting thoughts.

repression   A DEFENSE MECHANISM, operating unconsciously, that banishes unacceptable ideas, fantasies, AFFECTS, or IMPULSES from consciousness or that keeps out of consciousness what has never been conscious. The repressed material may sometimes emerge in disguised form. Often confused with the conscious mechanism of suppression.

S

separation anxiety   The sense of discomfort that a child feels when experiencing or being threatened by a separation from an attachment figure. This is a normal stage of development that indicates a strong primary attachment. It typically develops between ages 10 and 15 months. These concerns may preoccupy children up to age 3 years. If the concerns persist or arise later and are of clinical significance, they may indicate a separation ANXIETY disorder.

sociopath   An unofficial term for *antisocial personality.* See PERSONALITY DISORDER.

splitting   A mental mechanism in which the self or others are viewed as all good or all bad, with failure to integrate the positive and negative qualities of the self and others into cohesive images. Often the person alternately idealizes and devalues the same person.

stupor   Marked decrease in reactivity to and awareness of the environment, with reduced spontaneous movements and activity. It can be seen as a type of CATATONIC BEHAVIOR in schizophrenia, but it can also be observed in neurological disorders.

sublimation   A DEFENSE MECHANISM, operating unconsciously, by which instinctual drives, consciously unacceptable, are diverted into personally and socially acceptable channels.

substitution   A DEFENSE MECHANISM, operating unconsciously, by which an unattainable or unacceptable goal, emotion, or object is replaced by one that is more attainable or acceptable.

superego   In psychoanalytic theory (see PSYCHOANALYSIS), that part of the PERSONALITY structure associated with ethics, standards, and self-criticism. It is formed by identification with important and esteemed persons in early life, particularly parents. The supposed or actual wishes of these significant persons are taken over as part of the child's own standards to help form the conscience. See also EGO.

support group   A network of individuals who give courage, confidence, and help to one another through empathy, INSIGHT, and constructive feedback. In psychiatry, these groups are especially helpful for patients with substance use disorders and for family members of patients with a psychiatric disorder.

supportive psychotherapy   A type of therapy in which the therapist–patient relationship is used to help patients cope with specific crises or difficulties that they are currently facing. Supportive therapy avoids, rather than encourages, the development of TRANSFERENCE NEUROSIS. It employs a range of techniques, depending on the patient's strengths and weaknesses and the particular problems that are currently distressing. These techniques include listening in a sympathetic, concerned, understanding, and nonjudgmental fashion; providing factual information that may counter a patient's unrealistic fears; setting limits and encouraging the patient to control or relinquish self-destructive behavior and to give ATTENTION to more constructive action; and facilitating dis-

Index

Page numbers printed in **boldface** type refer to tables or figures.